DATE DUE

POLYURETHANES
in
Biomedical Applications

Nina M. K. Lamba
Kimberly A. Woodhouse
Stuart L. Cooper

CRC Press
Boca Raton   Boston   London   New York   Washington, D.C.

Acquiring Editor: Felicia Shapiro
Project Editor: Albert W. Starkweather
Cover design: Denise Craig

Library of Congress Cataloging-in-Publication Data

Catalog record is available from the Library of Congress

This book contains information obtained from authentic and highly regarded sources. Reprinted material is quoted with permission, and sources are indicated. A wide variety of references are listed. Reasonable efforts have been made to publish reliable data and information, but the author and the publisher cannot assume responsibility for the validity of all materials or for the consequences of their use.

Neither this book nor any part may be reproduced or transmitted in any form or by any means, electronic or mechanical, including photocopying, microfilming, and recording, or by any information storage or retrieval system, without prior permission in writing from the publisher.

The consent of CRC Press LLC does not extend to copying for general distribution, for promotion, for creating new works, or for resale. Specific permission must be obtained in writing from CRC Press LLC for such copying.

Direct all inquiries to CRC Press LLC, 2000 Corporate Blvd., N.W., Boca Raton, FL 33431.

Trademark Notice: Product or corporate names may be trademarks or registered trademarks, and are used only for identification and explanation, without intent to infringe.

© 1998 by CRC Press LLC

No claim to original U.S. Government works
International Standard Book Number 0-8493-4517-0
Printed in the United States of America 1 2 3 4 5 6 7 8 9 0
Printed on acid-free paper

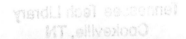

The Authors

Nina M. K. Lamba, Ph.D. graduated with a B.S. (Honors) degree in Applied Chemistry from Aston University, Birmingham, U.K. in 1991. She subsequently was awarded a doctorate in Bioengineering from the University of Strathclyde, Glasgow, U.K. in 1994. Her doctoral research was conducted under the supervision of Professor J. M. Courtney, and focused on the evaluation of blood–biomaterial interactions. Her current research is on leukocyte interactions with polyurethanes. She has co-authored seven publications on the subject of blood-contacting biomaterials, two chapters on cellular interactions with artificial surfaces, and is a member of the Royal Society of Chemistry. Dr. Lamba currently is working as a post doctoral Research Fellow in the Department of Chemical Engineering at the University of Delaware.

Kimberly A. Woodhouse, Ph.D., a registered professional engineer, received a bachelors degree in Engineering from McGill University, Montreal, Ontario, Canada, in 1979. She then spent 10 years in private sector manufacturing, working in chemical engineering and production. She received a Ph.D. in Chemical Engineering from McMaster University, Hamilton, Ontario, Canada under the supervision of Dr. J. L. Brash in 1993. At present she is an assistant professor at the University of Toronto in the Department of Chemical Engineering and Applied Chemistry, and is Associate Chair of Undergraduate Studies. Her current research is in tissue engineering, specifically polymeric/tissue based wound dressings for chronic ulcers and burns. In 1997, Dr. Woodhouse received the Engineering Excellence medal from the Professional Engineers of Ontario, for contributions to the field of engineering.

Stuart L. Cooper, Ph.D., received a B.S. degree in Chemical Engineering at M.I.T. in 1963 and then attended graduate school at Princeton University. Immediately after earning his doctorate, Dr. Cooper joined the faculty at the University of Wisconsin as an assistant professor and later was elevated to professor. In 1988, he was named the Paul A. Elfers Professor of Chemical Engineering. In January 1993, Dr. Cooper left the University of Wisconsin to become dean of the College of Engineering at the University of Delaware, where he also holds the H. Rodney Sharp Professorship in the Department of Chemical Engineering.

Dr. Cooper has published more than 300 papers in the fields of polymer science and biomaterials. In 1987, he won the Clemson Award for Basic Research of the Society for Biomaterials and the Materials Engineering and Sciences award of the American Institute of Chemical Engineers. He has co-edited two ACS Advances in Chemistry Series Volumes: Vol. 176, *Multiphase Polymers*, (1979), with G. M. Estes, and Vol. 199, *Biomaterials: Interfacial Phenomena and Applications*, (1982), with N. A. Peppas, A. S. Hoffman, and B. D. Ratner. He edited two other volumes, *The Vroman Effect*, (VSP, 1992) and *Polymer Biomaterials in Solution as Interfaces and as Solids*, (VSP, 1995), both with co-editors C. H. Bamford and T. S. Tsuruta. He also published a book, *Polyurethanes in Medicine*, (CRC Press, 1986) with co-author Michael Lelah and, in 1989, was a co-founding editor of the *Journal of Biomaterials Science, Polymer Edition*. In 1993, he was selected a Founding Fellow of the American Institute of Medical and Biological Engineering. Dr. Cooper is a Fellow of the American Physical Society and the American Institute of Chemical Engineers. He served as president of the Society for Biomaterials 1996–1997, and was elected International Fellow of the Society in 1996. He also is an active member of the American Chemical Society and The American Society for Artificial and Internal Organs.

Preface

Polyurethane elastomers are a family of segmented block copolymers that has found important application in medicine. The focus of this book is the use of polyurethanes in implanted medical devices. This book has been written primarily as an updated version of the highly successful monograph, *Polyurethanes in Medicine* by Michael D. Lelah and Stuart L. Cooper, published by CRC Press in 1986. In writing this book, we have broadened the scope of the subject, recognizing the widening horizon of biomaterials science, and the interdisciplinary nature of bioengineering.

The first five chapters deal with concepts in polymeric science, polyurethane synthesis and chemistry. The fabrication and processing of polyurethanes also is discussed, and commercially available biomedical polyurethanes are reported. Structure–property relationships and physical characterization of polyurethane materials are described. The section ends with a discussion of the surface characterization and surface properties of polyurethanes, as it is at the tissue/biomaterial interface that many of the biological reactions occur.

The last five chapters discuss the biological responses to implanted polymers. The introductory chapter on host responses is followed by a brief summary of test procedures and guidelines for biological testing. Literature pertaining to protein adsorption, blood responses and soft tissue interactions with polyurethanes is reviewed. There also is a discussion of the biodegradation and calcification of implanted materials. The penultimate chapter reviews the applications of polyurethanes in biomedical applications, with sections discussing the performance of polyurethanes in cardiovascular, artificial organ, soft tissue, and genito–urinary applications, among others. The book concludes with an assessment of the current status and the future direction of polyurethanes in medicine.

We are aware most readers will be relatively unfamiliar with some areas covered by this book. Therefore, preliminary and introductory information has been included to allow a reader new to the field of biomaterials to understand the underlying principles, and to appreciate the reviews and discussions in each chapter and how these issues relate to the use of synthetic materials in medical devices. By examining issues in the use of medical devices through consideration of one class of material, the polyurethanes, we believe this book will be of value to materials scientists, life scientists, engineers and clinicians, whether they are working in an academic, clinical or industrial environment. It also is designed to be a comprehensive literature review for the serious researcher in the field.

Stuart L. Cooper would like to acknowledge the work of many of his graduate students whose work is heavily referenced throughout this book. Support of this work over the years by the National Institutes of Health, National Science Foundation, American Heart Association and the Johnson & Johnson Focused Giving Program, was vital to building up a core of information which could be expanded into this book on polyurethane biomaterials.

Nina M. K. Lamba
Kimberly A. Woodhouse
Stuart L. Cooper
June 1997

Contents

Chapter 1 — Introduction
    I. Biomaterials 1
    II. Biocompatibility..1
    VIII. Biomedical Polymers 1
    IV. Organization 2
References 3

Chapter 2 — The Chemistry of Polyurethane Copolymers
    I. Introduction 5
    II. History of Polyurethane Copolymers 6
    III. Polyurethane Copolymers..6
    IV. Synthesis of Polyurethanes 8
        A. Isocyanate Chemistry 9
        B. Allophanate Reaction 11
        C. Biuret Formation 11
        D. Acylurea 12
        E. Isocyanurate Formation 12
        F. Uretidione Formation 12
        G. Carbodiimide Formation 12
        H. Catalysts 13
        I. Synthesis Media 14
    V. Raw Materials in Polyurethane Copolymer Synthesis...14
        A. Isocyanates 14
        B. Polyols 15
        C. Chain Extenders 15
    VI. Linear Polyurethane Elastomer Synthesis 17
    VII. Crosslinked Polyurethane Copolymers...17
    VIII. Polyurethane Modification 18
        A. Bulk Modification of Polyurethanes..20
        B. Surface Modification of Polyurethanes 21
Summary 23
References 23

Chapter 3 — Polyurethane Processing and Survey of Biomedical Polyurethanes
    I. Introduction 27
    II. Processing of Polyurethanes..27
        A. One-Dimensional Processes..27
        B. Two-Dimensional Processes 29
        C. Three-Dimensional Processes 31
            1. Foams 31
            2. Tubing 32
                a. Extruded Tubing 32
                b. Solvent Cast Tubing 33
                c. Porous and Fibrous Tubing 33

   3. Balloons, Bladders, and Other Devices 34
    a. Solvent Casting...34
    b. Molding..36
 III. Sterilization 36
  A. Steam Sterilization 36
  B. Ethylene Oxide Sterilization 36
  C. Radiation 37
 IV. Commercial and Experimental Polyurethanes 37
References 39

Chapter 4 — Bulk Characterization and Structure-Property Relationships of Polyurethanes

 I. Introduction 43
  A. States of Order and Thermal Transitions of Polymers..43
  B. Intermolecular Bonding in Polymers...48
  C. Mechanical Behavior 48
   1. Viscoelasticity..50
   2. Hysteresis 50
  D. Molecular Weight 51
 II. Structure of Polyurethanes..53
  A. Microphase Separation...53
   1. Thermodynamics of Phase Separation..53
   2. Kinetics of Microphase Separation...54
  B. Morphological Models of Block Copolymers 55
  C. Molecular Orientation in Polyurethanes..57
  D. Hydrogen Bonding 61
  E. Crosslinking..62
  F. The Effect of Polyurethane Chemistry on Physical Properties 63
   1. Isocyanate 63
   2. Polyols 64
   3. Chain Extenders 65
 III. Characterization of Polyurethanes..65
  A. Gel Permeation Chromatography 66
  B. Infrared Spectroscopy 66
  C. Differential Scanning Calorimetry...68
  D. Dynamic Mechanical Thermal Analysis 72
  E. Electron Microscopy 74
  F. Stress-Strain Properties and Ultimate Tensile Strength 78
   1. Tensile Properties 80
   2. Tensile Stress Hysteresis...82
   3. Fatigue Testing 82
  G. Solubility Tests...84
  H. Permeability and Extractability 84
  H. Electrical Properties 85
Summary 86
References 86

Chapter 5 — Surface Characterization of Polyurethanes

 I. Introduction 91
 II. Surface Energy and Surface Tension..91

      A. Contact Angles 94
      B. Contact Angle Measurement..95
      C. Contact Angle Hysteresis 97
  III. Attenuated Fourier Transform Infrared Spectroscopy (ATR–FTIR) 98
      A. ATR–FTIR Analysis of Polyurethanes 99
  IV. Surface Spectroscopic Techniques..100
      A. X-ray Photo-Electron Spectroscopy (XPS) 100
      B. Secondary Ion Mass Spectrometry (SIMS)..101
      C. Surface Spectroscopic Studies of Polyurethanes..102
  V. Surface Morphology 108
  VI. Surface Electrical Properties...111
Summary 111
References 112

Chapter 6 — Introduction to Host Responses
  I. Introduction 115
  II. Protein Adsorption 115
      A. The First Event..115
          1. Kinetics of Protein Adsorption 117
          2. Equilibria and Isotherms 118
          3. Protein Adsorption onto Biomaterials 119
      B. Coagulation System 122
      C. Fibrinolytic System 122
  III. Cells, Extracellular Matrix, and Cellular Interactions 124
      A. Platelets 124
      B. Erythrocytes..124
      C. Leukocytes..127
      D. The Extracellular Matrix 129
      E. Cell Receptors and Mediators...130
          1. Cell Adhesion Molecules 130
          2. Cytokines...130
      F. Hemostasis and Thrombosis 130
      G. The Inflammatory Response 133
      H. Foreign Body Response 135
      I. Wound Healing..136
          1. Proliferation of Fibroblasts 136
          2. Wound healing and Scar Contracture 137
  IV. Immune Response...138
      A. Innate Immunity 138
      B. Complement System 138
      C. Adaptive Immunity 140
Summary 140
References 142

Chapter 7 — Host Responses to Polyurethanes
  I. Introduction 147
  II. Assessment of Host Biomaterial Interactions 147
      A. *In Vitro* testing..147
      B. *Ex Vivo* testing 148
      C. *In Vivo* testing 148

        D. Clinical Testing 150
        E. Guidelines For Biological Testing Of Materials 150
    III. Protein Adsorption Onto Polyurethanes 150
        A. Albumin..151
        B. Fibrinogen 152
        C. Fibronectin..154
        D. Vitronectin 154
        E. Lipoproteins..154
        F. Coagulation System 154
        G. Fibrinolytic System 155
        H. Complement System 155
        I. The Vroman Effect...155
    IV. Cellular Responses to Polyurethanes...158
        A. Platelets 158
        B. Leukocytes..161
        C. Thrombus Formation..161
        D. Soft Tissue Interactions..164
        E. Neointima Formation on Polyurethanes 167
        F. Immunological Response to Biomaterials 169
        G. Infection..169
            1. Staphylococcus Epidermidis 170
            2. Gram Positive Bacteria 170
Summary 170
References 171

Chapter 8 — Degradation of Polyurethanes
    I. Introduction 181
    II. Mechanisms of Biodegradation 181
        A. Hydrolysis 181
        B. Oxidation 181
            1. Auto-oxidation...183
            2. Metal Catalyzed Oxidation 183
        C. Chemical Degradation..185
        D. Sterilization 185
        E. Biological Catalysis of Degradation 185
            1. Enzymes 185
            2. Cells...186
            3. Surface Cracking 187
        F. Environmental Stress Cracking..187
        G. Impact of Polyurethane Structure on Biodegradation 189
            1. Soft Segment 189
            2. Hard Segment..190
        H. Other Mechanisms of Biodegradation 194
        I. Implant Location 194
    III. Toxicity and Carcinogenicity 195
    IV. Calcification of Polyurethanes 197
    V. Biodegradable Polyurethanes 199
Summary 200
References 200

Chapter 9 — Polyurethanes in Biomedical Applications

- I. Introduction 205
- II. Cardiovascular Applications 205
  - A. Catheters 205
  - B. Pacemaker Lead Insulation 208
  - C. Vascular Prostheses 211
  - D. Heart Valves 219
  - E. Cardiac Assist Devices 222
    - 1. Left Ventricular Assist Devices 223
    - 2. Intraaortic Balloon Pumps 224
- III. Artificial Organs 226
  - A. Artificial Heart 226
  - B. Hemodialysis 227
  - C. Artificial Lung/Blood Oxygenation 228
  - D. Hemoperfusion 228
  - E. Artificial Pancreas 229
  - F. Blood Tubing 229
  - G. Blood Filters 229
- IV. Tissue Replacement and Augmentation 230
  - A. Breast Implants 230
  - B. Wound Dressings 231
    - 1. Types of Wounds 231
    - 2. Occlusive and Semiocclusive Dressings 232
    - 3. Wound Dressings and Infection 238
  - C. Facial Reconstruction 238
  - D. Adhesives 239
- V. Other Applications 239
  - A. Artificial Ducts 239
  - B. Contraceptives 240
  - C. Controlled Drug Delivery 240
  - D. Penile Prostheses 240
  - E. Miscellaneous 241
- References 241

Chapter 10 — Summary and Future Perspectives 255

List of Abbreviations 257

Index 259

1 Introduction

I. BIOMATERIALS

A biomaterial is a nonviable material used in a medical device, intended to interact with biological systems.[1] Biomaterials may be used singularly to replace or augment a specific tissue, or in combination to perform a more complex function, e.g., in organ replacement.[2] Biomedical materials include metals, ceramics, pyrolytic carbon materials, composites and polymers. Of these groups, polymers represent the largest class.

There are three fundamental properties that a biomaterial should possess; mechanical strength, a functional characteristic, and biocompatibility.[3] The functional characteristic is required so that the material has the specific property to perform the required task. Mechanical strength is required to retain an adequate level of performance. Biocompatibility is considered in more detail in the next section.

II. BIOCOMPATIBILITY

The interactions between polymers and the biological environment are not yet fully understood. The definition of biocompatibility has evolved over the years from one of biological inertness, to acceptance that some degree of interaction between the biomaterial and the host is inevitable and may actually be beneficial. A widely accepted definition of biocompatibility is taken to be the ability of a material to perform with an appropriate host response in a specific application.[1] This definition recognizes that the degree of biocompatibility required of a biomaterial depends very much on the application.

Biocompatibility can be considered in terms of blood compatibility (hemocompatibility) and tissue compatibility (histocompatibility). Blood compatibility is less well defined than biocompatibility, and there is no widely accepted definition.[4] It is often defined as what should not occur, including thrombosis, destruction of formed elements, and complement activation. Histocompatibility encompasses the lack of toxicity, and excessive tissue growth around an implant. It is unlikely that there will be one biomaterial that will work equally well in all applications. This is due to the large range of mechanical and functional requirements of biomaterials, as determined by the specific application and the host tissues.

III. BIOMEDICAL POLYMERS

A large number of polymers have been used in biomedical applications. During the 1930s, materials available for medical use were limited to those that were naturally available. Developments in polymer science opened up the variety of materials that were available. Since the mechanical properties of these synthetic polymers resembled those of biological tissues more closely than, for example, metals, wood and glass, they were readily introduced as biomaterials. Another contributory factor to the increased use and application of biomaterials was the development of antibiotics, which improved the survival rates of patients, increasing the need for prosthetic devices. Advances in surgery and medicine have been responsible for, and will continue to create a demand for biomaterials, both with respect to the need for new materials and their scope of application.

TABLE 1
Use of plastics in medical and pharmaceutical applications

Polymer Family	Usage, mm lbs, 1989
Polyvinylchloride (PVC)	480
Polystyrene	340
Low density polyethylene (LDPE)	320
High density polyethylene (HDPE)	250
Polypropylene (PP)	175
Polycarbonate (PC)	60
Thermoplastic polyesters	45
Acrylics	40
Silicones	25
Nylon	20
Acrylonitrile Butadiene Styrene (ABS)	15
Thermoplastic polyurethanes (TPUs)	10
All others	50
Total	1830

From Szycher, M. "Medical/Pharmaceutical markets for medical plastics." In *High Performance Biomaterials,* Szycher M., Ed. Technomic, Lancaster, 1991. With permission.

Polymers that are used in medical applications include naturally occurring materials such as natural rubber and cellulose. Synthetic biomaterials include silicone rubber (SR), polyvinylchloride (PVC), Nylon®, polytetrafluoroethylene (PTFE), polyethylene terephthalate (PET) and of course the polyurethanes. The current amounts of polymeric materials used in medical and pharmaceutical applications are presented in Table 1.[5]

Plasticized PVC is by far the most common polymeric biomaterial, due to its use in disposable medical devices, including blood storage bags, infusion sets and blood tubing. Polyurethanes account for very little of the total amount of polymers used for medical and pharmaceutical applications. This does not reflect the diversity of their applications and their relative success as a biomaterial. Polyurethane elastomers combine excellent mechanical properties with good blood compatibility, which has favored their use and development as biomaterials, particularly as components of implanted devices.

IV. ORGANIZATION

The first part of this book is designed to introduce the reader to concepts in polymer science, polyurethane chemistry, and the mechanical and surface properties of polyurethane elastomers. Chapter 2 explores the synthesis of polyurethane elastomers, their chemistry, and methods of bulk and surface modification. Chapter 3 contains a review of polymer processing, relevant to the fabrication of medical devices and a survey of biomedical polymers. It must be noted that in recent years, a number of these materials have been withdrawn from the medical implant marketplace and are no longer commercially available. Despite this, consideration of the chemistry, properties and performance has been given to these materials throughout the book, as they constitute some of the most widely studied polyurethanes for biomedical applications. Chapter 4 contains an examination of the microphase structure of the polyurethanes, and consideration of their physical properties. Characterization of the mechanical properties of the polyurethanes also is discussed. Chapter 5 contains an review of the surface characterization and properties of polyurethanes.

Introduction

The second half of the book contains an introduction to the biological systems that contribute to the host response to implanted biomaterials. After a brief discussion of the biological assessment of materials, Chapter 7 presents a review of the biological interactions with polyurethanes, including plasma protein adsorption, blood compatibility and soft tissue interactions of polyurethanes. Chapter 8 discusses the biodegradation of polyurethanes, reviewing the current understanding of toxicity of polyurethanes and their stability in the biological environment. Calcification of polyurethane devices also is considered. Chapter 9 reviews the more common applications and performance of polyurethanes as medical devices. Cardiovascular, artificial organs, tissue augmentation and genito-urinary applications are reviewed. A discussion on the future direction of polyurethanes and the field of biomaterials in general completes the book.

REFERENCES

1. Williams D. F., Ed. *Definitions in Biomaterials.* Elsevier Science Ltd., 1987.
2. Friedman D. W., Orland P. J. and Greco R. S. "History of Biomaterials." In *Implantation Biology — The Host Responses and Biomedical Devices,* Ed. Greco R. S. CRC Press, Boca Raton, FL, 1994: 1.
3. Courtney J. M., Lamba N. M. K., Gaylor J. D. S., Ryan C. J. and Lowe G. D. O. "Blood-contacting biomaterials: bioengineering viewpoints." *Artif. Organs,* 19:852, 1995.
4. Ratner B. D. "The blood compatibility catastrophe." *J. Biomed. Mater. Res.,* 27:283, 1993.
5. Szycher M. "Medical/Pharmaceutical markets for medical plastics." In *High Performance Biomaterials,* Ed. Szycher M. Technomic, Lancaster, PA, 1991: 3.

2 The Chemistry of Polyurethane Copolymers

I. INTRODUCTION

Polymers are a class of high molecular weight materials, with a structure that is characterized by "building blocks" of repeat units or monomers. The monomers react together to form long chains of repeating chemical units. The polymer chains that result may be linear or form a branched or three-dimensional network. Polymers can be classified in a number of ways, for example, according to whether they are of natural origin, or synthetic. Naturally occurring polymers include polysaccharides, cellulose, silk and natural rubber. Common synthetic polymers include polyethylene, polystyrene, polyvinylchloride, polyesters, polytetrafluoroethylene, polycarbonates, and the polyurethanes. Polymers also can be classified according to chemical composition, chemical structure, physical state, thermal behavior and application. Classification on the basis of chemical composition of the polymer considers the elemental composition and types of monomer residues within the chain. The chemical structure considers the stereoregularity of the polymer, and the placement of side chains, which also is referred to as the tacticity of a polymer. The physical structure of the material also can be used, to classify materials as crystalline or amorphous, indicating the state of order of the molecules, or to indicate whether or not the polymer chains are branched as opposed to linear. The thermal behavior of the polymer also can categorize polymers as either thermoplastic or thermosetting, which is an important consideration in processing. The ultimate application of the material also can be used to classify polymers.

Other criteria for polymer classification include the number or type of repeat units that are present in a polymer chain. In some cases polymers are composed of a single repeat unit, and such materials are referred to as homopolymers. Examples of homopolymers are polyvinylchloride and polyethylene. Heteropolymers, or copolymers as they often are called, contain more than one monomer residue within the polymer chains. Different types of heteropolymers exist, and are depicted in Figure 1. The precise sequence of the individual monomers influences the chemistry and physical nature of the material. Alternating copolymers consist of alternating residues. Block copolymers consist of several units of one type followed by a number of units of another residue within the main chain of the polymer. Graft copolymers consist of blocks of one residue as a side chain on a backbone of a different polymer. There are many excellent texts on polymeric materials, encompassing polymer synthesis and structure-property relationships of polymers, in which aspects of polymer structure, classification and chemistry are discussed in detail; the reader is directed towards these books for further information.[1-7]

Polyurethanes are a family of heterogeneous polymers; they contain the urethane linkage (Figure 2), analogous to the carbamate group in organic chemistry, within the polymer chains. Urethane groups usually do not constitute the majority of the functional groups within a polyurethane. It is the ability to incorporate other functional groups into the polymer network that contributes to the range of properties exhibited by polyurethane materials. Consequently, the properties of polyurethanes range from rigid hard thermosetting materials to those of much softer elastomers. Generally, thermoplastic polyurethanes, which comprise the most important group for implantable devices, have very high tensile strength, toughness, abrasion resistance, and resistance to degradation, in addition to biocompatibility that has sustained their use as biomaterials.

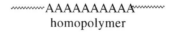

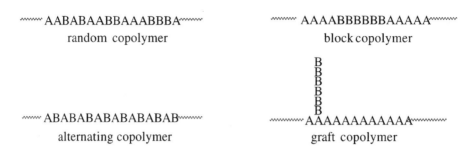

FIGURE 1   Types of polymer structure.

FIGURE 2   Urethane chemical structure.

II. HISTORY OF POLYURETHANE COPOLYMERS

Until the 1920s and 1930s the few industries that depended on polymeric materials were based on natural or modified natural materials. It was not until the 1930s that the science of polymers began to emerge, and the major growth of the technology of synthetic polymers came even later. The initial step that led to the worldwide interest in polyurethanes was taken by Otto Bayer of I. G. Farbenindustrie, Leverkusen, Germany, in 1937. This work that led to the discovery of the polyurethanes was performed in order to synthesize novel materials that were not covered by the polyamide patents of Nylon materials, held by Carothers at E. I. du Pont de Nemours & Co. The first materials synthesized by Bayer were prepared via reactions between diamines and aliphatic diisocyanates. These produced polyurea materials that were infusible and strongly hydrophilic and could not compete with the polyamides, particularly in fiber applications. Further work with aliphatic diisocyanates and glycols produced materials with properties that were more amenable to use in fibrous applications. Synthesis of materials with high-molecular weight glycols and aromatic diisocyanates yielded the first polyurethane elastomers. A brief summary of the highlights in the developments of polyurethanes are presented below in Table 1. Further details on the history of polyurethanes are available.[8,9]

Polyurethanes are employed in a broad range of uses and applications, including machinery, transport, furnishings, textiles, paper-making, packaging, adhesives and sealants, and medicine.[10] The outstanding mechanical properties and biocompatibility of the polyurethanes makes them some of the most promising synthetic biomaterials. These properties will be discussed throughout the course of this book.

III. POLYURETHANE COPOLYMERS

Polyurethane copolymers are an important subclass of the family of thermoplastic elastomers. They are composed of short, alternating polydisperse blocks of soft and hard segments, as shown in Figure 3. The soft segment is typically a low glass transition temperature (T_g) polyether, polyester

TABLE 1
Major developments in commercial polyurethanes

Year		Reference
1937	First application for polyurethane patent — I. G.Farbenindustrie	11
1938	First U.S. patent application — Rinke et al.	12
1941	Reaction of diisocyanates and glycols	13
1947	First rigid foams (Bayer)	
1952	First flexible polyurethanes	14
1954	Lycra® patent — Langerak	15
1955	Patent for Estane®	16
1957	Polyether urethanes foams commercially available	
1958	Thermoplastic polyurethanes (TPU)s discovered (Commercialized in 1961)	
1960	US Lycra® patent awarded	17
1972	Biomer® (Lycra T-126 with a new name)	18
1977	Pellethane® family of materials introduced	
1979	Second generation aliphatic polyurethanes disclosed	

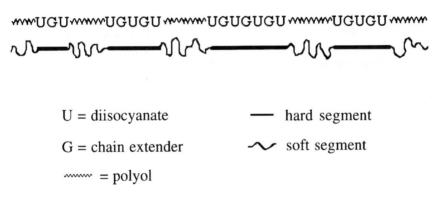

FIGURE 3 Segmented polyurethane structure.

or polyalkyldiol, generally of molecular weight 400–5000. The hard segment is usually a high glass transition temperature, possibly semicrystalline aromatic diisocyanate, linked with a low molecular weight chain extender. Polyurethanes are generally synthesized with chain extenders consisting of low molecular weight diols or diamines which produce additional urethane or urethane–urea segments respectively. The polyurethanes exhibit a broad range of physical properties, due to the options available in selecting the chemistries and molecular weights of the various components, and the ratios in which they are reacted. The properties range from very brittle and hard materials to soft, tacky, viscous ones. The polyurethane linkage itself can be considered as a mixed amide ester of carbamic acid; thus its high temperature properties lie between those of polyesters and polyamides.

The molecular structure of the polyurethanes must be taken into account when trying to understand and explain their physical behavior. There exists a degree of immiscibility between the hard urethane segments and the soft polyol segments, which means that although macroscopically polyurethanes are isotropic, microscopically polyurethanes are not structurally homogeneous. So although there is some degree of mixing of the soft and hard segments, phase separation of the two segments occurs, producing a structure that can be considered as hard segment domains dispersed in a soft segment matrix. The resultant two-phase micro-domain structure exhibited by the polyurethanes is responsible for their superior physical and mechanical properties, and is believed to contribute to their biocompatibility.

The term polyurethane implies that the monomer from which the polyurethane is synthesized is a urethane, and that the urethane structure is the predominant group. This is misleading, as urethane groups are not contained within the precursors, but instead are formed during polymerization; other functional groups also may be present, usually outnumbering the urethane groups. Other groups that may be present include ether, allophanate, urethane, urea, biuret, carbodiimide, isocyanurate and acylurea, as well as aliphatic chains and aromatic rings.[10,19] Through various steps in the synthesis of a polyurethane, the stiffness, crystallinity and flexibility of the polymer, and the ability of the polymer chains to orient, bond intermolecularly and chemically crosslink can be influenced.

The domain structure of polyurethanes and their scope for structural diversity creates a wide variety of uses and applications for these materials. The physical and mechanical properties can be designed and controlled at various stages during synthesis. Polyurethanes combine flexibility with high strength, wear resistance and a degree of hardness. In the following section, an introduction to the principles of polyurethane synthesis are presented. More detailed information can be found in a number of books; texts by Hepburn and Wirpsza are highly recommended.[10,19]

IV. SYNTHESIS OF POLYURETHANES

Methods of polymer synthesis generally fall into two categories: addition polymerization and condensation polymerization. Addition polymerization occurs when unsaturated monomers react through stages of initiation, propagation and termination. The monomers used often are simple molecules with a double bond, and once a double bond is broken in the initiation step, the reaction will usually proceed rapidly until the concentration of unreacted monomers is low. In most cases, addition occurs without creation of a side product. Condensation or step-growth polymerization occurs when bifunctional molecules react in a stepwise fashion to produce a linear chain of monomer residues. It is analogous to condensation reactions between low molecular weight reactants. A small molecule, such as water or carbon dioxide is usually eliminated. The method of polymer synthesis can influence the structure of the final material, including the molecular weight distribution of the polymer chains and the degree of branching of the chains. Addition polymerization can be used to synthesize homopolymers and copolymers. The precise type of copolymer formed, i.e., random, alternating, or block, is determined by the reaction conditions and concentration and reactivity ratios of the monomers. The final molecular weight and molecular weight distribution of the polymer is more difficult to control than in condensation polymerization, although the use of chain transfer agents may help. Control of the reaction can be gained through the selection of anionic polymerization methods, and under certain conditions, a nearly monodisperse distribution of linear molecules may be synthesized. Condensation polymerization also is used to prepare copolymers. Bifunctional monomers can be used to prepare linear polymers; monomers that are trifunctional or higher can be used to produce branched chains and three-dimensional crosslinked polymer networks.

Polyurethane polymerization reactions contain features of both addition and condensation polymerization. Although no small molecule is eliminated during polymerization, the reaction between the diol and the diisocyanate can be classified as a condensation reaction. The kinetics of the polymerization reaction more closely resemble those of condensation polymerization than addition polymerization. Some textbooks refer to this type of condensation polymerization, where no condensation product is formed, as polyaddition or rearrangement polymerization.[7] Commercially, polyurethanes can be synthesized via a "one-step" process or multistep syntheses.

The one step process is the quickest and easiest of the manufacturing techniques. A difunctional or multifunctional liquid isocyanate and liquid diol are mixed in a mold, and allowed to react. A lightly crosslinked structure can be synthesized with careful selection of the precursors. Curing of the material from a one-step procedure produces an elastomer. Synthesis via more than one step

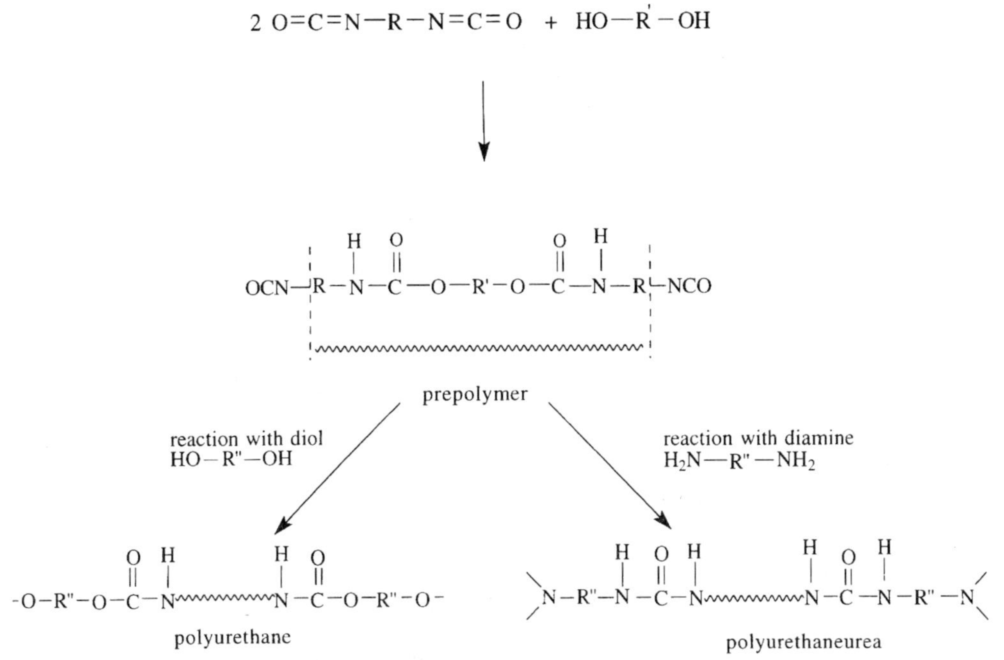

$$2\ O{=}C{=}N-R-N{=}C{=}O\ +\ HO-R'-OH$$

$$OCN-R-N(H)-C(=O)-O-R'-O-C(=O)-N(H)-R-NCO$$

prepolymer

reaction with diol HO—R"—OH

reaction with diamine H_2N—R"—NH_2

—O—R"—O—C(=O)—N(H)—~~~~~N(H)—C(=O)—O—R"—O—

polyurethane

$\rangle$N—R"—N(H)—C(=O)—N(H)—~~~~~N(H)—C(=O)—N(H)—R"—N$\langle$

polyurethaneurea

FIGURE 4 Two-step polyurethane synthesis. First Step: prepolymer synthesis from a diisocyanate and dihydroxy compound. Second step: chain extension.

imparts greater control over the chemistry of the reaction, influencing the structure, physical properties, reactivity and processability of the finished product; hence multistep synthetic routes are preferred.

The most common method for synthesis, particularly of biomedical polyurethanes, consists of two steps, and is commonly referred to as the prepolymer method. The first step involves synthesis of a prepolymer from the diol in excess diisocyanate to produce an isocyanate terminated molecule (Figure 4). The prepolymer generally has a low molecular weight, but can be as high as 15,000–20,000, and is either a viscous liquid or a low melting solid. Some prepolymers can be stabilized with 0.01–0.1% acid chloride and stored. Subsequent reaction of this prepolymer with a diol or diamine chain extender constitutes the second step, which produces a multi-block copolymer of the $(AB)_n$ type. Depending on the conditions used, side reactions that create allophanate and biuret links may occur.

A. Isocyanate Chemistry

Isocyanates are fundamental starting materials for the polyurethanes. The isocyanate group is very reactive, and exists in a number of canonical forms, as shown below in Figure 5.

The electron distribution of the isocyanate group means that the species can react with either electron donors or electron acceptors. Thus there are a large number of possible reagents, including other isocyanate groups. Most reactions of isocyanates involve addition at the $N = C$ double bond. Aromatic isocyanates are generally more reactive than aliphatics, as the electron-withdrawing nature of the benzene ring makes the isocyanate carbon more susceptible to nucleophilic attack. Electron-donating substituents near the isocyanate carbon will reduce the rate of reaction of the isocyanate. The presence of bulky side groups in the ortho- position on aromatic isocyanates, or branched or bulky substituents on aliphatic molecules will sterically hinder the approach of electron donors, and reduce the rate of reaction. In diisocyanates, the rate of reaction of the second isocyanate group

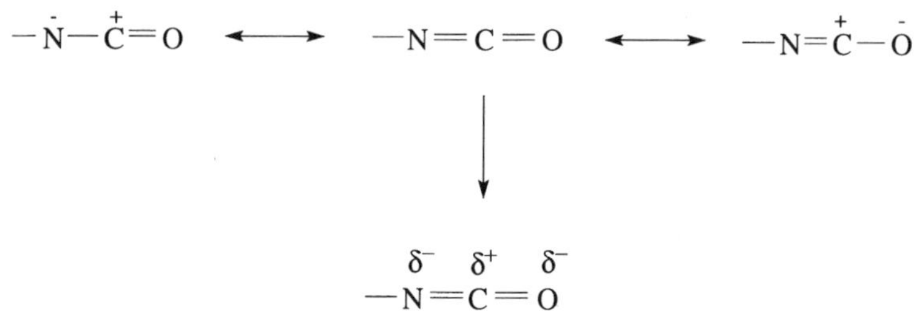

$$-\overset{-}{N}-\overset{+}{C}=O \longleftrightarrow -N=C=O \longleftrightarrow -N=\overset{+}{C}-\overset{-}{O}$$

$$\downarrow$$

$$\overset{\delta^-\ \ \delta^+\ \ \delta^-}{-N=C=O}$$

FIGURE 5 Resonant structures of isocyanates.

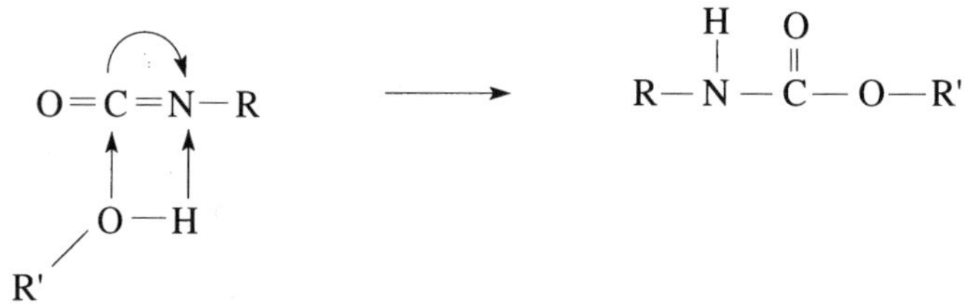

FIGURE 6 Urethane formation.

is slower than that of the first group, although this difference is reduced if the isocyanate groups are separated by an aliphatic chain or aromatic rings.

The primary reaction for polyurethane synthesis is the reaction of the isocyanate group with an hydroxy terminated molecule (Figure 6). Primary alcohols react about three times faster than secondary alcohols, and about 200 times faster than tertiary alcohols. The size of the side groups on higher alcohols sterically hinders the approach of the isocyanate, reducing the rate of reaction.

The reactivity of the isocyanate group also promotes reactions with other functional groups, which enhances the diversity of polyurethane copolymers. Some of these reactions are shown in Figure 7. The isocyanate group also is able to react with the newly formed functional groups in the polymer, if the isocyanate is present in excess concentration. These reactions can be utilized in order to obtain a crosslinked structure. Isocyanates also react readily with water. The presence of water in the reaction medium during synthesis can lead to the production of unstable carbamic acids which then decompose to amines. Carbon dioxide gas is liberated, producing a foam. The amine can then react with an isocyanate group to form a urea group. Through mechanisms such as these, and additional steps in processing and manufacturing, the final properties of the polymer can be influenced by selecting the starting materials and the synthetic route. In polyurethane synthesis, control of the molar ratios of chain extender, polyol and isocyanate is very important in determining the final properties of the polymer, and can be exploited in order to control and design the properties of the material.

Polymer networks can be consolidated through crosslink formation, which involves increasing the strength of interactions between polymer chains. The ultimate crosslink is a primary covalent bond. Such crosslinks are extremely strong and stable, and cannot be broken once formed. Other types of intermolecular bonds such as hydrogen bonds form weaker interactions between the urethane groups and the ether or ester links, and may serve to promote microphase separation of the materials.

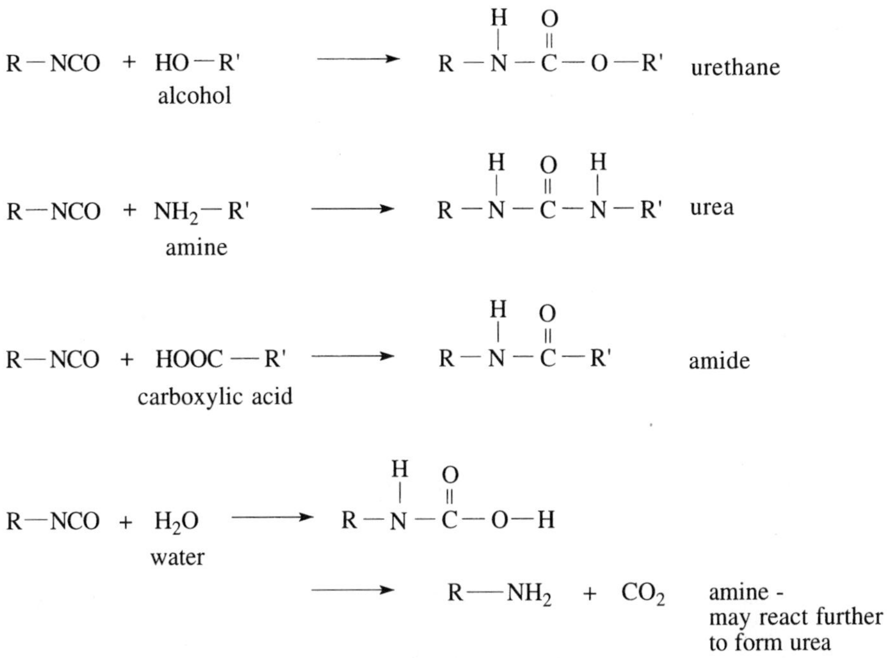

$$R-NCO + HO-R' \longrightarrow R-\underset{H}{\overset{|}{N}}-\overset{O}{\overset{\|}{C}}-O-R' \quad \text{urethane}$$
alcohol

$$R-NCO + NH_2-R' \longrightarrow R-\underset{H}{\overset{|}{N}}-\overset{O}{\overset{\|}{C}}-\underset{H}{\overset{|}{N}}-R' \quad \text{urea}$$
amine

$$R-NCO + HOOC-R' \longrightarrow R-\underset{H}{\overset{|}{N}}-\overset{O}{\overset{\|}{C}}-R' \quad \text{amide}$$
carboxylic acid

$$R-NCO + H_2O \longrightarrow R-\underset{H}{\overset{|}{N}}-\overset{O}{\overset{\|}{C}}-O-H$$
water

$$\longrightarrow R-NH_2 + CO_2 \quad \text{amine - may react further to form urea}$$

FIGURE 7 Reactions of isocyanates commonly used in polyurethane synthesis.

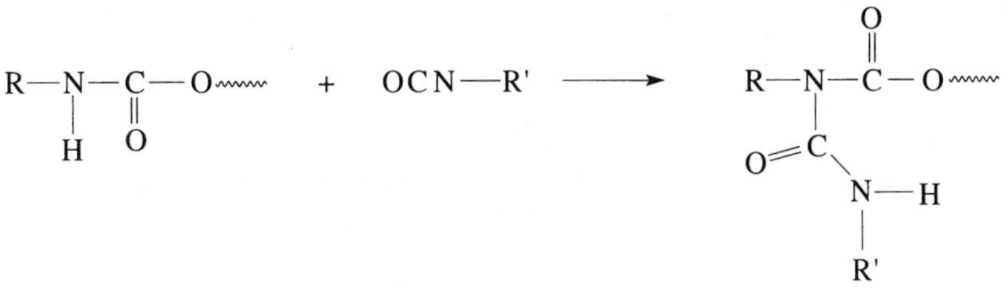

$$R-\underset{H}{\overset{|}{N}}-\overset{O}{\overset{\|}{C}}-O\sim + OCN-R' \longrightarrow R-\underset{\underset{O=C}{|}}{\overset{|}{N}}-\overset{O}{\overset{\|}{C}}-O\sim$$
$$\underset{R'}{\overset{|}{N}}-H$$

FIGURE 8 Allophanate formation.

B. ALLOPHANATE REACTION

This reaction occurs when excess isocyanate is present. The urethane group donates an active hydrogen on the nitrogen atom which reacts with the isocyanate (Figure 8). Allophanate bonds are thermally labile and will dissociate at elevated temperatures.

C. BIURET FORMATION

In this reaction, between a urea group and an isocyanate group, the urea group donates an active hydrogen to the isocyanate (Figure 9).

A terminal isocyanate group also can react with other urethane or urea groups to produce a branched or crosslinked polymer structure. Biuret links are more stable than allophanate links, but still are thermally labile and will dissociate at high temperatures.

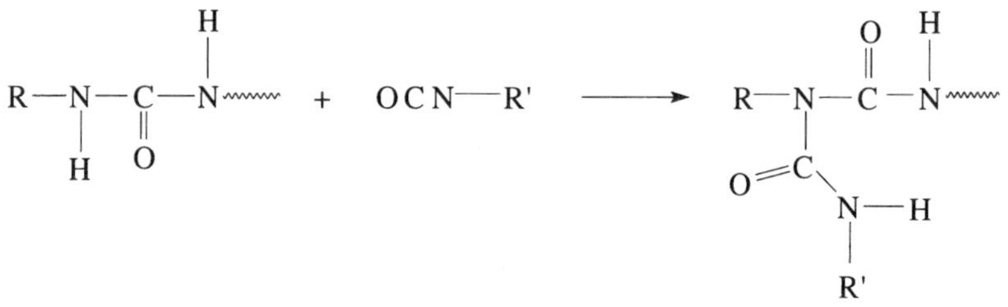

FIGURE 9 Biuret formation.

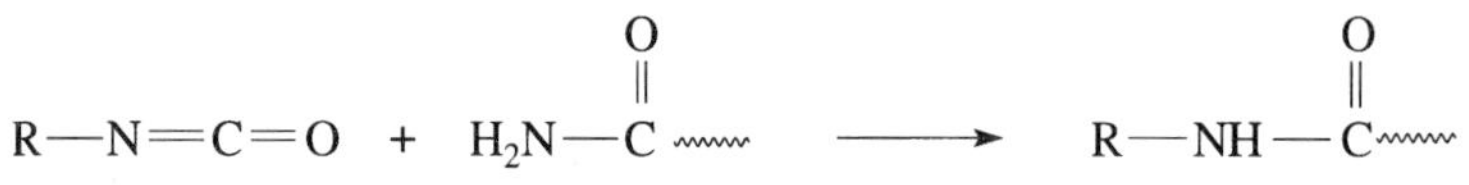

FIGURE 10 Acylurea formation.

D. ACYLUREA

This is an intermolecular interaction between an amide and an isocyanate, producing an acylurea group (Figure 10).

All of the above reactions can occur during the synthesis of polyurethane elastomers. The following reactions are possible during polymer synthesis, under special circumstances.

E. ISOCYANURATE FORMATION

The formation of isocyanurate groups essentially occurs through trimerization of isocyanate groups (Figure 11). Excess isocyanate in the reaction mixture is required. Under certain conditions, the isocyanate groups associate to form cyclic trimers. These isocyanurates are thermally stable and isocyanurate formation is irreversible. This method of crosslinking can be used to produce heat stable and flame resistant polyurethanes and is typically used in the manufacture of rigid polyurethane foam systems designed for high temperature applications.

F. URETIDIONE FORMATION

Dimerization of isocyanate groups also can occur, although it has only been reported to occur with aromatic isocyanates (Figure 12). These dimer structures breakdown at temperatures above 150°C.

G. CARBODIIMIDE FORMATION

Isocyanates also may react to produce carbodiimides, as shown in Figure 13. These groups are formed at high temperature and are thermally stable at temperatures in excess of 200°C. Carbodiimide groups in an elastomer can act as proton scavengers and thus their presence offers resistance to hydrolysis.

The above reactions of polyurethanes are very important in determining the final properties of the polymer, and some often are actively encouraged during polymer synthesis and processing. Additionally, other structures such as such as polymers or biological molecules can be grafted onto the polyurethane backbone, through displacement of the urethane hydrogen atom, or coupling via diisocyanate bridges. This allows modification of polyurethane bulk and surfaces in order to alter interfacial reactions. Surface modification can be employed to retain the mechanical properties of the material. Examples of surface modification will be discussed in later in this chapter.

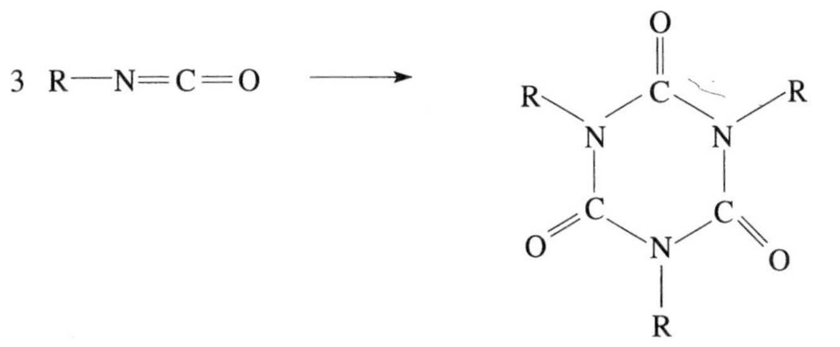

3 R—N=C=O ⟶ [isocyanurate ring structure]

FIGURE 11 Isocyanurate formation via isocyanate trimerization.

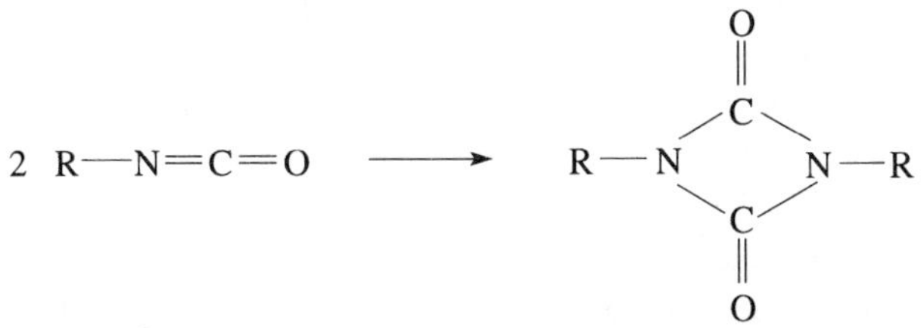

2 R—N=C=O ⟶ [uretidione ring structure]

FIGURE 12 Dimerization of isocyanates to produce uretidiones.

2 R—N=C=O ⟶ RN=C=NR + CO_2

FIGURE 13 Carbodiimide formation.

The reaction temperature can influence the balance between polymer chain extension and crosslink formation in the polymer network through these side reactions. Up to temperatures of approximately 50°C, reaction of the isocyanate with hydroxy groups predominates. As the reaction temperature rises towards 150°C, the crosslinking steps and branching reactions become more important, as the polymer undergoes further reactions. Above 150°C, allophanate and biuret links will be broken and aromatic polyurethanes will start to degrade. Aliphatic polyurethanes will start to degrade at 220°C. Decomposition products include free isocyanate, alcohols, free amines, olefins and carbon dioxide. Degradation of the polyurethane soft segments also may occur. Degradation of polyurethanes is discussed in Chapter 8. Isocyanate reactions are exothermic, and since polymers generally have low thermal conductivity, heat transfer is slow. Thus, the temperature can rise appreciably during the course of the reaction, influencing the course of polymerization and ultimately affecting the physical properties of the polymer.

H. Catalysts

Although isocyanates react readily with linear polyols, the rate of reaction decreases rapidly as the size of the substituents on the higher alcohols increases. Thus, catalysts are required to facilitate polyurethane formation. Catalysts for the isocyanate and alcohol reaction are mild and strong bases, such as sodium hydroxide, sodium acetate and triamines, and metals especially tin compounds. Commonly used catalysts include tertiary amines, for example tri-ethylene diamine 1,4 diazo(2,2,2)bicyclooctane (DABCO). Tertiary amines may be modified to contain hydroxy groups, so that they can form hydrogen bonds with the polymer, effectively reducing their volatility and odor. Tertiary amines promote the reaction of the isocyanate group with hydroxy groups and water.

TABLE 2
Relative reactivity of reaction of isocyanate groups with hydroxyl groups

Catalyst	Concentration/g 100 g^{-1}	Relative activity
DABCO	0.1	130
DABCO	0.2	260
DABCO	0.3	330
Dibutyltin dilaurate	0.1	210
Dibutyltin dilaurate	0.5	670
Tin (II) caprylate	0.1	540
Tin (II) caprylate	0.3	3500
DABCO + dibutyltin dilaurate	0.2 + 0.1	1000
DABCO + tin (II) caprylate	0.3 + 0.3	4250

From Wirpsza Z. *Polyurethanes: Chemistry, Technology and Applications.* (1st ed.): Ellis Horwood, London, 1993.

Organometallic compounds, such as ferric acetylacetonate or cobalt naphthenate also promote reaction of the isocyanate group. The best catalysts, however, for the formation of urethane links are organotin compounds. Relative activities of the reaction between isocyanate and water with different catalysts are presented in Table 2.[20]

Organotin compounds will promote the reaction of isocyanates with diols in preference to reaction with water. Dibutyltin dilaurate and stannous octoate are widely used in polyurethane synthesis, as they are readily soluble in the reaction medium, are not very volatile, and have a low odor. Dibutyltin dilaurate and tin dicarboxylate are approximately ten times more efficient than tertiary amines at promoting the reaction between isocyanates and hydroxy groups. Catalysts with large side groups are generally less efficient, due to steric hindrance, and some latent organotin compounds exist. Organotin catalysts will also promote biuret and urea crosslinking reactions, but not isocyanurate formation. Strong bases will promote biuret, allophanate and isocyanurate reactions. A mixture of tertiary amines and organotin compounds can be used, in order to gain a balance between the chain extension and crosslinking steps of polyurethane formation.

I. Synthesis Media

Laboratory or experimental syntheses of polyurethanes are generally performed via bulk or solution polymerization. The choice of solvent may affect both the rate of an uncatalyzed reaction or the effectiveness of the catalyst. In general, solvents that readily complex with the compound containing the active hydrogen or catalyst (for example, by hydrogen bonding or dipole moment interactions) will result in a slower reaction than solvents that cannot readily associate with reactants or the catalyst. Common solvents used in synthesis include N,N-dimethylacetamide (DMA), dimethylformamide (DMF), tetrahydrofuran (THF), and dimethylsulfoxide (DMSO). In most commercial production, however, solvent free bulk polymerization techniques are used. This difference in synthesis conditions alters both the rate and yield of the various reactions.

V. RAW MATERIALS IN POLYURETHANE COPOLYMER SYNTHESIS

A. Isocyanates

Both aliphatic and aromatic isocyanates can be used to synthesize polyurethanes. The presence of an aromatic isocyanate in the hard segment produces a stiffer polymer chain with a higher melting point. The two most commonly used isocyanates in polyurethane synthesis are toluene diisocyanate (TDI) and methylene *bis* (p-phenyl isocyanate) or 4,4′-diphenylmethane diisocyanate (MDI). TDI is less expensive than MDI, but MDI has superior reactivity, and polymers based on MDI may possess better physical properties. TDI is usually prepared as an isomeric mixture of 2,4-TDI and 2,6-TDI. MDI is crystallizable while 2,4-TDI does not crystallize in the solid state. Other aromatic diisocyanates, such as naphthalene diisocyanate (NDI) and 3,3′ bitoluene diisocyanate (TODI) also can result in high-performance polymers, but at a higher cost than MDI based materials. Typical aliphatic isocyanates include 1,6-hexane diisocyanate (HDI), isophorone diisocyanate (IPDI), and methylene bis (p-cyclohexyl isocyanate) (H_{12}MDI). Because aromatic diisocyanates and polymers made from them are somewhat unstable toward light and become yellow with time, aliphatic isocyanates have found wider use in coating applications, than aromatic containing materials. In addition to greater light stability, polyurethanes based on aliphatic isocyanates possess increased resistance to hydrolysis and thermal degradation. Unfortunately, this is sometimes accompanied by a decrease in the mechanical properties of the material. The chemical structures of commonly used diisocyanates used in polyurethane synthesis are shown below, in Figure 14.

B. Polyols

Polyols available for elastomer synthesis include polyesters, polyethers, polycarbonates, hydrocarbons and polydimethylsiloxanes. The most commonly used polyols are polyether or polyester based compounds of molecular weight 400–5000. Primary alcohols will react readily with isocyanates at temperatures of 25–50°C. Secondary and tertiary alcohols are less reactive than primary alcohols by factors of 0.3 and 0.005 respectively. The flexible polyol comprises the soft segment matrix in which the hard segments are dispersed. Commonly used polyols are shown in Figure 15.

Traditionally, polyurethanes have been produced with polyester and polyether soft segments. Polyurethanes synthesized from polyesters possess relatively good physical properties; however, they are susceptible to hydrolytic cleavage of the ester linkage. Polyether-based polyurethanes exhibit a relatively high resistance to hydrolytic cleavage, when compared with polyester urethanes, and are favored for use in applications where hydrolytic stability is required. The polyether that results in a polyurethane with the best physical properties is polytetramethylene oxide (PTMO or PTMEG). Urethanes prepared with this soft segment show a level of mechanical strength comparable to that of polyester polyurethanes and possess relatively good hydrolytic stability and water resistance.[21] Polyethylene oxide-based materials swell in water due to the hydrophilic nature of the soft segments. Polypropylene oxide-based polyurethanes offer greater hydrolytic resistance, but possess lower physical properties. When environmental stability is a major concern, polyalkyl glycols offer an alternative to the relatively less stable polyether and polyester polyurethanes.

Hydrogenated polybutadiene and polyisobutylene-based polyurethanes show excellent resistance to light and thermal degradation and hydrolysis.[22,23] Unfortunately, the synthesis of these materials is difficult, and the physical properties of the resulting polymers are poor relative to those of conventional polyurethanes. The use of polydimethylsiloxane glycol (PDMS) as a soft segment leads to polyurethanes with improved low-temperature properties. The glass transition temperature of PDMS is about –123°C which allows the use of these materials at low temperatures.

C. Chain Extenders

Chain extenders can be categorized into two general classes of aromatic diols and diamines, and the corresponding aliphatic diols and diamines. In general, aliphatic chain extenders yield softer materials than aromatic chain extenders. Commonly used chain extenders are shown in Figure 16. Chain extenders are used to extend the length of the hard segment, and increase the hydrogen-bond density and the molecular weight of the polyurethane. Trifunctional or higher chain extenders also act as branching or crosslinking agents. The reaction of equimolar quantities of macroglycol and

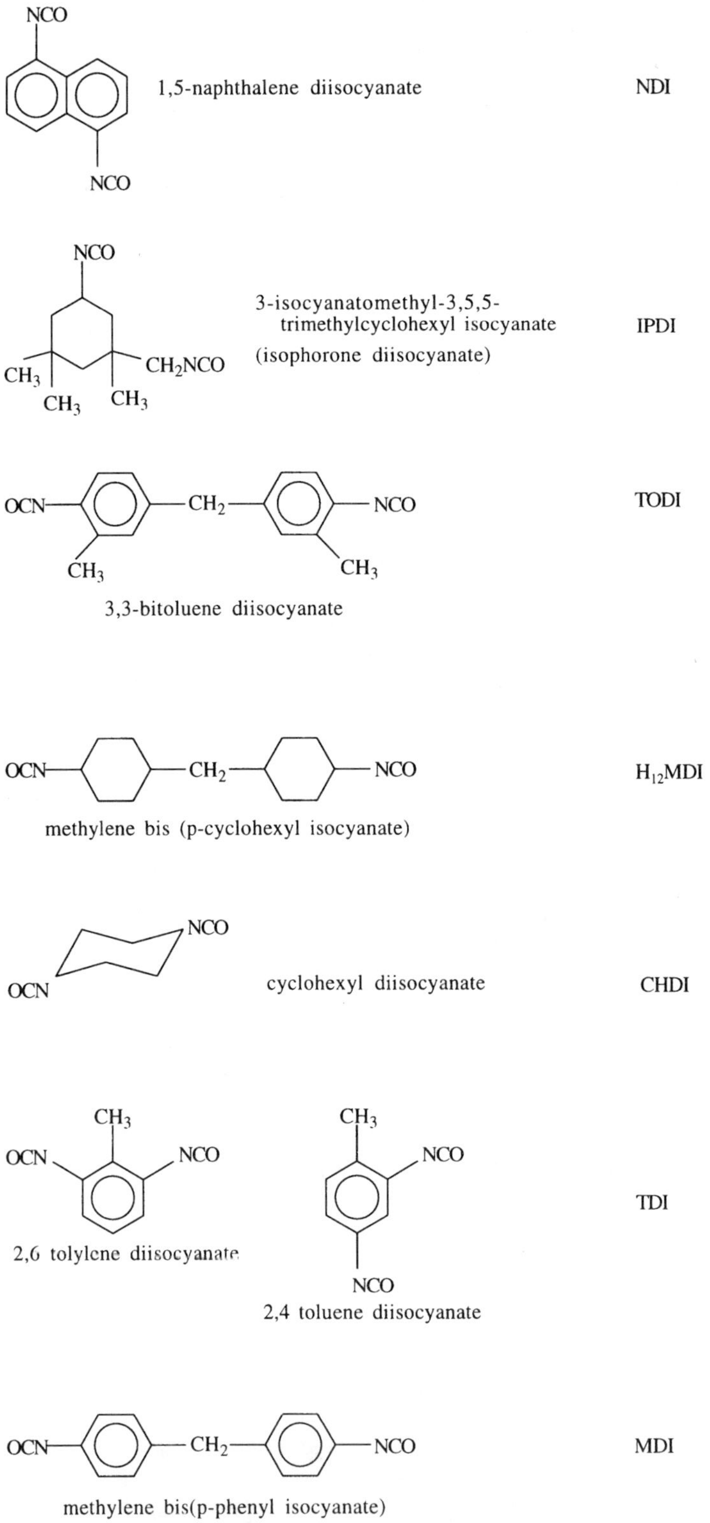

FIGURE 14 Some commonly used isocyanates.

diisocyanate generally results in a polymer that may not exhibit microphase separation and may possess poor physical properties. Common commercial chain extenders include 1,4-butanediol (BD), ethylene diamine (ED), 4,4′ methylene bis (2-chloroaniline) (MOCA), ethylene glycol (EG), and hexanediol (HD). MOCA is not used in polyurethanes for biomedical applications, as it has been shown to be carcinogenic in rats.

Diamine chain extenders react rapidly and vigorously with isocyanates to produce urea groups, and the resultant urea groups can produce a polymer crosslinked with biuret links. These polymers set so rapidly that their use is limited to one-step reaction injection molding processes. Diamines with large substituent groups that sterically hinder the approach to the isocyanate group find more application, as do amines with neighboring groups that reduce the reactivity of the amine. Such compounds are still fairly reactive, but provide more time for processing operations to be performed. Amine reactivity also can be reduced by complexing the amine with acids or various metal salts. Glycol extended polyurethanes are more flexible and less strong than the amine-extended analogs. Cyclic extenders increase the strength of the material compared with their linear analogs. Mixtures of chain extenders also can be used.

VI. LINEAR POLYURETHANE ELASTOMER SYNTHESIS

Linear polyurethanes are synthesized using bi-functional reagents such as 1000 or 2000 molecular weight polyols and aromatic diisocyanates. A low molecular weight chain extender is employed and in order to prevent crosslink formation, the polyurethane synthesis may be performed at temperatures below 80°C to inhibit allophanate and biuret formation. The lack of crosslinks in the network means that such polyurethanes are melt or solvent processable and are classified as thermoplastic.

Noncrosslinked polyurethanes are synthesized using linear dihydroxy polyester or polyether compounds and excess diisocyanate to form the prepolymer. The prepolymer is then reacted with the chain extender in exact molar proportions calculated from the free isocyanate present. Control of the precise molar ratio of isocyanate groups and chain extender reduces the availability of free isocyanate groups for crosslinking. Such polyurethanes are widely used as thermoplastics, and as coatings and adhesives and they can be applied by melt and solution techniques. The polymers can be dissolved in polar solvents such as tetrahydrofuran (THF) and dimethylformamide (DMF).

In order to prepare a crosslinked polyurethane, an excess of isocyanate is used in the chain extension step, so that on heat-curing, side reactions such as allophanate and biuret formation occur. The amount of crosslinking is relatively small, as it is dependent on the number of free isocyanate groups, so long curing conditions may be needed to attain the required level of crosslinking. These polyurethanes are insoluble after curing, and are more often used in speciality applications.

The properties are determined by the length and structure of the segments, the stoichiometric ratio of the components, and the degree of branching. For optimal mechanical strength, the ratio of isocyanate groups to hydroxy groups should be 1.0–1.1. If it is less than 1.0, the molecular weight and hence the mechanical strength of the material decreases, as does the hardness, resilience, maximum elongation and compressibility of the material. A more detailed discussion on how the chain chemistry affects the physical properties of the polymer is presented in Chapter 4.

VII. CROSSLINKED POLYURETHANE COPOLYMERS

Crosslinked polyurethanes contain a significant number of bonds that bind the polymer chains intermolecularly. The ultimate crosslink is a primary covalent bond. Such crosslinks are extremely strong and stable. Other types of intermolecular bonds form weaker links. Allophanate and biuret groups dissociate at higher temperatures as do intermolecular hydrogen bonds between hard segments. crosslinked polyurethanes are traditionally created by using tri-functional, or higher, isocyanates,

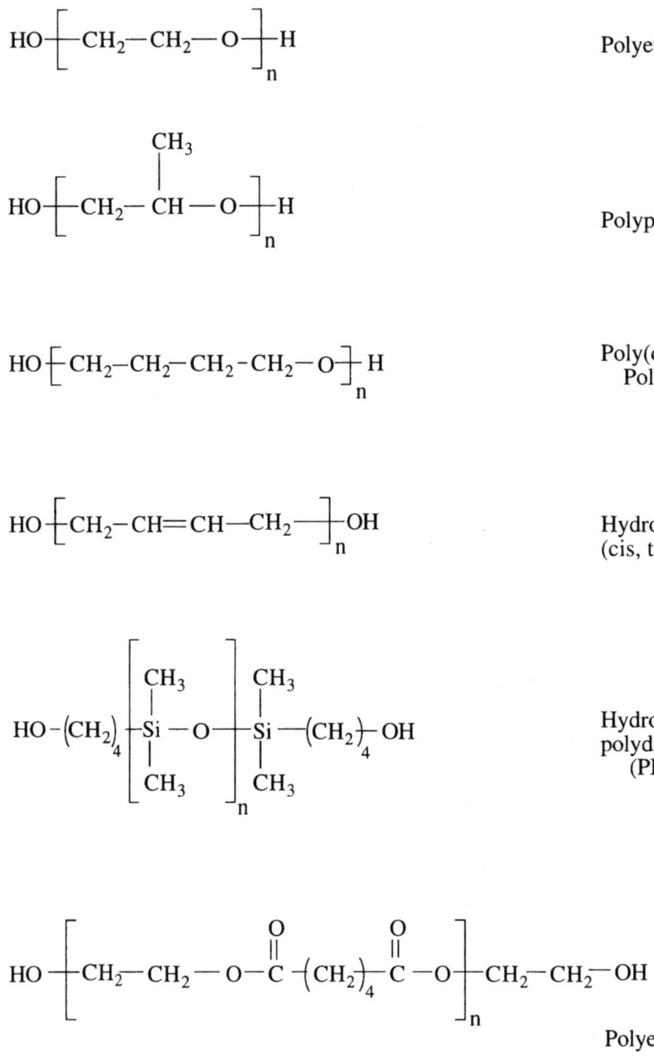

HO─[CH₂─CH₂─O]ₙ─H   Polyethylene oxide (PEO)

HO─[CH₂─CH(CH₃)─O]ₙ─H   Polypropylene oxide (PPO)

HO─[CH₂─CH₂─CH₂─CH₂─O]ₙ─H   Poly(oxytetramethylene)glycol, (PTMEG)
Poly(tetramethylene)oxide, (PTMO)

HO─[CH₂─CH=CH─CH₂]ₙ─OH   Hydroxy terminated poly 1,4-butadiene
(cis, trans and 1,2 isomers not shown)

HO─(CH₂)₄─[Si(CH₃)₂─O]ₙ─Si(CH₃)₂─(CH₂)₄─OH   Hydroxybutyl terminated polydimethylsiloxane (PDMS)

HO─[CH₂─CH₂─O─C(=O)─(CH₂)₄─C(=O)─O─CH₂─CH₂]ₙ─OH   Polyethylene adipate

FIGURE 15 Some commonly used polyols.

polyols and chain extenders. These materials generally have poorer physical properties than the linear polyurethanes due to disruption of the microphase separation.

Crosslinked polyurethanes can be used as flexible foams or cast elastomers. Flexible foams can be fabricated by selecting long, Y-shaped triols. Rigid foam polyurethanes can be made by using short chain polysaccharidic hexols as crosslinking agents. Diamines, 1,4 butanediol, or water can be used for the chain extension reactions. As mentioned previously, control of the molar ratios of chain extender, polyol and isocyanate is critical in determining the final properties of the polymer, and can be employed in order to control the properties of the material. Foam production is considered in more detail in Chapter 3.

VIII. POLYURETHANE MODIFICATION

Much effort in biomaterials development has been directed towards chemical modification of biomaterials in order to enhance their biocompatibility, as thrombosis and infection associated with

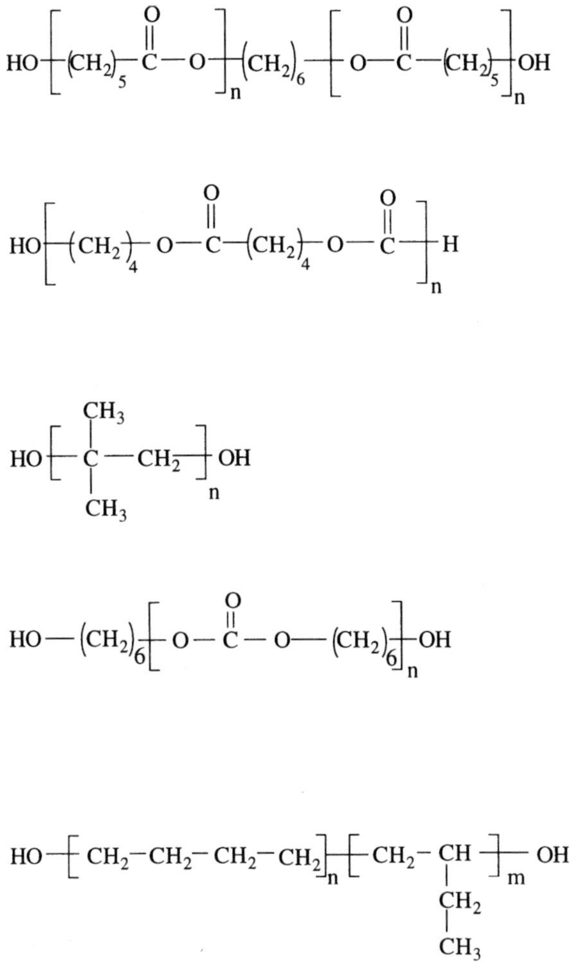

Polycaprolactone

Polytetramethylene adipate

Hydroxy terminated polyisobutylene

Polyhexamethylene carbonate glycol

Hydrogenated polybutadiene

FIGURE 15 (continued)

medical implants are problematic. Polymeric biomaterials in particular lend themselves to modification through the options available in polymer synthesis and manufacture. Synthetic approaches to enhance the biocompatibility have encompassed bulk and surface modification of polymers. Bulk modification is achieved through the employment of different reagents from which the polymer is synthesized, or chemical modification of the whole polymer after polymerization from the constituent monomers. Surface modification can be achieved through a number of routes including bulk modification or surface derivation, and is performed once the device is formed. One major advantage that surface modification offers above bulk modification is the opportunity to retain the material's mechanical characteristics, which are intimately related to the chemical composition of the bulk, while altering the interfacial characteristics of the material. These advantages may be offset once a material is produced commercially, by increasing the number of processing steps and technological requirements, and may even prevent production at a commercial level. Surface modification of polymers include the incorporation of other polymers, ionic groups, and grafting of biological molecules, such as anti-thrombotic agents, anti-platelet agents, peptides, proteins and enzymes. Many of these modifications have been applied to polyurethane elastomers. Bulk modification and surface modification of polyurethanes are discussed further below.

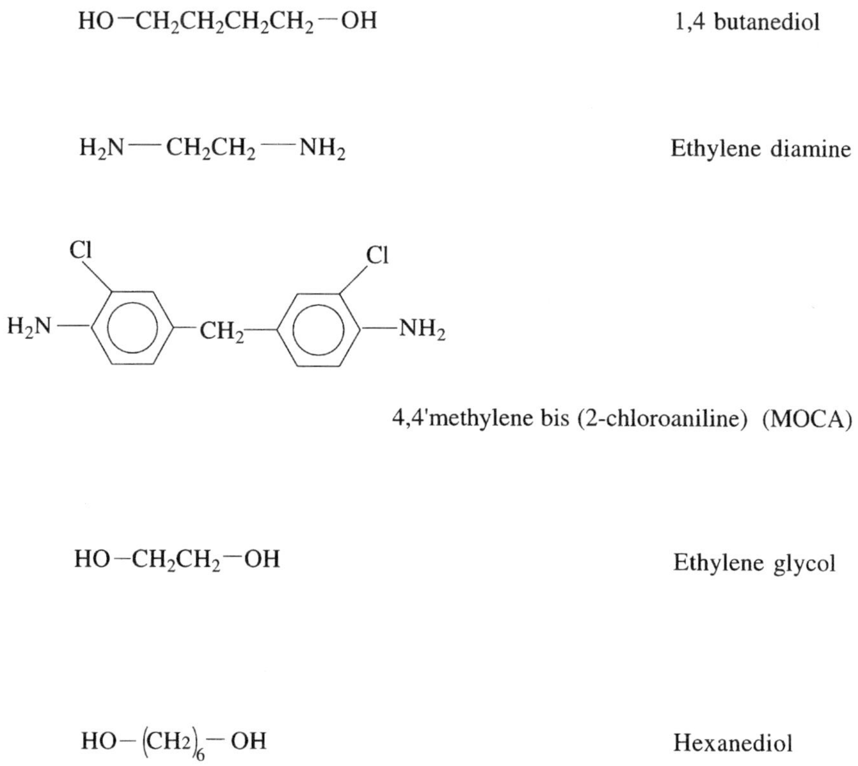

HO—CH₂CH₂CH₂CH₂—OH   1,4 butanediol

H₂N—CH₂CH₂—NH₂   Ethylene diamine

4,4'methylene bis (2-chloroaniline) (MOCA)

HO—CH₂CH₂—OH   Ethylene glycol

HO—(CH2)₆—OH   Hexanediol

FIGURE 16 Typical chain extenders.

A. BULK MODIFICATION OF POLYURETHANES

As shown in this chapter, the ability to select different reagents provides a number of synthetic options in polyurethane synthesis. The chemistry of the reagents can be chosen so that specific groups can be incorporated into the structure. These groups can modify the biological performance, or can provide sites for further modification to improve biocompatibility. Such modifications include altering the chemical structure of the diisocyanate, soft segment or chain extender, and this approach has been illustrated earlier in this chapter. Other possible routes include derivatization of a polyurethane to incorporate specific chemical groups. The incorporation of ionic groups in polyurethanes has been performed; Cooper and coworkers have incorporated sulfonate, carboxyl, and tertiary amino groups, in order to change the physicochemical nature of the surface.[24-28] These modifications were achieved through alterations in hard segment or soft segment chemistry, or by abstraction of the urethane hydrogen and reaction with an appropriate compound. Figure 17 shows a reaction scheme for the sulfonation of polyurethanes through substitution of the urethane hydrogen. This method is not limited to the inclusion of ionic groups but also has been used to attach alkyl chains to polyurethanes.[29]

Santerre et al.[30] have altered the biological properties of polyurethanes by incorporating a biphenyldisulfonic acid (BDDS) chain extender in a polyurethane, in order to incorporate sulfonate groups into the polyurethane. The incorporation of additives such as antioxidants that will migrate or 'bloom' to the surface is another means of modifying the surface of polymers. Surface-modifiying additives consisting of surface active, high molecular weight copolymers have been added to polyurethanes to alter the surface characteristics of the material.[31] Harvey et al. have bound a plasminogen activator to a polyurethane surface by incorporating a water-insoluble surfactant

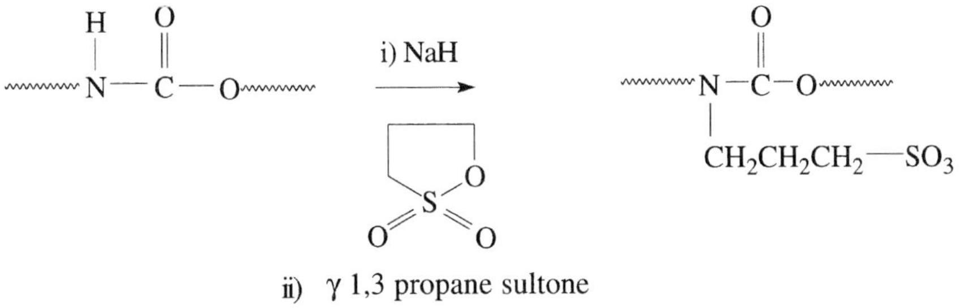

FIGURE 17 Sulfonation of polyurethane at the urethane group.

(tridodecylmethylammonium chloride, TDMAC) into the material.[32] Tissue plasminogen activator (tPA) was adsorbed onto the surface and bound electrostatically. The blooming of additives to the surface is not unusual in polymeric materials, and with respect to the biomedical polyurethanes, the migration of processing additives to the surface has been observed. This is discussed in more detail in Chapter 5.

B. Surface Modification of Polyurethanes

Surface modification of biomaterials is an important method for the improvement of biomaterial performance. Although the surface chemistry and physicochemical properties of polymers can be modified through alterations in bulk chemistry, which ultimately affect the surface characteristics, this can sometimes compromise the mechanical performance of the material, as the mechanical and physical properties of polymers are strongly related to their chemical structure. As discussed in Chapter 1, both the mechanical and interfacial characteristics of biomaterials are fundamental factors of biocompatibility. Thus, surface modification of polyurethanes offers a route by which the interfacial properties can be altered with little or no effect on the mechanical performance.

Techniques to alter the surface chemistry of polyurethanes include bulk modification, surface treatment after bulk modification, and surface treatment alone. This last category can be divided further into physical and chemical grafting. Techniques and examples of bulk modification of polyurethanes have been discussed above. However, the bulk composition of a polyurethane can be modified to incorporate some functional groups, which are then reacted with other reagents once the surface has been formed. Lin *et al.* modified a polyurethane to contain carboxyl groups, which were subsequently reacted with peptides to promote cell attachment.[27] Fibrinolytic agents have been attached to lysine derivatized polyurethanes,[33] and through the use of polymeric enzyme carriers.[34] Heparinized surfaces have been prepared through the synthesis of polyurethanes containing quaternary ammonium groups which electrostatically bind heparin.[35] Other materials that bind heparin through ionic interactions have shown good short term anticoagulant properties; however when heparin or other molecules are bound electrostatically to surfaces, they can be slowly released into the blood. This can be used as a means of obtaining controlled release of pharmaceutical agents. Covalent attachment of molecules can help overcome leaching from the surface; however attachment of the molecules is more difficult and may affect the biological activity of the molecule. The heparinization of polyurethanes has been achieved through chemical grafting, usually incorporating a spacer molecule such as polyethylene oxide,[36] and polyamido amine chains.[37] A more detailed review on the heparinization of polyurethanes is available.[38]

Covalent attachment of polymers or pharmaceutical agents to the polymer surface also has been achieved through the use of diisocyanate bridges, such as $H_{12}MDI$. This can react with urethane, hydroxy or amine groups at the polyurethane surface resulting in the formation of covalent bonds. The unreacted functional groups also can react with hydroxy or amine groups on other molecules. This procedure is depicted in Figure 18. A large number of molecules have been grafted

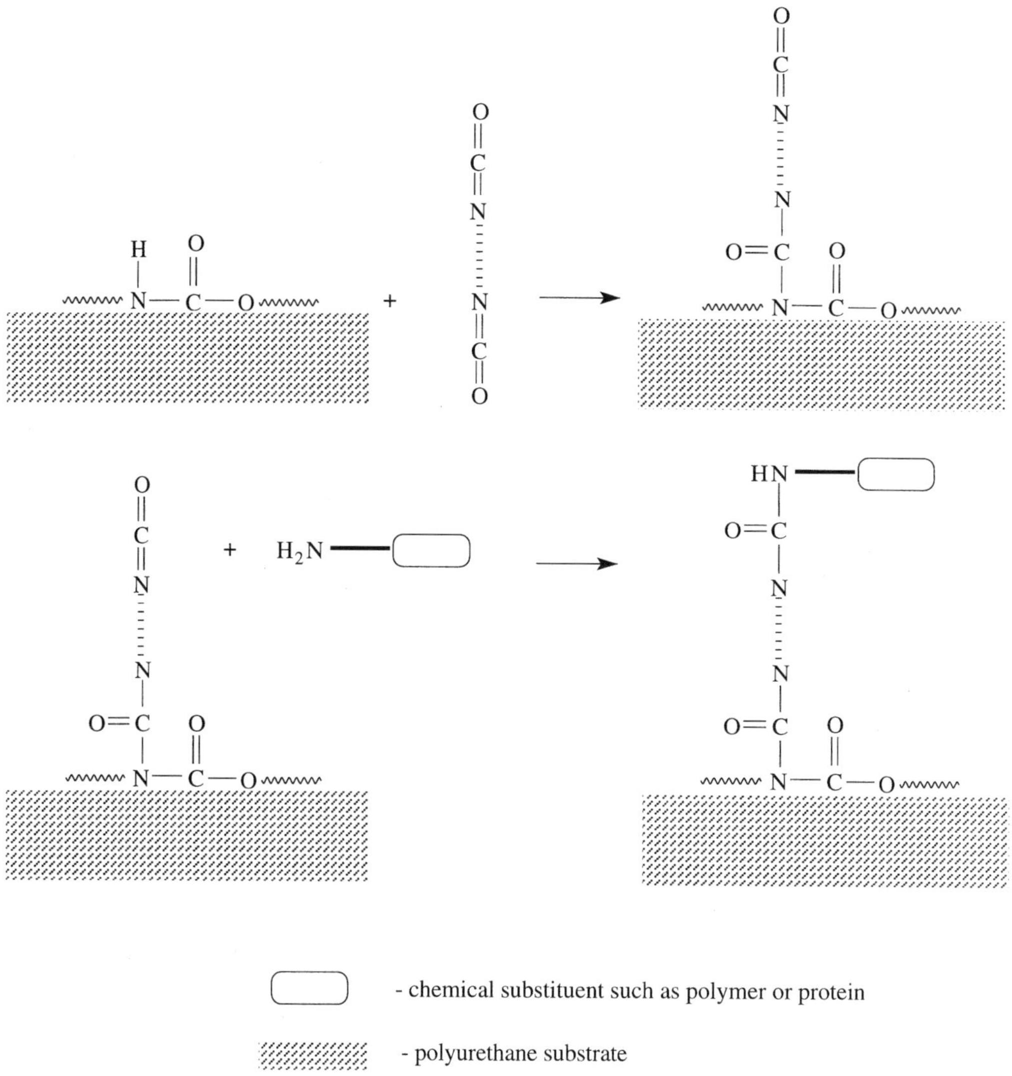

FIGURE 18 Surface modification of polyurethanes via diisocyanate bridges.

to the surface in this manner including polyethylene oxide (PEO), albumin, PEO-heparin and albumin-heparin complexes, prostacyclin (a naturally occurring anti-platelet aggregating agent),[39,40] and thrombomodulin.[41]

Graft photopolymerization can be used to provide a coating onto a polyurethane substrate. This technique has been used to graft polyvinyl pyrrollidone (PVP), N-vinyl pyrrollidone (NVP), polyethylene glycol (PEG), polyhydroxyethyl methacrylate (HEMA), and polyacrylamide onto polyurethanes. Bamford and Middleton also have grafted hydrophilic monomers on to polyurethane surfaces.[42] Radiation induced grafting of HEMA and other methacrylates onto polyurethane elastomers also has been achieved.[43] More recently, Aldenhoff and Koole modified dipyridamole,[44] an inhibitor of platelet activation, to contain photopolymerizable groups, and successfully grafted the structure onto a polyurethane surface.

Another technique for polymer surface modification is the application of plasma glow discharge technology. In this context, plasma refers to a partially ionized gas, composed of electrons, ions, free radicals, photons, as atoms or molecules either in their ground state or an excited state.[45] The surface to be treated is exposed to a highly reactive gas plasma. The technique can be used to apply thin coatings of material onto substrates, or to etch surfaces to make them more wettable. Due to the high reactivity of the plasma, polymerization between the plasma constituents and the substrate occurs at the interface. Plasma glow discharge techniques generally have a depth penetration of approximately 400Å. Polyurethanes have been treated with glow discharge techniques, using sulfur dioxide, introducing ionic sulfonate groups at the surface. Acetone, methanol and formic acid plasmas can be used to deposit carbonyl, methyl, and carboxyl groups respectively. Plasma desposition has been used to introduce functional groups at the surface which have then been used to immobilize albumin,[46] heparin,[47] enzymes,[48] and antibiotics,[49] on polyurethane surfaces.

SUMMARY

It can be seen that polyurethane synthesis contains a diverse range of synthetic options. The chemistry of polyurethane elastomers can be varied through the chemistry of the diisocyanate, the polyol, the chain extender and the ratios in which these are reacted. The chemistry ultimately affects the mechanical and the biological properties of the finished material. The range of synthetic options is further enhanced by the possibilities offered through derivatization of the polymer. As discussed in this chapter, polyurethanes can be functionalized via chemical modification of the bulk, or by chemical modification and grafting of the surface, once the material has been formed into a shape. Options also exist for modification of bulk and surface properties of polyurethanes, through blending with other polymers, construction of composite materials, and the use of additives, such as those used to assist polyurethane melt processing.

REFERENCES

1. Flory P. J. *Principles of Polymer Chemistry.* Cornell University Press, Ithaca, NY, 1953.
2. Cowie J. M. G. *Polymers: The Chemistry and Physics of Modern Materials.* International Textbook, Aylesbury, UK, 1973.
3. Allcock H. R. and Lampe F. W. *Contemporary Polymer Chemistry.* Prentice-Hall, Englewood Cliffs, NJ, 1981.
4. Billmeyer F. W. *Textbook of Polymer Science.* Wiley, New York, NY, 1984.
5. Rodriguez F. *Principles of Polymer Systems.* (4th Ed.): Hemisphere Publishing, NY, 1996.
6. Sperling L. H. *Introduction to Physical Polymer Science.* (2nd Ed.): Wiley, New York, 1992.
7. Brydson J. A. *Plastics Materials.* (6th Ed.): Butterworth Scientific, London, UK, 1995.
8. Saunders J. H. and Frisch K. C. *Polyurethanes: Chemistry and Technology.* Interscience, New York, 1962.
9. Wright P. and Cumming A. P. C. *Solid Polyurethane Elastomers.* Maclaren & Sons, London, 1969.
10. Wirpsza Z. *Polyurethanes: Chemistry, Technology and Applications.* (1st Ed.): Ellis Horwood, London, 1993.
11. Bayer O. "The diisocyanate polyaddition process (polyurethanes). Description of a new principle for building up high-molecular compounds." *Angew. Chem,* A59:257, 1937.
12. Rinke H., Schild H. and Siefken W. U.S. Patent 2,511,544. 1938.
13. Lieser T. U.S. Patent 2,266,777. 1941.
14. Hochtlen A. *Kunstoffe,* 42:303, 1952.
15. Langerak E. O., Prucino L. J., and Remington W. R. U.S. Patent 2,692,893. Du Pont, 1954.
16. Schollenberger C. S., Scott H. and Moore G. R. "Polyurethane VC. Virtually crosslinked elastomer." *Rubber World,* 137:549, 1958.
17. Steuber N. U.S. Patent 2,929,804. 1960.
18. Boretos J. W. "Tissue pathology and physical stability of a polyether elastomer on three-year implantation." *J. Biomed. Mater. Res.,* 6:473, 1972.
19. Hepburn C. *Polyurethane Elastomers.* (2nd Ed.): Elsevier Applied Science, London, 1992.
20. Baker J. and Gaunt J. J. "The mechanism of the reaction of aryl isocyanates with alcohols and amines. II. The base catalyzed reaction of phenylisocyanate with alcohols." *Chem. Sci.,* 9:19, 1949.

21. Frisch K. C. "Recent advances in the chemistry of polyurethanes." *Rubber Chem. Technol.*, 45:1442, 1972.
22. Brunette C. M., Hsu S. L., and MacKnight W. J. "Structural and mechanical properties of polybutadiene-containing polyurethanes." *Polym. Eng. Sci.,* 21:163, 1981.
23. Speckhard T. A., Strate G. V., Gibson P. E., and Cooper S. L. "Properties of isobutylene-polyurethane block copolymers. I. Macroglycols from ozonolysis of an isobutylene isoprene copolymer." *Polym. Eng. Sci.,* 23:337, 1983.
24. Lelah M. D., Pierce J. A., Lambrecht L. K., and Cooper S. L. "Polyether-urethane ionomers: surface property/*ex vivo* blood compatibility relationships. *J. Coll. Interf. Sci.,* 104:422, 1985.
25. Okkema A. Z., Visser S. A., and Cooper S. L. "Physical and blood-contacting properties of polyurethanes based on a sulfonic acid-containing diol chain extender." *J. Biomed. Mater. Res.* 25:1371, 1991.
26. Grasel T. G. and Cooper S. L. "Properties and biological interactions of polyurethane anionomers: effect of sulfonate incorporation." *J. Biomed. Mater. Res.,* 23:311, 1989.
27. Lin H.-B., Sun W., Mosher D. F., Garcia-Echeverria C., Schaufelberger K., Lelkes P. I., and Cooper S. L. "Synthesis, surface and cell adhesion properties of polyurethanes containing covalently grafted RGD-peptides." *J. Biomed. Mater. Res.,* 28:329, 1994.
28. Goddard R. J. and Cooper S. L. "Polyurethane cationomers with pendant trimethylammonium groups. 2. Investigation of the microphase separation transition." *Macromolecules,* 28:1401, 1995.
29. Grasel T. G., Pierce J. A., and Cooper S. L. "Effects of alkyl grafting on surface properties and blood compatibility of polyurethane block copolymers." *J. Biomed. Mater. Res.,* 21:815, 1987.
30. Santerre J. P. and Brash J. L. "Methods for the covalent attachment of potentially bioactive moieties to sulfonated polyurethanes." *Macromolecules,* 24:5497, 1991.
31. Ward R. S., Litwak P., White K. A., Robinson J., Yilgor I., and *Riffle J. S. BPS-215M: A new polyurethaneurea for biomedical devices: Developments and* in vivo *testing in the Pierce-Donachy VAD.* 13th Annual Meeting of the Society for Biomaterials. New York. 1987: 259.
32. Harvey R. A., Kim H. C., Pincus J., Trooskin S. Z., Wilcox J. N., and Greco R. S. "Binding of tissue plasminogen activator to vascular grafts." *Thromb. Haemost.,* 61:131, 1989.
33. Woodhouse K. A. and Brash J. L. "Adsorption of plasminogen to lysine-derivatized polyurethane surfaces." *Biomaterials,* 13:1103, 1992.
34. Ryu G. H., Park S., Kim M., Han D. K., Kim Y. H., and Min B. "Antithrombogenicity of lumbrokinase-immobilized polyurethane." *J. Biomed. Mater. Res.,* 28:1069, 1994.
35. Ito Y., Sisido M., and Imanishi Y. "Synthesis and antithrombogenicity of polyetherurethaneurea having quaternary ammonium groups in the side chains and of the polymer/heparin complex." *J. Biomed. Mater. Res.,* 20:1017, 1986.
36. Park K. D., Okano T., Nojiri C., and Kim S. W. "Heparin immobilization onto segmented polyurethaneurea surfaces — effect of hydrophilic spacers." *J. Biomed. Mater. Res.,* 22:977, 1988.
37. Azzuoli G., Barbucci R., Benvenuti M., Ferruti P., and Necentini M. "Chemical and biological evaluation of heparinized poly(amide-amine) grafted polyurethane." *Biomaterials,* 8:61, 1987.
38. Eloy R., Belleville J., Rissoan M. C., and Baguet J. "Heparinization of medical grade polyurethanes." *J. Biomater. Appl.,* 2:475, 1988.
39. Bamford C. H., Middleton I. P., and Satake Y. "Grafting and attachment of anti-platelet agents to poly(ether-urethanes)." *Polymer Prepr.,* 25:27, 1984.
40. Joseph G. and Sharma C. P. "Prostacyclin immobilized albuminated surfaces." *J. Biomed. Mater. Res.,* 21:937, 1987.
41. Kishida A., Ueno Y., Fukudome N., Yashima E., Maruyama I., and Akashi M. "Immobilization of human thrombomodulin onto poly(ether urethaneurea) for developing antithrombogenic blood-contacting biomaterials." *Biomaterials,* 15:848, 1994.
42. Bamford C. H. and Middleton I. P. "Studies on functionalizing and grafting to poly(ether-urethanes). *Eur. Polym. J.,* 19:1027, 1983.
43. Jansen B. and Ellinghorst G. "Modification of polyetherurethane for biomedical application by radiation induced grafting. I. Grafting procedure, determination of mechanical properties and chemical modification of grafted films." *J. Biomed. Mater. Res.,* 19:1085, 1985.
44. Aldenhoff Y. B. J. and Koole L. H. "Studies on a new strategy for surface modification of polymeric biomaterials." *J. Biomed. Mater. Res.,* 29:917, 1995.

45. Gombotz W. R. and Hoffman A. S. "Gas-discharge techniques for biomaterial modification." In *CRC Criticial Reviews in Biocompatibility.* CRC Press, Boca Raton, Florida, 1987:
46. Joseph G. and Sharma C. P. Note: "Platelet adhesion to surfaces treated with glow discharge and albumin." *J. Biomed. Mater. Res.,* 20:677, 1986.
47. Kang I.-K., Kwon O. H., Lee Y. M., and Sung Y. K. "Preparation and surface characterization of functional group-grafted and heparin-immobilized polyurethanes by plasma glow disharge." *Biomaterials,* 17:841, 1996.
48. Danilich M. J., Kottke-Marchant K., Anderson J. M., and Marchant R. E. "The immobilization of glucose oxidase onto radio-frequency plasma-modified poly(etherurethaneurea)." *J. Biomater. Sci., Polym. Ed.,* 3:195, 1992.
49. Mittelman M. W., Sahi V. P., Soric I., and Sodhi R. N. S. *Antimicrobial activity of remote plasma modified polyurethane against biofilm bacteria.* Fifth World Biomaterials Congress. Toronto, Canada. 1996: 257.

3 Fabrication and Processing of Polyurethanes

I. INTRODUCTION

In order for a polyurethane to be used as a medical device it must be formed into the appropriate shape and size for a specific application. Fabrication can be considered to be the physical, mechanical, or thermal manipulation of the polymer in order to attain this form. Although fabrication of polyurethanes usually starts with the polymer, it can begin with the monomers or pre-polymers. Thus, polyurethane processing is frequently based on the use of low molecular weight liquid prepolymers which are easy to handle at reasonably low pressure. Advantage is taken during processing of the rapid reactions which characterize polyurethane polymerizations to convert these precursor monomers and prepolymers into solid end products.

In the first step of fabrication, the polymer may be mixed or compounded with additives that are required for the device application or that may be needed to aid processing. These additives can include plasticizers, fillers, pigments, antioxidants, UV light stabilizers and mold release agents. Polymer processing may require the mixing of powders, pellets, or polymer melts, that involve high operating and capital costs. Fortunately for the researcher or medical device manufacturer, biomedical polyurethanes can usually be synthesized at reasonable cost on a bench scale. It is important to note, however, that the additives can impact not only the cost but also the host response to the biomaterial. Full evaluation of the additives' effects on the performance and tissue response are important aspects of qualifying polyurethanes or any other biomaterial for a given application. The polyurethane elastomers used in many biomedical applications can be produced by casting, by roll mills and by injection molding and are frequently produced using the two step prepolymer process. For general information on polyurethane processing the reader is referred to the Polyurethane Handbook by Oertel.[1]

II. PROCESSING OF POLYURETHANES

A. ONE-DIMENSIONAL PROCESSES

One dimensional processes include coatings and adhesives. In the application of coatings and adhesives the most important dimension is usually the thickness of the coating. Coating may be performed at room temperature, using a simple solution dipping technique or by spray coating. Hot coating techniques include hot-melt, fluidized bed, and electrostatic powder coating. The fluidized bed method can be used where the polymer is a reactive powder.

In solvent coating, the choice of solvent is extremely important. Often solution viscosity, which is controlled by polyurethane molecular weight and solution concentration, is of primary importance in these processes. Generally, it is desirable to work at maximum concentrations to minimize the use of solvent. There are only a few solvents that are suitable for dissolving polyurethanes. These are listed in Table 1 with some of their properties.[2-4]

Polyurethanes require relatively polar solvents for solubilization. An important consideration in the choice of the solvent to be used for fabrication is the boiling point. Tetrahydrofuran (THF) is a useful solvent for coating because of its low boiling point and thus lower evaporation time. Unfortunately, the most effective solvents for solubilizing polyurethanes are either toxic, carcinogenic, mutagenic, or teratogenic.[4] Thus, these solvents need to be handled with care. It also is important

TABLE 1
Common solvents of polyurethanes and some physical properties

Solvent	Boiling Pt (°C)	Melting Pt (°C)	Specific Gravity at 0°C	Viscosity at 20°C (cp.)
N-N Dimethylacetamide (DMA)	165	−20.00	0.937	—
Dimethylformamide (DMF)	153	−60.48	0.949	—
Dimethylsulfoxide (DMSO)	189	18.4	1.101	—
Tetrahydrofuran (THF)	64–65	−65	0.889	0.486
m-cresol	202	11.5	1.034	20.8
Methyl ethyl ketone (MEK)	79.6	−86.35	0.805	0.423 (15°C)
Toluene	110.62	−95.0	0.867	0.590

From Lelah, M.D. and Cooper, S.L. *Polyurethanes in Medicine,* CRC Press, 1986. With permission.

that all the solvent be removed from the finished material before it is used as an implant. This requires carefully controlled drying operations and extensive washing with water where possible.

The first step in solvent casting is the preparation of the substrate. Because most of the solvents for the polyurethanes are rather polar in nature it is necessary to treat the substrate in order to both clean the substrate and improve its wettability by the polymer solution. The substrate surface, which may be metal or polymer, may be cleaned with a surfactant solution or degreased with liquid THF, acetone, or vapor phase isopropanol. The wettability of the substrate by the solution directly influences the quality of the coating. It is sometimes necessary to etch the surface to improve wettability. This may done using either a liquid etching or a plasma etching process. Liquid etching techniques include the use of chromic acid, aqueous sodium hydroxide and fuming sulfuric acid.[5] Optimum etching conditions need to be established because at high concentrations and temperatures and long etching times most liquids used are capable of dissolving, swelling, or degrading the substrate. Chromic acid etching is a popular technique and has been used to prepare both polyethylene and glass surfaces for subsequent coating with biomedical polyurethanes.[6] It is necessary, however, to remove inorganic chromium-containing deposits from the etched surface prior to coating, usually with a nitric acid wash.

Considerable interest has been generated in using electrical discharge in various gases for the surface treatment of polymeric substrates.[5,7] Etching is dependent on the plasma conditions such as gas pressure, substrate temperature, electric field and current densities, and system geometry. Oxygen plasma generation is popular, and the two electric discharges that have been used extensively for plasma etching are glow discharges and arcs.[8] The plasma normally heats the substrate and cooling is sometimes necessary to prevent thermal degradation of the substrate.

The next stage in the solvent casting fabrication technique is the actual coating process. This may be a static dipping contact, or may involve the flow of coating solution over the substrate. Solution concentration, contact time, and temperature will affect the thickness of the final coating. Evaporation or removal of the solvent after contact is controlled by system temperature, pressure, drying gas flow rate, and solvent boiling point. The evaporation rate will affect the composition and structure of the coating, especially for very thin coatings. For the segmented polyurethanes, the rate of evaporation can affect phase separation of the final coating thereby altering the physical and chemical properties of the surface. A slow evaporation rate will allow for pseudo-equilibrium to be established during evaporation. The nonequilibrium conditions achieved during rapid evaporation (for example under high vacuum, spin-coating or high gas flow rates) may result in unusual bulk and surface morphologies of the typically phase-separated hard and soft polyurethane segments. Optimization of both contact and evaporation, with suitable examination of the properties of the coating are necessary to ensure the generation of a coating with the desired characteristics.

Plasma polymerization is another technique that is used to coat materials. In recent years it has been gaining in its use in many applications. In this technique a polymer film is laid on a substrate through the use of ionized gaseous plasmas or monomer gases.[9] In glow-discharge polymerization, the substrate to be coated onto the surface can be made the anode of an electrical discharge over a potential of several thousand volts. The material deposited onto the surface typically forms a highly adherent and tightly crosslinked film. The drawback to this process is that the characteristics of the film and the reactions that will occur in the plasma often are difficult to predict and reproducibility can be a problem. Time dependent changes in surface chemistry also occur after processing due to surface reorganization and further reaction of unstable groups on the treated surface.[10-11] Treatment of polyurethane surface by plasma polymerization has been reported by a number of researchers.[10,12-16]

Coatings are used to modify the surface of a biomaterial. A more recent strategy for surface modification of materials is the addition of surface-modifying additives or SMAs. These materials are added during fabrication of the polymeric material and will rise to the surface. SMAs are designed to reduce the interfacial surface energy of the material by using low molecular weight block co-polymers. One block is compatible with the bulk material and the other is incompatible and of lower surface energy. The first "anchors" the SMA into the bulk, the second lowers the interfacial energy.

B. TWO-DIMENSIONAL PROCESSES

The two-dimensional fabrication processes include extrusion, the production of fibers, and lamination. In extrusion a material is forced through a die that shapes the profile. Continuous flow of material results in a long shape of constant cross section. Figure 1 shows the cross section of a typical extruder, which is essentially a screw conveyer carrying cold plastic pellets forward, and compacting and melting them in the compression section using heat from external heaters and from the friction of viscous flow.[17] Extrusion is used for the fabrication of tubing, rods, flat film, and sheeting. However, extrusion of polyurethanes containing high hard segment contents is not always a preferred method of fabrication for polyurethanes as they may undergo some degradation before they flow at high temperatures. There are and have been notable exceptions including the Estanes® (B.F. Goodrich), Pellethanes® (Upjohn Co., New Haven, CT), and extruded grade Biomer® (Ethicon Inc., Somerville, NJ).

Fiber spinning is another example of a two-dimensional fabrication process. Spandex is the generic name given to elastic fibers that contain at least 85% segmented polyurethane. The method used to spin polyurethane fibers depends on the reactivity between the chain extender and the isocyanate.[18] If the degree of reactivity is low, for example if a diol chain extender is used, then melt polymerization or melt spinning techniques can be applied. Melt spinning is the same as melt extrusion, where a fiber is formed in an extrusion-type process. This cannot generally be used for polyurethaneureas. If the chain extender has a higher reactivity with isocyanate groups, then solution techniques are favored.

The manufacture of spandex fibers may employ a reactive method as follows:[19] The liquid prepolymer with two or three isocyanate groups is fed under pressure through a filter and nozzle into a bath containing a diamine dissolved in toluene, or other nonsolvent for the polyurethane. As the prepolymer enters the bath, chain extension occurs, and a polyurethaneurea skin is formed on the surface. Unreacted polyurethane causes the filaments to stick to one another, forming thicker fibers. Maturation is said to occur as the diamine diffuses through the filaments, continuing to react with isocyanate groups within the core of the filament. The fibers are dried in an oven, to evaporate the solvent. This method of production yields fibers comprised of a number of filaments of irregular cross-sectional area. Alternatively, fibers may be dry or wet spun. In dry spinning a pump is used to feed a polymer solution through a spinneret into a heated chamber. The spinneret may have a number of holes. As the solvent evaporates, filaments are produced, and these are drawn into fibers.

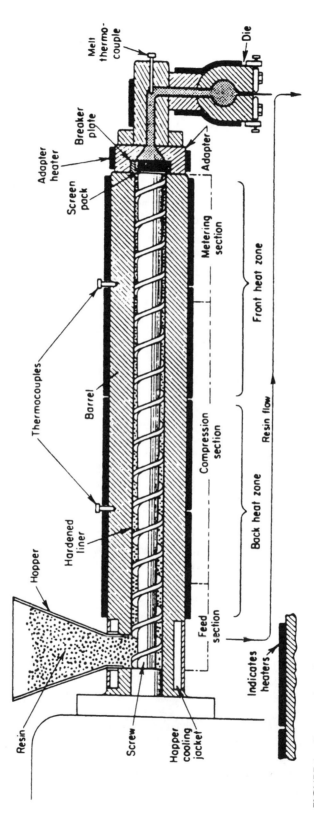

FIGURE 1 Cross section of a typical extruder. From *Petrothane Polyolefins A Processing Guide*, 3rd Edition. Ed., U.S. Industrial Chemicals Co., New York, 1965.

Fabrication and Processing of Polyurethanes

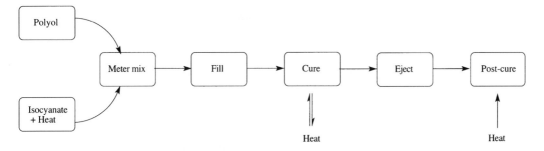

FIGURE 2 Typical RIM process unit operation.

Solvent evaoration and recovery are important in this process. In wet spinning the polymer is precipitated in an immiscible liquid such as water, after passing the polymer solution through a spinneret. Wet spinning requires lower financial investment than dry spinning, but the resulting fibers typically have irregular cross-sectional area and rougher surfaces than fibers produced by dry spinning.

The third technique is lamination, where thin sheets of the same polymer, or alternating materials in composites, are layered together. The production of laminates usually involves machining operations such as rolling on mandrels for the production of curved surfaces. Laminates also can be produced during extrusion.

C. Three-Dimensional Processes

In molding operations pressure and heat are usually applied to make the polymer flow into a preferred form. Dimensional stability of the molded polymer is then achieved by cooling. Thermoplastic polyurethanes have to be cooled to below the melt point, T_m, or the hard segment glass transition temperature, T_g before being removed from the mold. Injection molding is a process for producing molded samples in cyclical fashion by carrying out each step in a separate zone of the same apparatus. The rapidity with which the isocyanate-polyol reaction takes place in the synthesis of polyurethanes has been used to advantage in reaction injection molding (RIM). In the typical RIM process (Figure 2) the two components are mixed by high-pressure injection (impingement mixing) into a special chamber and almost immediately injected into a closed, low pressure mold (Figure 3).[20] Both cellular (foam) and solid molded parts can be obtained using RIM. RIM technology is used very extensively in the automobile industry for the production of polyurethane bumpers and fascia and for the production of rigid structural foams for use in furniture and in electrical equipment housing.

Other three-dimensional fabrication processes include sheet forming, vacuum forming, post forming, cold forming, weaving, knitting and machining. Polyurethane elastomers are not easily machinable.[21] In the following sections we examine some of the processes used to form polyurethane into foams, tubing, balloons, and bladders.

1. Foams

Polyurethane foams can be categorized as soft, rigid or semirigid and are crosslinked in structure. In order to obtain the cell-like structure of foams, additional components may be required in their manufacture. In addition to catalysts, these additives may include surfactants, blowing agents and fillers, pigments or dyes. Foams also may be classed as closed cell or open cell. Closed cell foams have cellular structures in which each cell is completely enclosed by a membrane. They are typically produced in processes where some pressure is maintained during the cell formation. Open cell foams, which have interconnecting pores, often are made during free expansion processes.

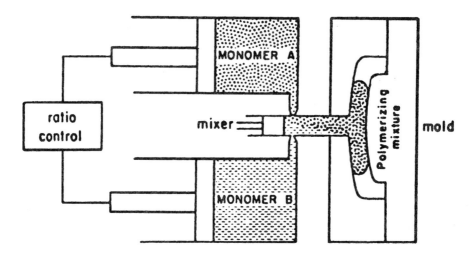

FIGURE 3 Schematic diagram of the RIM Process. From Lelah, M.D. and Cooper, S.L. *Polyurethanes in Medicine*, CRC Press, Boca Raton, FL, 1986. With permission.

Surfactants are required in foam production in order to control the bubble size, which is achieved through control of surface energy. Surfactants also can promote mixing of components that may otherwise be partially immiscible. They also serve to stabilize bubble nuclei in the liquid reaction mixture, preventing bubbles coalescing into fewer, larger bubbles. Furthermore, they control the fluidity of the polymer in the expansion step, as the bubbles are formed. Ionic compounds were originally used as surface active agents in polyurethane foam manufacture. Current agents are nonionic organosilicon-polyether copolymers, which are particularly good at creating closed-cell structures.

The major blowing agent for polyurethane foams is carbon dioxide. This can be generated within the reaction mixture using a controlled amount of water and excess isocyanate. In some instances, the water may be introduced in the form of hydrated salts or molecular sieves. As descirbed in Chapter 2, the reaction of isocyanate with water leads to the formation of a urea group, with the liberation of carbon dioxide. The rigidity of the foam can be controlled by the chain flexibility and foam density by the amounts of carbon dioxide generated. If a lighter foam is required, then a physical blowing agent also may be used. In the past, the most commonly used agents were the chlorofluorocarbons (CFCs). Due to their environmental impact on the stratospheric ozone layer, their use in many applications including foam production has been decreased and alternatives have been sought and introduced. The use of CFCs is scheduled to be eliminated in the U.S. by 2000. Replacements for CFCs in foam production include hydrofluorocarbons, liquid carbon dioxide and formic acid. Lighter foams can be produced by reducing the pressure of the mixture, but this increases the complexity of the manufacturing process. Air also can be used, although constant mixing is required.

2. Tubing

a. Extruded tubing

Extrusion techniques have been used for the fabrication of polyurethane tubing. The Pellethane®2363 family has been used in pacemaker lead insulation and other tubular applications in the biomedical field. The extrusion equipment for the processing of Pellethane is similar to that used for flexible PVC.[22] Other polyurethanes that are capable of being extruded into tubing form are the Estane family and Extrusion Grade Biomer.[23] Basic concepts in extrusion are described by Rodriquez.[9]

b. Solvent cast tubing

The most straightforward way to fabricate a nonporous tubing with a polyurethane inner surface is by using commercially available extruded tubing of polyethylene or polyvinyl chloride and then solvent casting a thin film of polyurethane on the inner surface of the extruded tubing. The composite tubing, which can then be used as a vascular prosthesis or for *in vitro* testing, will have a surface characteristic of polyurethane, but mechanical properties characteristic of the extruded substrate polymer. An important consideration is the complete removal of the solvent. This is accomplished by extended drying in a nitrogen gas stream followed by drying in vacuum, preferably at moderate temperature. The tubing is then washed extensively with water. The choice of the solvent influences the rate of drying.

Another solution casting technique utilizes the casting of a polymer solution over an appropriate mold, such as a mandrel, followed by solvent evaporation in a forced draft oven. Sometimes this step is followed by heat-setting in order to provide dimensional stability. This method can be performed in a single pass for thin-walled tubing or repeated in order to build up thicker-walled tubing.[24-25] One method of application of a polymer solution on a mandrel involves slow spinning of the mandrel horizontally on a lathe and solution spinning polymer fibers onto the mandrel in a sequence of layers.[25] Another method utilizes a dipping technique in which the mandrel is slowly dipped in, and then removed from the polymer solution. If this process is performed in a vacuum or in a forced air environment the process can be cyclical, leading to a thick coating of polymer on the mandrel. The mandrel can be inverted to provide a coating with even thickness at all longitudinal positions. Teflon® (E. I. du Pont de Nemours & Co.) is a useful mandrel material as it has a very low surface tension and aids in the release of the polymer. The application techniques described above can be used for the fabrication of other components in addition to tubing. Complete removal of the solvent is important both from the requirement for dimensional stability of the final product and also, as most of the solvents are water soluble, it is important not to have solvent extraction when the device contacts tissue. Lamination techniques have been used to produce anisotropic vascular prostheses.[26]

c. Porous and fibrous tubing

For compliance matching between host vessels and vascular prostheses, it is desirable to fabricate tubing with mechanical properties that match those of the natural vessels. Natural vessel compliance is higher than that obtainable in nonporous polyurethanes due to the relatively high modulus of polyurethanes. One method of overcoming this problem is to fabricate a porous polyurethane tubing. Dryer *et al.*[27] in 1960, used polyurethane foam to replace canine aorta. These grafts consisted of a two- to four-mm thick sponge-like polyurethane. Lyman *et al.*[28] developed a technique for the precipitation of a solution of a copolyether urethane urea material onto a mandrel by controlled solvent-nonsolvent exchange using DMF as the polymer solvent and water as the nonsolvent. White *et al.*[29] developed a controlled microporous graft using the replamineform process. In this method tubular prostheses are fashioned using a machined template of the microporous calcite spines of sea urchins (Figure 4). Liquid phase polymer components are then pressure injected into the calcite and polymerized *in situ*. The calcite is then dissolved using hydrochloric acid, leaving the polymer as a microporous tube having a mirror image pore-to-solid structure of the original calcite.

Nonwoven spinning processes have been used to fabricate porous polyurethane tubing for biomedical applications. Annis *et al.*[30] fabricated 10 mm I.D. grafts by a process of electrostatic spinning. The MDI-based polyurethane was dissolved in THF and the solution ejected from a syringe into the region of an electrostatic field formed by charging a steel mandrel to –20 kV. Fibers drawn from the solution were collected on the rotating mandrel to produce the elastic tube. Leidner and coworkers developed an alternative approach in which a solution of Pellethane® 2363-75D in DMF was extruded through fine orifices.[31-32] The resulting fibers were stretched and wrapped on a rotating mandrel. Since the fibers still contained solvent on reaching the mandrel, fiber to fiber bonding occurred resulting in a stable, helically wound porous tube. Hess *et al.*[33] also manufactured a fibrous polyurethane microvascular prosthesis by spraying liquid polyurethane directly on rotating

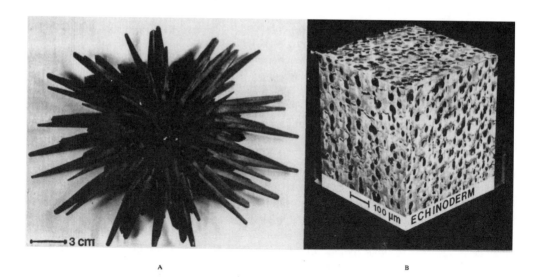

FIGURE 4 Echinoderm (A) with composite scanning electron microscope photographs showing the three-dimensional pore network characteristic of the calcite (CaCO$_3$) spines (B). From White, R.A. Weber, J.N., and White E.W., *Science*, 176,922, 1972.

mandrels.[34] The elasticity and anisotropy or the resultant tubing could be varied by changing the orientation of the synthetic fibers by varying the angle and rate of translation of the spraying jets and the rotating mandrel.

All the spinning techniques described have the advantage that the average porosity and pore sizes can be varied and controlled over a broad range. In addition, pore size and porosity can be changed by varying the thickness of the graft to control permeability. The grafts can be fabricated with suitable anisotropic properties by varying the angle of the fiber wrapping on the rotating mandrel. This high degree of variability and control of the physical and mechanical properties of the graft is important in the design of an artificial vessel, allowing different devices to be made for different animal species and prosthesis locations.

One of the novel tube forming methods includes the Flotation-Precipitation method where a polymer solution of known concentration is sprayed onto a flowing water surface. The polymer precipitates out of the solution and is transferred to a rotating mandrel lying flush with the flowing surface. The precipitated polymer forms multilayers of randomly oriented fibers resulting in a porous tube that can be used as a blood conduit.

3. Balloons, Bladders, and Other Devices

Blood or tissue contact surfaces in biomedical devices can be classified as to whether the surface is flexible or whether it is rigid. Balloons and pump bladders are examples of moving, flexing surface, while pump and device housing may be considered to be rigid contact surfaces. Both classes of surfaces can be fabricated by either solvent casting or molding techniques. In the next two sections the fabrication of polyurethane devices other than tubing by either solvent casting or molding techniques will be described.

a. Solvent casting

The process of solvent casting of devices is similar to that for the fabrication of tubing by solvent-casting techniques. Solvent-cast methods have been used for the processing of polyurethane intra-aortic balloons, which consist of one or more chambers supported on a perforated catheter tube with a suitable tip.[35] A mandrel was molded onto a catheter with tip in place and followed by dip coating with Estane 5710-F1 and 5707-F1 polyetherurethanes to form an integral film of uniform coating on the tip and along the entire length of the catheter. Rigidax®, a eutectic water dispersible inorganic salt, was used as the mandrel material, primarily due to its compatibility with the Estanes. This process was not useful for other elastomers because these polyurethanes were only soluble in DMSO or DMF, solvents which attack Rigidax. Fabrication difficulties were overcome by adopting a two stage process in which the balloon envelope was made separately from the catheter and tip. In this process paraffin wax mandrels were fabricated in a RTV silicone rubber mold. The balloon film was then formed on the mandrel by repeated dipping in a polyurethane solution (Figure 5).

Lyman et al.[36] used a solution casting technique to fabricate a hemispherical heart from a copolyetherurethane. The diaphragm and outer housing were formed over a polished aluminum mold. Multiple dipping of the mold into the polymer solution was used to obtain proper thickness. Each coating was dried for 15 min. at 90°C in a forced convection oven. Tubing and other connections were welded to the mold by applying a number of coats of the polyurethane solution. Phillips et al.[37] describe the fabrication of seam-free sacs for blood pumps and left-ventricular-assist devices using Biomer® A mold of Epolene® CIO mold wax (Eastman Chemical) was prepared from a replica mold of aluminum. The wax mold was dipped in Dow Corning #236 air drying dispersion to prepare a smooth, glossy mold surface. The mold was then dipped five to seven times in a Biomer® solution in DMA, and then dried at 140 to 160°F. The wax mold was then crushed and removed from the polyurethane sac. Phillips also discusses methods for the multiple immersion technique in solution casting. A first method utilizes a vertical dipping procedure where the mandrel should be inverted after each dip to avoid thickness variation in the final product. For molds that are cylindrical in the radial direction, the mandrel can be rotated in a horizontal position while slowly being immersed in the polyurethane solution. A third technique is used to fabricate planar

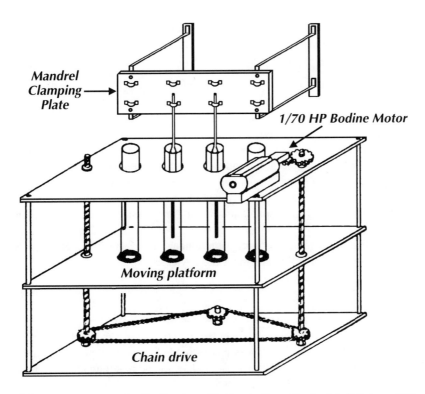

FIGURE 5 Laboratory apparatus for dip forming of balloons. From Brash, J.L. Fritzinger B.K. and Bruck S.D. *J. Biomed Mater. Res.*, 7,313, 1973.

diaphragms or sheets.[37] A disc of the appropriate shape is mounted on the head stock of a lathe. A contoured doctor blade is then brought in within 0.2 mm of the disc while the polymer solution is applied with a syringe. The disc is rotated while the doctor blade is slowly retracted. Mandrels or discs for this application have been fabricated from aluminum and coated with release agents such as tetrafluoroethylene or silicone mold release.

A prime consideration in solvent casting is cleanliness. Airborne and solution-contained impurities may affect the quality of the fabricated device and its surface structure. Filtered air should be used during the dipping and drying stages.[38]

b. Molding

Some polyurethane elastomers can be fabricated into useful biomedical devices by traditional thermoplastic molding methods. Tecoflex®-HR (Thermo Electron Corp., Waltham, MA) is an aliphatic polyurethane that can be cast using liquid molding techniques.[22,37] The procedure consists of preparing the prepolymer and curative, mixing, and finally injecting into a specially designed mold. The polymer is cured initially in the mold and then post-cured after its removal. Important consideration in molding include proper mold design, temperature control, the design of the mold charging system, and proper preparation of the prepolymer and curative system.[38] All the urethane contact surfaces should be coated with a Teflon based mold release agent. This provides the releasing properties necessary for removal of the cured polyurethane. Polyurethanes tend to adhere well to uncoated metallic surfaces.

The emphasis of the above discussions has been on the fabrication of a smooth, molded device. There is interest in the used of flocking techniques to establish textured surfaces for tissue-and blood contacting purposes.[39]

III. STERILIZATION

In order for a polyurethane to be used in medical applications it must be sterilized to minimize the risk of infection. There are generally three types of sterilization agent used for biomedical implants; steam, ethylene oxide (EtO) and radiation. Each has its advantages and disadvantages.

A. STEAM STERILIZATION

Steam sterilization or autoclaving was the earliest method applied to biomaterials and is still used for many materials, although it is not typically used for polyurethanes. The sterilization is achieved by exposing the material to saturated steam at 121°C. This requires a pressurized chamber and the process usually lasts between 15 minutes and three hours, although longer times will be used if the entire implant cannot achieve a temperature of 121°C. For this method of sterilization to be successful all parts of the material being sterilized must be contacted by the steam.

Steam sterilization is used in hospitals and laboratories because of its speed, simplicity and lack of toxicity. It is primarily used to sterilize metal instruments and solutions for intravenous injection. Its main disadvantage for use with polyurethane materials is the high temperature, which may soften the polymer, potentially deforming the device.

B. ETHYLENE OXIDE STERILIZATION

Ethylene oxide (EtO) is a liquid below 11°C and, in contrast to steam sterilization is a low pressure, low temperature sterilization method. Used either on its own or in combination with oxygen, nitrogen or a chlorofluorocarbon (CFC), ethylene oxide is toxic, explosive and flammable. It represents a significant occupation health and safety hazard and handling costs are high. Care must be taken to remove all traces of the EtO from the implant after sterilization, as residual traces of EtO in medical devices are problematic.[40-41] An evaluation of different sterilization protocols was recently performed. The author concluded that despite the problems of residual EtO in the material, EtO sterilization was one of the best methods to sterilize polyurethanes.[42]

EtO sterilization is run under a partial vacuum at 30–50°C, 40–90% humidity and an EtO concentration of 600–1200 mg/l. The samples are typically sterilized in gas permeable packaging and the vacuum used must be compatible with the material. After a sterilization cycle of anywhere from two to 48 hr, the chamber will be re-pressurized with air and several cycles of fresh air will be used to eliminate the EtO. It also may be necessary to further aerate the material outside the chamber to be completely assured of removing the EtO.

Although used extensively to sterilize many different kinds of medical device because it is efficient and compatible with many materials, recently industry has been looking for different methods because of the occupational health and safety issues associated with EtO sterilization. The residuals of sterilization which include EtO itself, and ethylene glycol are toxic and exposure for personnel to EtO itself is limited to less than 1ppm (time weighted average)/day (OSHA regulations, U.S.A.). In addition, the use of CFCs is an remains an environmental concern and North American legislation will require different mixtures to be used in the future.

C. Radiation

In this method of sterilization, ionizing radiation from either cobalt-60 isotope or accelerated electrons generated by machine is delivered in a uniform dose throughout the material. Cobalt-60 radiation is widely used. It is simple, rapid and effective for those materials which are not sensitive to radiation. Polyurethanes have shown some degradation when gamma radiation has been used and PTFE is extremely sensitive to radiation. In cobalt-60 sterilization the material is placed in a sealed irradiator and passed by the unshielded source via conveyor. The system is designed to expose all parts of the material to be sterilized to an uniform dosage of radiation. Both the minimum and maximum levels are monitored. Although relatively simple and safe to use, cobalt-60 sterilization requires a large capital outlay and continual renewal of the isotope source and associated waste disposal. It can require long processing times.

In electron beam sterilization an accelerator is used to generate electrons and the material is passed under the beam to accumulate the dose. Because the electrons do not have the penetration depth of gamma rays, this method cannot be used with thick materials and cobalt-60 is used instead. This method has the advantage that it does not require a radioactive isotope. However, it also requires large capital expenditures to set up.

There are other sterilization techniques being investigated to overcome the short comings of EtO and radiation sterilization. These new methods include low temperature gas plasma and gaseous ozone. To date, these have not been used in major commercial installations.

IV. COMMERCIAL AND EXPERIMENTAL POLYURETHANES

The following section is intended to provide a brief overview of commercially produced polyurethanes. Not all of the polyurethanes presented in the following table (Table 2) are currently available. Some of the more prominent biomedical polyurethanes have been withdrawn from use in medical devices in response to potential product liability lawsuits. Notably, Biomer has been withdrawn totally from biomedical use, and the use of Pellethane has been restricted to implantation periods that do not exceed 29 days. However, as some of the more established polyurethanes are no longer available for medical use, smaller manufacturers are producing comparable materials, intended as substitutes. For example, BioSpan (The Polymer Technology Group Incorporated, Emeryville, CA) is being marketed as a direct replacement for Biomer.[43]

Table 2 demonstrates again that polyurethane is really a term to describe a class of materials, rather than an elastomer with specific chemistry. The table below contains information on the polyurethane composition, with respect to the soft and hard segment components. Processing aids

TABLE 2
Commercial biomedical polyurethanes

Polyurethane	Description (Possible Formulation)	Uses
Biomer (Ethicon)	Family of polyetherurethane ureas At least two chemically distinct forms Solution Grade originally from Ethicon Soft segment: 2000 MW PTMO Isocyanate: MDI Chain extender: Diamines, primarily ethylene diamine Extrudable Grade: Chain extender: Water	Bladders, chamber coatings, catheters Extrudable No longer available
BioSpan	PTMO/MDI/mixed diamine chain extenders, DPMA and DMA, antioxidants	
Cardiothane 51 (Avcothane)	Mixture of polyetherurethane and polydimethylsiloxane	Artificial hearts, intra-aortic balloons blood conduits
Cardiomat Family	Similar to Biomer	
Pellethane (Dow Chemical)	Series of thermoplastic elastomers Based on PTMO/MDI/1,4 butanediol can be fabricated by injection molding	Pacemaker leads, blood bags
ChronoFlex AL	Aliphatic (HMDI), polycarbonate, BD	
ChronoFlex AR	Aromatic, polycarbonate, amine	
ChronoFlex C (CardioTech International Inc.)	Aromatic, urethane/urea	
Corplex (Corvita Corp.)	PTMO/MDI/BD	
Corethane (Corvita Corp.)	Polycarbonate based polyurethane	Cardiovascular applications
Tecoflex (Thermedics)	Aliphatic from hydrogenated MDI/PTMO 1,4 butanediol	Wound dressings
Mitrathane (PolyMedica)	MDI/PTMEG/EDA Polyether urethane urea similar to Biomer	
Rimplast	Silicone urethanes, aliphatic and aromatic esters and ethers	
Toyobo TM5	PTMO/MDI/Propylene diamine	LVAD
Vialon (Becton Dickinson Polymer Research, Sandy, UT)	PTMO/MDI/BD	Catheters
Estane (Goodrich)	Polyesterurethane Formulation varies	Cardiovascular, wound dressings
Enka PUR 817	Polyetherurethane	Vascular prostheses
Enka PUR 923	Polyetherurethane with polydimethylsiloxane	
Enka PUR 947	Polyesterurethane	
Enka PUR 981 (ENKA AG)	Polyesterurethane	
Comfeel Ulcus (Coloplast Inc)	Carboxymethylcellulose backed by a polyurethane film	Hydrocolloid wound dressing
Viasorb (Sherwood)	Cotton polyester pad within a polyurethane sleeve	Composite dressing
Bioclusive	Transparent polyurethane film with acrylic	Semiocclusive/occlusive

TABLE 2 (continued)
Commercial biomedical polyurethanes

Polyurethane	Description (Possible Formulation)	Uses
(Johnson and Johnson)	adhesive	wound dressings
Blisterfilm (Cheseborough Ponds)	Polyurethane dressing with perimeter adhesive	Composite Dressing
Opsite (Smith and Nephew)	Polyurethane film, polyvinylether adhesive	Occlusive wound dressing Donor sites, partial thickness Wound dressings
Tegaderm (3M)	Polyurethane film, acrylic adhesive	Wound dressings
Epigard	Bilayer dressing with outer membrane and inner layer of reticulated polyurethane foam	Wound dressings full thickness wounds
Lyofoam (Acme United Corp.)	Foam	Wound dressings
Omiderm (Omikron Science)	Acrylamide and hydroethyl methacrylate bonded to polyurethane	Wound dressings Initial burn dressing
Microthane	Polyester foam Polyadipate oligomers, TDI	Used in Meme breast implant
Surethane (Cardiac Control Systems)	MDI/PTMEG,EDA,DAMCH,PDMS/Soln Polyether urethane urea	

are an important part of any fabrication procedure, but information on the nature and percentage constitution is not always readily available. Processing steps also may inadvertently introduce low levels of contaminants into the material. The presence of small quantities of processing aids or mold release agents can influence the bulk and the surface properties. Batch-to-batch variation in the composition of materials is possible, and this has been observed in Biomer. Studies of batch variation and contamination are discussed in detail in Chapter 5.

REFERENCES

1. Oertel G. *Polyurethane Handbook.* (2nd Ed.): Hanser/Gardner Publications Inc., Cincinnati, OH., 1993.
2. Brandrup J. and Immergut E. H., Ed. *Polymer Handbook.* New York: Interscience, 1975:
3. Weast R. C. *CRC Handbook of Chemistry and Physics.* CRC Press, Boca Raton, FL.
4. Sax N. I. *Dangerous Properties of Industrial Materials.* (5th Ed.): Van Nostrand, New York, 1979.
5. Mijovic J. S. and Koutsky J. A. "Etching of polymeric substances: a review." *Polym. Plast. Technol. Eng.,* 9:139, 1977.
6. Lelah M. D., Lambrecht L. K., Young B. R., and Cooper S. L. "Physicochemical characterization and *in vivo* blood tolerability of cast and extruded Biomer." *J. Biomed. Mater. Res.,* 17:1, 1983.
7. Hollahan J. R. and Bell A. T. *Techniques and Applications of Plasma Chemistry.* John Wiley & Sons, New York, 1974.
8. Dundas P. H. and Thorpe M. L. "Economics and technology of chemical processing with electric field plasmas." *Chemical Eng.,* 76:123, 1969.
9. Rodriguez F. *Principles of Polymer Systems.* (4th Ed.): Hemisphere Pub. Corp., New York, 1996.
10. Giroux T. A. and Cooper S. L. "Surface characterization of plasma-derivatized polyurethanes."*J. Appl. Polym. Sci.,* 43:145, 1991.
11. Lin J.-C., Ko T.-M., and Cooper S. L. "Polyethylene surface sulfonation: surface characterization and platelet adhesion studies." *J. Coll. Interf. Sci.,* 164:99, 1994.

12. Gombotz W. R. and Hoffman A. S. "Gas-discharge techniques for biomaterial modification." In *CRC Critical Reviews in Biocompatibility*. CRC Press, Boca Raton, FL, 1987:
13. Sterret T. L., Sachdeva R., and Jerabek P. "Protein adsorption characteristics of plasma treated polyurethane surfaces." *J. Mat. Sci., Mat. Med,* 3:402, 1992.
14. Danilich M. J., Kottke-Marchant K., Anderson J. M., and Marchant R. E. "The immobilization of glucose oxidase onto radio-frequency plasma-modified poly(etherurethaneurea)." *J. Biomater. Sci., Polym. Ed.,* 3:195, 1992.
15. Ulubayram K. and Hasirci N. "Properties of plasma-modified polyurethane surfaces." *Colloids Surf. B: Biointerfaces,* 1:261, 1993.
16. Mittelman M. W., Sahi V. P., Soric I., and Sodhi R. N. S. *Antimicrobial activity of remote plasma modified polyurethane against biofilm bacteria*. Fifth World Biomaterials Congress. Toronto, Canada. 1996: 257.
17. *Petrothene Polyolefins: A Processing Guide*. U.S. Industrial Chemicals Co., 1965.
18. Allport D. C. and Janes W. H. *Block Copolymers*. John Wiley & Sons, New York, 1973.
19. Wirpsza Z. *Polyurethanes: Chemistry, Technology and Applications.* (1st Ed.): Ellis Horwood, London, 1993.
20. Lee L. J. "Polyurethane reaction injection molding: process, materials and properties." *Rubber Chem. Technol.,* 54:542, 1980.
21. Boretos J. W. Machining of plastics. In *Medical Engineering,* Ed. Ray, C. D. Year Book Medical, Chicago, 1974: Chapter 91.
22. Ulrich H., Bonk H. W., and Colovos G. C. "Synthesis and biomedical applications of polyurethanes." In *Synthetic Biomedical Polymers: Concepts and Applications,* Ed. Szycher M, Robinson, W. J. Technomic, Lancaster, PA, 1980:
23. Lelah M. D., Pierce J. A., Lambrecht L. K., and Cooper S. L. "Polyether-urethane ionomers: surface property/*ex vivo* blood compatibility relationships." *J. Coll. Interf. Sci.,* 104:422, 1985.
24. Lyman D. J., Searle W. J., Albo D., Bergman S., Lamb J., Metcalf L. C., and Richards K. "Polyurethane elastomers in surgery." *Int. J. Polym. Mater.,* 5:211, 1977.
25. Boretos J. W. *Procedures for the fabrication of segmented polyurethane polymers into useful biomedical prostheses*. National Institutes of Health, 1968.
26. Kardos J. L., Mehta B. S., Apostolou S. F., Thies C., and Clark R. E. "Design, fabrication and testing of prosthetic blood vessels." *Biomater., Med. Dev., Artif. Organs,* 2:387, 1974.
27. Dryer B., Akutsu T. and Kolff W. J. "Aortic grafts of polyurethane in dogs." *J. Appl. Physiol.,* 15:18, 1960.
28. Lyman D. J., Fazzio F. J., Voorhees H., Robinson G., and Albo D. "Compliance as a factor affecting the patency of a copolyurethane vascular graft." *J. Biomed. Mater. Res.,* 12:337, 1978.
29. White R. A., Weber J. N., and White E. W. "Replamineform: a new process for preparing porous ceramic, metal and polymer prosthetic materials." *Sci.,* 176:922, 1972.
30. Annis D., Bornat A., Edwards R. O., Higham A., Loveday B., and Wilson J. "An elastomeric vascular prosthesis." *Trans. Am. Soc. Artif. Intern. Organs,* 24:209, 1978.
31. Leidner J., Wong E. W. C., McGregor D. C., and Wilson G. J. "A novel process for the manufacturing of porous grafts: process description and product evaluation." *J. Biomed. Mater. Res.,* 17:229, 1983.
32. Wilson G. J., MacGregor D. C., Klement P., Lee J. M., Nido P. J. d., Wong E. W. C., and Leidner J. "Anisotropic polyurethane nonwoven conduits: a new approach to the design of a vascular prosthesis." *Trans. Am. Soc. Artif. Intern. Organs,* 29:260, 1983.
33. Hess F., Jerusalem C., and Braun B. "A fibrous polyurethane microvascular prothesis. Morphological evaluation of the neo-intima." *J. Cardiovasc. Surg.,* 24:509, 1983.
34. Planck H. *Entwicklung einer testilen Anterienprothese mit faserforminger struktur* [Dissertation]. University of Stuttgart, 1980.
35. Brash J. L., Fritzinger B. K., and Bruck S. D. "Development of block copolyether-urethane intra-aortic balloons and other medical devices." *J. Biomed. Mater. Res.,* 7:313, 1973.
36. Lyman D. J., Kwan-Gett C., Swart H. H. J., Bland A., Eastwood N., Kawai J., and Kolff W. J. "The development and implantation of a polyurethane hemispherical artificial heart." *Trans. Am. Soc. Artif. Intern. Organs,* 17:456, 1971.

37. Phillips W. M., Pierce W. S., Rosenberg G., and Donachy J. H. "The use of segmented polyurethane in ventricular assist devices and artificial hearts." In *Synthetic Biomedical Polymers — Concepts and Applications,* Ed. Szycher M., Robinson W. J. Technomic, Westport, CT, 1980: 39.
38. Poirier V. "Fabrication and testing of flocked blood pump bladders." In *Synthetic Biomedical Polymers — Concepts and Applications,* Ed. Szycher M., Robinson W. J. Technomic, Westport, CT, 1980: 73.
39. Lelah M. D. and Cooper S. L. *Polyurethanes in Medicine.* CRC Press, Boca Raton, FL, 1986.
40. Dolovich J., Marshall C. P., Smith E. K. M., Shimizu A., Pearson F. C., Surgona M. A., and Lee W. "Allergy to ethylene oxide in chronic hemodialysis patients." *Artif. Organs,* 8:334, 1984.
41. Ansorge W., Pelger M., Dietrich W., and Baurmeister U. "Ethylene oxide in dialyzer rinsing fluid: effect of rinsing technique, dialyzer storage time and potting compound." *Artif. Organs,* 11:118, 1987.
42. Shintani H. "The relative safety of gamma-ray, autoclave and ethylene oxide gas sterilization of thermosetting polyurethane." *Biomed. Instrument. Technol.,* 29:513, 1995.
43. Ward R. S. *BioSpan Segmented Polyurethane.* The Polymer Technology Group, 1995.

4 Structure and Physical Characterization of Polyurethanes

I. INTRODUCTION

When co-monomers of small size assemble into a random copolymer with a fairly uniform structure, the polymer formed can be considered to be homogeneous, so that the composition and structure of the material is the same throughout the bulk. When a copolymer is prepared from two monomers to produce a polymer with long sequences of each monomer i.e., a block copolymer (see Chapter 2), these sequences will tend to phase separate into domains or microphases. This manifests itself in the physical properties, which often display characteristic features of the individual components. Polyurethanes are block copolymers, that are considered to consist of domains of 'hard' segment that are dispersed in a 'soft' segment matrix. The hard segments are derived from the diisocyanate and the chain extender; the soft segment matrix consists of the polyol. Phase separation occurs in polyurethanes and is believed to account for their physical characteristics, including their high tensile strength and modulus. It also has been proposed that the microphase structure is a contributory factor to the blood compatibility of polyurethanes.

An understanding of the structure-property relationships in polyurethanes offers the potential to synthesize a material with a specific set of properties, enhancing performance for a given application. The physical properties of polyurethane materials can vary tremendously, and contribute to the broad range of applications in which polyurethanes are used. These properties are determined by a number of factors, including the molecular weight and chemistry of the soft segment, the diisocyanate and the chain extender, interactions between the hard and soft phases, and the degree of crystallinity within the material. In this chapter, an overview of the morphology and properties of polymers will be given. Polyurethane materials will then be considered, with emphasis on the phase separated nature of these materials, the molecular structure of these microdomains and how physical properties can be influenced through polyurethane synthesis. Finally, the mechanical and physical properties of polyurethanes will be discussed, and some of the more commonly used characterization techniques will be outlined. Examples of biomedical polyurethanes are utilized where possible.

A. STATES OF ORDER AND THERMAL TRANSITIONS OF POLYMERS

Polymers are long chain molecules, and are capable of adopting numerous conformations through the rotation of valence bonds. If substituents are present on the backbone, there are a number of possible arrangements of these substituents. Tacticity is the name given to the arrangement of these groups within the extended polymer chain. Isotactic polymers have substituents on the same side of the polymer chain, whereas syndiotactic chains have substituent groups placed on alternate sides of the chain. Atactic polymers have no obvious repeating pattern so the substituent groups appear at random on either side of the chain. The various tactic forms of polypropylene are shown in Figure 1.[1] The tacticity of a polymer can influence the polymer's physical and mechanical properties by its effect on crystallization. Atactic polymers cannot usually crystallize; isotactic and syndiotactic polymers may do so under favorable conditions.

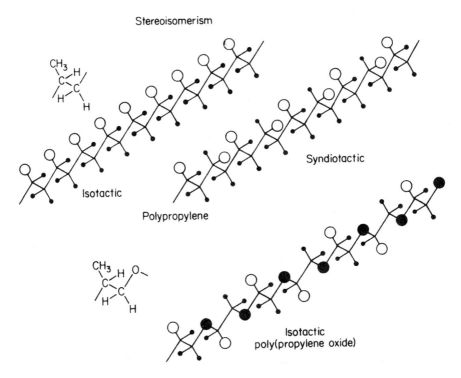

FIGURE 1 Schematic of stereoisomers of polypropylene. From *Principles of Polymer Systems*. Rodriguez, F. (4th Ed.): Hemisphere Pub. Corp., New York, 1996. Reproduced with permission. All rights reserved.

The flexibility of the polymer chain determines in part the conformations that the molecule can adopt; chain rotation and flexibility are required to enable packing of molecules and the formation of an ordered structure. Crosslinking of a polymer reduces the ability of a polymer to crystallize by restricting the conformations that the molecules can adopt. The ability of chains to associate with other molecules through the formation of intermolecular bonds, such as H-bonding and van der Waal's interactions also promote the formation of semicrystalline regions. The ability of polymer chains to pack efficiently in the solid state also is affected by steric factors.

The organization of molecules in the solid state determines many of the properties of the material. The ordering of polymer chains can be used to classify polymers as amorphous or semicrystalline. In amorphous materials, the polymer chains are entangled, with no apparent long range order. Semicrystalline polymers, in contrast, exhibit long range ordering of molecules.

Amorphous polymers exhibit a glass transition temperature, T_g. This is the temperature at which the polymer undergoes a change from a glassy, brittle material to a more elastic, rubbery material. This transition usually occurs over a small temperature range and is indicative of the onset of large scale rotation about the backbone of the polymer chain. It is influenced by factors that affect the movement of polymer chains and movement within individual polymer chains. The glass transition temperature varies widely with polymer structure. The softness and elasticity of a polymer can be interpreted as an indication of the motion of the polymer chains. When a material passes through its glass transition temperature, the polymer molecules have gained sufficient energy for rotation about the backbone which enhances mobility. If rubbery and elastic properties are required of a material for a given application, then the operating temperature should be above the glass transition temperature. Typical values of the glass transition temperature for a number of homopolymers are given in Table 1.[2]

Factors that influence the glass transition temperature include the flexibility of the polymer chain, and the presence of substituent groups on the polymer backbone. As the polymer chain must

TABLE 1
Glass transition temperatures (T_g) of common polymers

Polymer	T_g/°C
Polydimethyl siloxane (PDMS)	−123
Polyethylene	−93
Poly propylene	−20
Poly(oxyethylene)	−67
Polyacrylonitrile	5
Poly(4-methyl pent-1-ene)	29
Polyvinyl alcohol	85
Poly(vinyl chloride)	81
Poly(methyl methacrylate)	105
Polystyrene	100

Adapted from Cowie J.M.G. *Polymers: The Chemistry and Physics of Modern Materials*. International Textbook, Aylesbury, UK, 1973.

overcome an energy barrier to rotation in order to make the transition from a glassy material to a rubbery one, a highly flexible polymer backbone produces a material with a low glass transition temperature. C–O bonds rotate about the bond axis much more easily than C–C bonds, because the attached hydrogen atoms or other groups sterically hinder rotation about the C–C bond. This makes ether-containing chains more flexible than aliphatic hydrocarbon chains. Polyols that are used to prepare polyurethanes usually have a high degree of rotational freedom about the polymer backbone, producing a low T_g in the homopolymer. The presence of large bulky groups will elevate the T_g of a material, and polar side groups that promote interchain attraction will also reduce the mobility. The glass transition temperatures of typical polyurethane soft segment components are generally between −10 and −60°C.

The degree of crystallinity within a polymer can vary from a few percent (e.g., in mostly atactic commercial-grade poly(vinyl chloride)) to more than 90% (in highly linear polyethylene). No polymer is completely crystalline, due to the presence of lattice-defects that contain unordered, amorphous material. The tendency for a polymer to crystallize is enhanced by chain regularity, chain flexibility and the presence of repeat units that can pack together. Short side group substituents on the main polymer backbone can sterically inhibit crystallization, although long side groups may undergo side chain crystallization, producing a stiffer material. Highly linear and stereoregular polymers with a very low degree of branching tend to create highly crystalline structures.

Semicrystalline materials have a state of order within the material that can be detected by X-ray scattering or thermal analysis. The presence of crystalline regions within a polymer influences properties such as the tensile strength and stiffness, due to increased intermolecular associations through a reduction in the distance between chains. The ordering that occurs in a semicrystalline polymers can affect the ability of the amorphous component polymer backbone to rotate, resulting in a small rise in the glass transition temperature of the material. These crystallites produce regions that are harder, stronger and more chemically resistant than their amorphous counterparts. Semicrystalline materials typically exhibit higher modulus, strength, and creep resistance. For polymers which can crystallize to any extent there also exists a melting temperature, T_m, due to melting of the crystalline phase. The melting temperature of a polymer usually refers to the T_m of a highly crystalline polymer of very high molecular mass. Lattice defects and the sensitivity of the crystalline phases to thermal history often suppresses the observed T_m for a given polymer. Semicrystalline

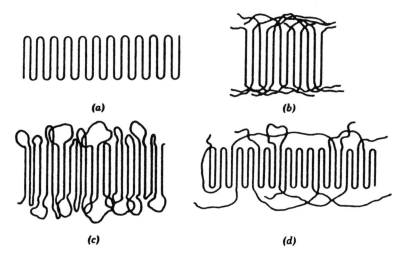

FIGURE 2 Two dimensional representation of polymeric lamellae: (a) sharp folds, (b) "switchboard model", (c) loose loops with adjacent reentry, (d) combination of several forms. From Lelah, M.D. and Cooper, S.L. *Polyurethanes in Medicine*, CRC Press, Boca Raton, FL, 1986. With permission.

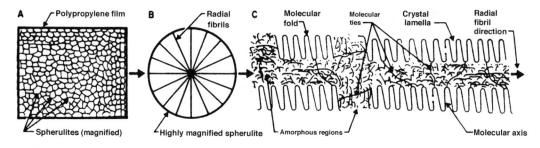

FIGURE 3 (A) Fully grown spherulites are shown macroscopically; (B) magnified view of spherulite shows idealized radial fibril structure; (C) magnified section of two fibrils shows chain-folding lamellae interconnected by tie molecules. From Fried J.R. *Plast. Eng.*, 3(6):49, 1982. With permission.

polymers with amorphous and crystalline regions usually possess both a T_g and a T_m. The melting point of the hard segment domains in a polyurethane can range from about 110 to more than 200°C.

Semicrystalline polymers actually consist of arrays of small crystals. Spherulites also may be formed, which grow radially from a point nucleus. The number and size of spherulites is critical in determining the final properties of a crystalline polymer. A representation of an ideal folded-chain crystal is shown in Figure 2a. The amorphous component of semicrystalline polymers resides in an interlamellar region hypothetically described by a switchboard model (Figure 2b) or by various loop conformations (Figures 2c and 2d). Crystallization is important in the polyurethanes, where both the hard segment and the soft segment may be semicrystalline.

The basic unit of crystalline polymer morphology is the crystalline lamella, shown in Figure 2. When crystallizable polymers such as polyethylene and isotactic polypropylene are cooled from the melt, growing crystallite lamellae are organized into radial lamellar fibrils contained within large spherulites, as shown in Figure 3. In most cases, chains fold with their chain axis oriented perpendicular to the radial (growth) direction. Regions between spherulites and between fibrils contain disordered polymer chains and chain segments which have been excluded from the ordered crystalline lamellae. The thickness of a lamella is in the order of 200Å while the spherulite is

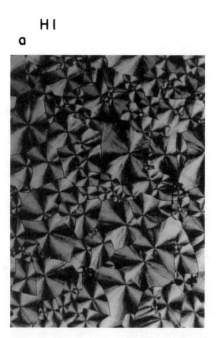

FIGURE 4 Maltese-cross shaped spherulites observed in an optical microscope between crossed polarizers.

typically several microns in size.[3] Spherulites are distinguished by their characteristic appearance in the polarizing microscope, where they are seen as birefringent areas sometimes possessing a dark Maltese cross pattern (Figure 4).

Many of the polymers used in biomedical applications have a viscoelastic response corresponding to one of the several curves illustrated in the modulus-temperature representation of Figure 5, if the temperature scale is shifted so that the T_g in Figure 5 coincides with that of the polymer of interest. Most materials considered to be rubbery have very low glass transition temperatures. Below the glass transition temperature, the modulus of all polymer families is typically 3×10^5 N/m^{-2} (4.5×10^5 psi). As the temperature of a linear polymer increases, a region is reached where the modulus drops three orders of magnitude and the polymer transforms from a glassy state to a material that is leathery in character. This glass transition region may be 5 to 10°C in breadth. As the temperature rises above T_g, the linear polymer softens. Viscous flow is inhibited by polymer chain entanglement until substantially higher temperatures are reached. Polymers A and C in Figure 5 are classified as thermoplastic materials. When such materials are heated sufficiently above their glass transition temperatures, they become fluid-like and may be processed. On subsequent cooling, the polymer becomes rigid again. Polymer C has a higher molecular weight and requires higher temperatures before flow can take place.

For a polymer to have useful properties above the T_g, two strategies can be employed. A low level of covalent cross linking can be incorporated into the polymer in order to make a rubbery network structure which has a low and largely temperature independent modulus above the T_g. The second strategy is to use a semicrystalline polymer. Between T_g and T_m there is a region of decreasing modulus with temperature where the more fluid amorphous segments are held together by crystalline regions. Semicrystalline polymers tend to be tough, ductile plastics whose properties are sensitive to processing history. However, crystallinity within a polymer can make polymer processing more difficult; higher temperatures may be required for melt processing, increasing the likelihood of significant thermal degradation of the polymer, and aggressive, high boiling-point solvents may be required for solution processing.

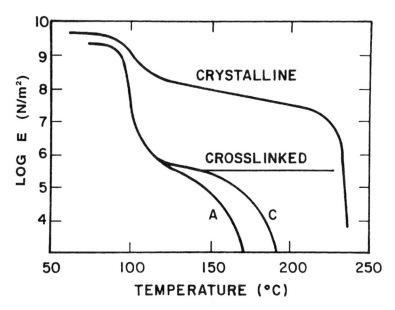

FIGURE 5 Modulus vs. temperature profiles for crystalline isotactic polystyrene, for polystyrene samples A and C, and for lightly crosslinked atactic polystyrene ($T_g = 100°C$). From Lelah, M.D. and Cooper, S.L. *Polyurethanes in Medicine*, CRC Press, Boca Raton, FL, 1986. With permission.

B. Intermolecular Bonding in Polymers

The presence of functional groups on the polymer molecules can influence the degree of intermolecular bonding in polymers. Secondary bonding such as van der Waals interactions, dipole-dipole-interactions and hydrogen bonds can contribute to the properties of the polymer. Strong interactions are promoted by the regular arrangement of atoms within the polymer chains, and the presence of polar groups. Intermolecular bonding in polymers can help to stabilize crystallites, and provides a driving force for crystallization and phase separation in block copolymers. The degree of interchain attraction may increase the density of the material and the tensile strength. Polyamides contain polar groups that can bond intermolecularly through dipole-dipole interactions and remain aligned. This is believed to account for the high tensile strength of Nylon and its success as a fiber. Intermolecular bonding in polymers also serves to increase the hardness, stiffness, modulus, solvent resistance and other physical properties, and to decrease the low temperature flexibility.

C. Mechanical Behavior

Mechanical tests of a material are performed in order to investigate a material's response to stress. The simplest of tests is the tensile test, where a stress is applied to a material to elongate it. The change in length of the specimen is recorded. The force is usually applied until the specimen breaks. The stress, σ, is defined as the applied force per unit area. The strain, ε, is the change in length induced by the applied force divided by the original length. Young's Modulus, E, is defined as stress divided by strain, within the elastic region. The tensile properties of polymers can be characterized by their deformation behavior or stress-strain response. Amorphous, rubbery polymers are soft, and extend reversibly. They exhibit low moduli when compared to semicrystalline polymers or polymers in the glassy state, and will extend up to several hundred percent. They also often exhibit an increase in stress prior to breakage as a result of strain-induced crystallization. This is caused by molecular orientation in the direction of the applied stress. The properties of polymers are rate and temperature dependent. Thus, if the elastomer of Figure 6 is deformed at higher rates, or at lower temperatures, then a series of stress-strain responses can be observed as depicted.

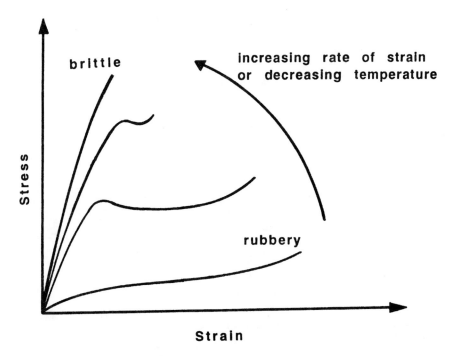

FIGURE 6 Tensile properties of polymers.

Glassy or semicrystalline materials behave elastically at low levels of strain, i.e., the specimen returns to its original dimensions once the load is removed. Beyond the elastic limit, the sample undergoes plastic deformation, and the material does not return to its original dimensions. Eventually the material will fail. The point just before breakage occurs is defined as the ultimate strength of the material. During loading, the freedom of motion of the polymer chains is retained, while the network structure of the polymer chains prevents flow and large-scale movements. For some semicrystalline materials, particularly spherulitic ones, the failure point may be defined as the stress point where large inelastic deformation, or yielding starts. The toughness of a material is related to the energy absorbed during loading and is proportional to the area under the stress-strain curve. The typical deformation behavior (stress-strain response) for an elastomer is shown as the bottom curve in Figure 6.

The fatigue behavior of polymers also is important in biomaterial evaluation, in applications where dynamic stresses are applied. This is particularly true for applications such as pacemaker lead insulation, prosthetic heart valves and the artificial heart where the materials are subjected to repeated flexing or loading and unloading. The materials used in these applications must be able to withstand many cycles of stress and unloading of deformation before failure. Fatigue is broadly defined as the degradation of mechanical and/or other polymer properties with time, due to repeated application of stress. Fatigue testing usually involves the measurement of structural failure after repeated loading; the applied load is smaller than that required for failure in a continuous loading experiment application. Figure 7 shows the stress-lifetime curves for three polyurethanes, with PPO, polyethylene adipate (PEA), and polytetramethyleneadipate (PTMA). Generally, the number of cycles that a material can withstand decreases as the size of the applied load increases. For some materials a minimum stress may exist below which failure of the material does not occur within a measurable number of cycles.

In general, polyurethane elastomers have superior modulus, tensile strength, tear strength, and abrasion resistance compared to even the highest quality natural rubber. However, the polyurethanes can exhibit substantial creep, stress-relaxation and stress hysteresis compared to other rubbery materials.

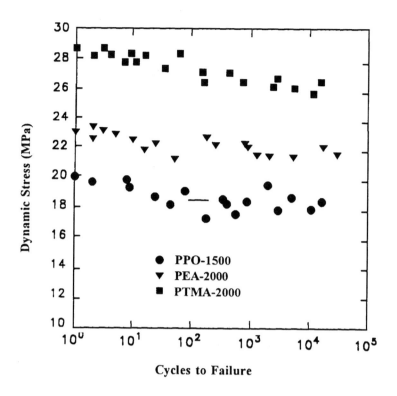

FIGURE 7 Fatigue testing of PPO (m.w. 1500), PEA (m.w. 2000), and PTMA (m.w. 2000) soft segment polyurethanes. From Myers, C. W., Ph.D. Thesis, University of Wisconsin–Madison, 1993.

1. Viscoelasticity

Viscoelasticity refers to the time-dependent mechanical properties of materials, which are usually exhibited by polymers. For ideal elastic materials, mechanical properties are adequately described by Hooke's Law, which states that the strain produced in the material is proportional to the stress and independent of the rate at which the stress is applied. For viscous liquids, mechanical behavior is described by Newton's Law; the stress is proportional to the rate of the applied strain. The mechanical properties of polymers are not adequately described by either of these limits, but fall between the two. Hence, materials that exhibit this type of behavior are said to be viscoelastic. Viscoelasticity can be measured through either creep or stress-relaxation measurements. Creep tests involve application of a constant load, while monitoring the elongation of the specimen over time. Creep is defined as the time-dependent extension which a material experiences under constant load. Stress-relaxation measurements record the stress required to hold a specimen at a fixed elongation. Stress-relaxation is observed if the load applied to material held at fixed elongation decreases. The viscoelastic behavior of a given polymer is a function of its chemical composition and the difference between the glass transition temperature and the test or service temperature. At a given temperature, a polymer with a low T_g exhibits a faster viscoelastic response than a polymer with a higher T_g.

2. Hysteresis

Hysteresis is the name given to the energy losses that occur in polymers when they repeatedly are loaded and unloaded. This can be observed in polymers, and is usually measured by examination of the different stress-strain curves generated when the sample is loaded and then unloaded. The area enclosed by the two curves is related to the energy that is dissipated during the stress-strain cycle. In an amorphous material, the carbon chain backbone of the polymer chain adopts a randomly coiled conformation. On application of stress, the chains will uncoil and either form crystalline regions, or be stretched out to significant orientation levels. On release of the stress the chains will once again coil up and return to the rubbery state. Such transitions and deformations are not instantaneous and there is a time lag before the original characteristics are recovered. Deformations are dependent on the rate of application of subsequent stress cycles. Significant hysteresis can lead to large temperature increases in cyclically deformed polymers.

D. Molecular Weight

Unlike their low molecular weight precursors, polymers cannot be assigned a precise molecular weight. Due to the random processes that occur during polymerization, polymers are produced with a range of molecular weights; the average molecular weight and the distribution of molecular weights around this average influences the physical properties of the material. Two average molecular weights are commonly used, the number average molecular weight ($\overline{M_n}$) and the weight average molecular weight ($\overline{M_w}$). These are defined as:

$$\overline{M_n} = \Sigma N_i M_i / \Sigma N_i$$

and

$$\overline{M_w} = \Sigma N_i M_i^2 / \Sigma N_i M_i$$

where N_i is the number of moles of species i, and
        M_i the molecular weight of species i.

A typical distribution of polymer molecular weight is shown in Figure 8. The ratio of $\overline{M_w}$ to $\overline{M_n}$ is referred to as the polydispersity index, and it provides an indication of the breadth of molecular weight distribution. The most probable value for ideally polymerized condensation polymers and some addition polymers is two, although values for commercial polymers may lie between 1.5 and 50. Special polymerization techniques can be used to reduce the polydispersity index to 1.1 or less. The molecular weight of a polymer influences the mechanical properties of the material, including the tensile strength, modulus and glass transition temperature. Generally, a polymer of high molecular weight has a higher modulus, tensile strength and slightly higher glass transition temperature than a polymer with a lower molecular weight. Polymers of high molecular weight are also more difficult to melt process. Most properties are asymptotic, and so an optimal molecular weight can be determined to enhance ease of manufacture and polymer performance. Figure 9 shows qualitatively the variation in properties with increasing molecular weight.

Typical linear polyurethane elastomers have number average molecular weights in the range 25,000 to 100,000 and weight average molecular weights from 50,000 to 300,000. In the case of the polyurethanes and other highly polar condensation polymers, the most rapid increase in properties occurs before about 20,000 number average molecular weight.

The polydispersity of the soft segments used in polyurethane synthesis is often small, (approximately 1.3) due to the ionic polymerization methods typically employed in polyether polyol synthesis. However, the polydispersity of the soft segment does not have a great effect on the final properties of the polyurethane. The polydispersity of the hard segment is influenced by a number of factors including the synthetic procedure and the degree of completion of the reaction. The two-step or prepolymer method of polyurethane synthesis appears to produce a narrower molecular weight distribution than the one-step method. The polydispersity of a polyurethane prepared via a one step method approaches two. It has been found that a decrease in the breadth of the hard-segment size distribution, either by use of a two-step synthesis method, or by using monodisperse crystallizable hard segments synthesized by a special stepwise process has the effect of significantly

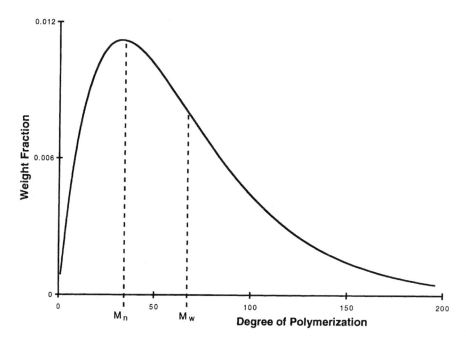

FIGURE 8 Distribution of molecular weights in a typical polymer.

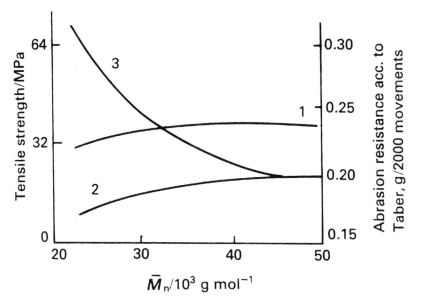

FIGURE 9 Thermoplastic polyurethane properties vs. molecular weight: 1-polyesterurethane tensile strength, 2-polyetherurethane tensile strength 3- abrasion resistance. From Wirpsza Z. *Polyurethanes: Chemistry, Technology and Applications.* (1st ed.): Ellis Horwood, London, 1993.

increasing the tensile modulus of a polyurethane.[4] Furthermore, it has been found that for a total chain molecular weight exceeding 25,000, the total molecular weight has little effect on the physical properties.[5] At sufficiently high molecular weight, the size, distribution and composition of the individual segments determine the macroscopic properties of the material.

II. STRUCTURE OF POLYURETHANES

The polyurethanes are segmented or block copolymers, consisting of alternating hard segments (which may be glassy or semicrystalline) and soft (elastomeric) chain segments. The microphase separation of these two chemically distinct components gives rise to the unusual and useful physical and mechanical properties of the polyurethanes. Various characterization techniques have been applied to study the micro-structure of these materials, and have provided information on the characteristics of polyurethanes. X-ray studies, thermal analysis, birefringence studies, analysis of the mechanical properties of polyurethanes, and electron microscopic studies strongly support the view that polyurethanes can be considered as possessing a microphase separated solid state structure. There is general agreement on the following:

1. The driving force behind the phase separation into hard and soft domains is the chemical incompatibility of the hard and soft segments.
2. The hard segments consist of urethane segments, and form glassy or semicrystalline domains.
3. The macroglycol soft segments form an amorphous or semicrystalline matrix in which the hard segments are dispersed at low-to-moderate hard segment content.
4. The hard domains act as multifunctional crosslinking sites and reinforcing filler, resulting in materials which possess high modulus and exhibit elastomeric behavior.

At low temperatures, the glass transition temperature (T_g) of the soft segment influences the mechanical properties of the polymer. At higher temperatures, either the glass transition temperature or the melting point (T_m) of the hard segments determines the point at which physical crosslinks dissociate. Factors that influence the degree of phase separation in polyurethane materials include hydrogen bonding between polymer chains, segment length, polarity and crystallizability, overall composition and mechanical and thermal history. In the following section, reasons for phase separation between the hard and soft segments will be discussed, and experimental evidence supporting the presence of microdomains will be presented.

A. MICROPHASE SEPARATION

In 1966, Cooper and Tobolsky compared the viscoelastic properties of linear polyesterurethanes with a styrene-butadiene-styrene triblock copolymer.[6] Both of these types of polymers demonstrated an unusually high plateau modulus which was not accompanied by covalent crosslinking or crystallinity. It was postulated that these properties arose from microphase separation or clustering of the hard and soft segments in the solid state. Evidence for the existence of such a two-phase microstructure using electron microscopy was collected but the data may have been artifactual.[7] Thomas and coworkers have since demonstrated the presence of a two-phase structure in a segmented polyurethane using electron microscopy.[8] An appreciation of the phase separated nature of the polyurethanes is most important when trying to understand factors that contribute to their solid-state properties.

1. Thermodynamics of Phase Separation

Polyurethanes are segmented block copolymers with an $(AB)^n$ structure, where A represents the hard block with a degree of polymerization, (number of repeat units, DP) of one to 10, and B represents the soft block which has a degree of polymerization in the range 15 to 30. Generally, the hard and soft segments of a polyurethane have a positive heat of mixing and are therefore incompatible. Thus, there is a tendency toward phase separation of the two components; however, the topology of the block copolymer molecules imposes restrictions on segregation, leading to microdomain formation.

Most theories on block copolymer microphase separation and the thermodynamics behind the process consider four factors; the Flory–Huggins solubility parameter χ, the degree of polymerization, conformational and steric constraints, and the weight fraction of the components.[9] The size and shape of the domains in block copolymers is influenced by conformation, entropy and interfacial energy. Thermodynamic theories for phase separation in block copolymers have been developed by Krause,[10–11] Meier,[12] Helfand,[13,14] and Le Grand.[15] Krause analyzed microphase separation from a strictly thermodynamic approach based on macroscopic variables, with an assumption of complete phase separation with sharp boundaries.[10,11] The model predicts that phase separation becomes more difficult as the number of blocks increases in a copolymer molecule of a given length.

The theories of Helfand *et al.*[13,14] included thermodynamic models of microphase separation. From a thermodynamic perspective, there is a positive surface free energy (see Chapter 5) associated with the interface between the A and B domains. Growth of the domains is favored, as a means of reducing the interfacial energy between the two phases. Furthermore, as a result of the tendency of the joints between the blocks of the copolymer to stay at the interfacial regions, there is a loss of entropy (decrease in randomness of the system) in two ways. One is attributable to the confinement of the urethane joints to the interface. The other has its origin in maintaining the virtually constant overall polymer density by the suppression of a vast number of polymer conformations. The equilibrium domain size and shape are a result of the balance of these three free-energy terms.

Le Grand developed a model to account for domain formation and stability based on the change in free energy that occurs between a random mixture of block copolymer molecules and a micellar domain structure.[15] This model also considers the interfacial boundary between the phases. It also is believed that the phase separation in amorphous block copolymers should be favored by high molecular weight, or a minimum number of individual blocks in each polymer chain. For block copolymers with a crystallizable component, the entropy and enthalpy of crystallization influences phase separation. Crystallization of either component and the formation of intermolecular hydrogen bonds can act as driving forces for phase separation. In addition to the effects of the number, size, and interactions of the copolymer blocks, temperature also can affect phase separation. A higher temperature will enhance phase mixing due to a decrease in the free energy of mixing of the system.

2. Kinetics of Microphase Separation

Analysis of the microphase separated nature of the polyurethanes has generally been considered from a thermodynamic perspective. However, a number of investigations using infrared spectroscopy, vibrational spectroscopy, differential scanning calorimetry (DSC) and scattering techniques have been applied to study the kinetics of phase separation in polyurethanes. The morphology of segmented copolymers following thermal treatment has been shown to be time dependent.[16–18] Increasing the temperature of a segmented copolymer induces phase mixing; subsequent cooling of the system causes phase separation into the original morphology. A finite amount of time is required to produce a given change in morphology, owing to kinetic and viscous effects.

Wilkes *et al.*[16–17] used Small Angle X-ray Scattering (SAXS) to study the time-dependent behavior of a polyesterurethane. Samples were heated briefly and then quenched. Changes in soft segment glass transition temperature, degree of phase separation and Young's Modulus as a function of time were recorded, implying that changes in the microdomain structure had occurred. Ophir and Wilkes also studied a series of polyesterurethanes with different degrees of crosslinking. The lightly crosslinked samples showed greater displacement from the original properties and came to equilibrium in a shorter time than more heavily crosslinked samples, indicating crosslinking to be a domain disruptive process which inhibits the transient response of morphology to change in temperature.

Other studies of the kinetics of phase separation in polyurethanes have shown that the separation of the hard and soft segments is rapid when compared with the ordering of the hard segments.[19] Chu *et al.*[20] studied the kinetics of phase separation in polyurethanes containing MDI/BD hard segments with either PTMO or PPO–PEO soft segments. A single relaxation time was calculated for the PTMO system, whereas behavior of the PPO–PEO polyurethane was best described by two relaxation times. The soft segments possess similar solubility parameters, but the PTMO based polyurethane showed better phase separation. This was attributed in part to kinetic factors. They postulate that the kinetics of phase separation are controlled by hard segment mobility, system viscosity and hard segment interactions. Tao et al.[21] studied the phase separation in thin films of polyurethanes containing a semirigid monodisperse hard segment of MDI and BD, and PPG soft segments. They concluded that the rigidity of the hard segment exerts a strong influence on phase separation in thin films. However, thin film morphology and kinetics of phase separation differs between from that of thick films, and thin films take longer to phase separate. Lee and Hsu showed that between the soft segment glass transition temperature and the hard segment domain dissociation temperature, the rate of phase separation is strongly dependent on temperature.[22]

B. Morphological Models of Block Copolymers

Segmented thermoplastic elastomers exhibit structural heterogeneity on the molecular, domain and, in some cases, on a large scale involving spherulitic texture. Each level of structural organization is studied by specific methods. Molecular sequence distributions can be studied by chemical methods, such as Nuclear Magnetic Resonance (NMR) or IR spectroscopy. Domain structures may be probed directly by electron microscopy, or more quantitatively by small-angle X-ray scattering (SAXS). Electron microscopy can provide direct information on domain structure under favorable conditions, but due to the small size of the hard segment domains (50 to 100 Å), interpretation of electron micrographs is difficult. A few investigators have observed microphase separation in certain polyurethane samples.[7–8,23] A polyetherurethane has been shown to have a larger degree of phase separation than the analogous polyesterurethane.[24]

An early model first proposed by Estes et al.[25] for the schematic representation of a two-dimensional cross-section of the domain structure in an undeformed polyurethane is shown in Figure 10. The shaded regions represent hard-segment domains which exist as an interconnecting network. Both phases are considered to be continuous and interpenetrating. The model also assumes that phase separation is not complete, so that some urethane blocks are dispersed in the rubbery matrix. The domain size in the direction of the chain axis is given as approximately 50Å, which agrees well with the calculated 55Å contour length for an average hard block.[26]. Early X-ray diffraction studies performed by Bonart and coworkers identified short-range order associated with hydrogen bonding, as depicted in Figure 11.[27] Further studies on strained specimens revealed that the urethane segments oriented perpendicular to the strain axis when the sample elongation was less than 200%. At higher elongations the soft segments were observed to crystallize, producing "force-strands," and the hard segments re-oriented into the direction of the stretch. The hard segments stagger in such a way as to produce a maximum number of hydrogen bonds between the N–H and C = O groups of adjacent segments. Upon annealing, this process is accelerated, resulting in the structure shown in Figure 11b. This morphology exhibits hard-segment orientation in the direction of elongation, and stress relaxed, disoriented soft segments. This restructuring of hard segments is related to stress softening and hysteresis phenomena characteristic of segmented polyurethanes. Based on these and other studies, Bonart et al. proposed models of molecular rearrangement with hard segment domains in segmented polyurethanes, and segmented polyurethaneureas. Domain structure was related to the mutual hard segment affinity, enhanced by molecular arrangements which allow formation of the maximum number of stress-free hydrogen bonds.

Wilkes and Yusek studied domain formation in polyesterurethanes using X-ray techniques.[28] They found that the domains were lamellar in shape with an average separation of 100 to 250Å. Higher spacings were obtained in samples with longer soft segments and higher urethane contents. The hard segments act as cross links, inhibiting stress-relaxation and inducing stress-crystallization of the soft segments which results in higher tensile strength. Upon heat setting the hard segments

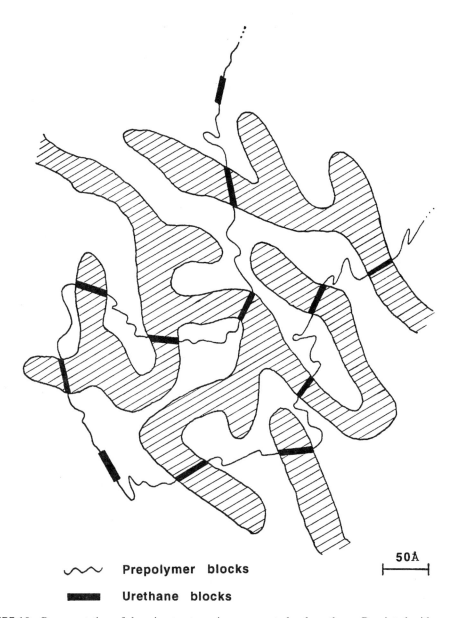

FIGURE 10 Representation of domain structures in a segmented polyurethane. Reprinted with permission from Estes G. M., Seymour R. W., and Cooper S. L. *Macromolecules,* 4:452, 1971. Copyright 1971 American Chemical Society.

break up and reform. The morphological model proposed in Figure 12 is of a polyurethane which has been stretched 200 to 400% and annealed at 60 to 100°C. It represents a summary of primary morphological features.

Blackwell and coworkers were able to interpret wide angle X-ray data of heat-set polyurethanes which defined the chain conformation and packing of hard segments in crystalline polyurethane elastomers.[3,29] The models are based on the structure of MDI-butanediol hard-segment analogs, and one view of the packing of the chains in the hard segment is shown in Figure 13. Planar zig–zag –CH_2–CH_2– sections connect successive diisocyanate units. The chains are linked together in stacks through C = O ... H–N hydrogen bonds which involve half of the urethane groups. Dielectric relaxation studies of segmented polyether and polyesterurethanes have been performed by North

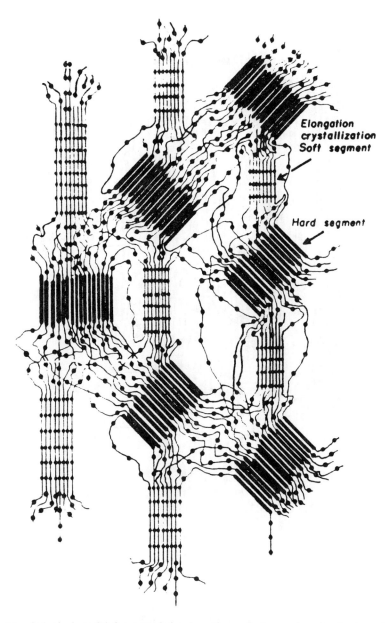

FIGURE 11 Morphological model for extended polyurethane elastomer domain structure; (a) structure at 200% elongation, (b) structure of material annealed at 500% elongation. From Bonart R. J. *Macromol. Sci. Phys.*, B2:115, 1968. With permission, Marcel Dekker, Inc.

et al.[30,31] They concluded that the MDI based materials contain nonspherical hard segment domains, with a diffuse phase boundary between the hard and soft segments.

C. MOLECULAR ORIENTATION IN POLYURETHANES

Molecular orientation in polyurethanes is important from both theoretical and practical viewpoints, as the measurement of orientation under strain not only provides a basis for establishing mechanisms of polymer deformation, but also contributes to a better understanding of structure-property relationships. A variety of experimental methods have been applied to the examination of the molecular orientation

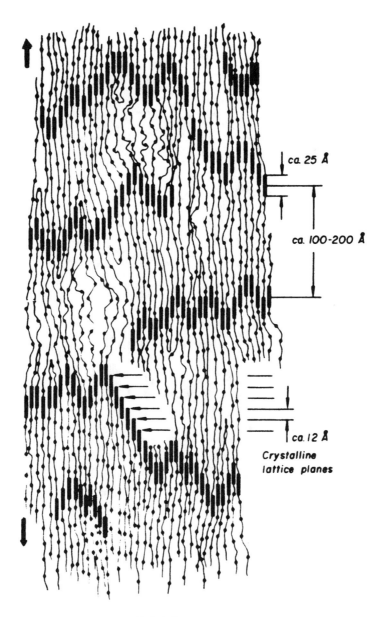

FIGURE 11 (continued)

response of polyurethanes under strain. These include small angle light scattering (SALS), small and wide angle X-ray scattering (SAXS and WAXS), birefringence, sound transmission, polarized fluorescence, polarized Raman scattering, and infrared dichroism. SALS, SAXS, and WAXS are essentially limited to study of the crystalline phase, while birefringence and sound transmission yield average orientation information. Infrared dichroism is a particularly useful technique for studying the orientation response of the hard and soft segments of segmented polyurethanes subjected to strain. Polarized infrared radiation is used to measure the orientation of particular chemical groups or bonds on the polymer chain by monitoring changes in the IR spectrum upon stretching.

Bonart and coworkers performed early studies on the orientation behavior of polyurethanes and polyurethane ureas using X-ray diffraction and infrared dichroism.[27,32] The polyether and polyester soft segments were found to orient in the direction of stretch. Hard-segment behavior

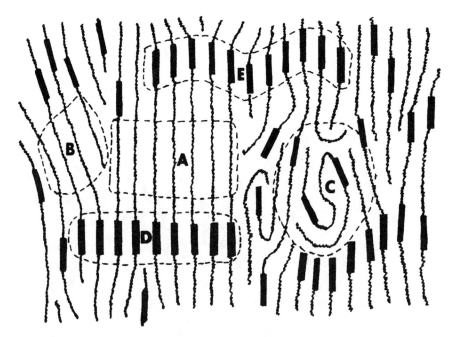

FIGURE 12 Morphological model of segmented polyurethane. (A) Stress-crystallized soft segment; (B) paracrystalline soft segment; (C) amorphous "solution" of hard and soft segments; (D) crystalline hard segment domains; (E) paracrystalline hard segment domains. From Wilkes, C.E. and Yusek, C.S. *J. Macromol. Sci. — Phys. B,* B7:157, 1973. With permission, Marcel Dekker, Inc.

was more complex. The aromatic urethane segments were found to orient perpendicular to the stretch direction at elongations below 200%. Further stretching resulted in orientation of the hard segments in the stretch direction. Estes *et al.* investigated noncrystalline polyether and polyester-urethanes and found that hard segments retained more orientation after removal of the stress than the soft segments.[25] Seymour *et al.*[33] extended Estes' conclusion using differential infrared dichroism. They found that a major change in orientation behavior with composition occurred at the point where the morphology changed from isolated hard domains to an interlocked structure.

Based on these and other studies, it may be concluded that segmental orientation in polyurethanes passes through three stages as hard-segment content increases.[34,35] At low hard-segment content, very little equilibrium orientation is retained in either the hard or soft segments. At somewhat higher hard-segment content, the hard segments retain significantly greater orientation. It has been suggested that this composition level represents the point where the morphology changes from isolated hard domains to the interconnecting structure mentioned earlier.[36] When the length of the hard segments is sufficiently great to permit microcrystallinity, spherulitic texture is observed and transverse orientation appears at low strains.

D. Hydrogen Bonding

Polyurethanes are extensively hydrogen bonded.[33,37-39] Hydrogen bonding involves the N-H group in urethane or urea groups as the donor, and the urethane carbonyl, the ester carbonyl (in polyesterurethanes), or the ether oxygen (in polyetherurethanes) as the acceptor. The relative amounts of hydrogen bonds between the hard and soft segments is determined by the degree of phase separation. Hydrogen bonding interactions are schematically portrayed in Figure 14 where the hydrogen bonds are represented by dotted lines. Increased phase segregation favors inter-urethane hydrogen bonding.

Hydrogen bonding is best examined using IR spectroscopy, although X-ray diffraction also is useful if the hard segments are crystalline. A number of researchers have examined hydrogen bonding and

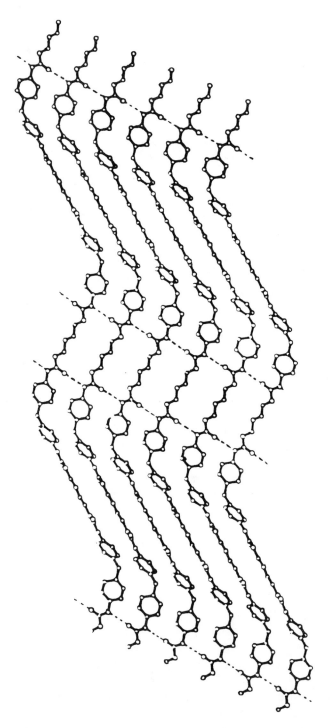

FIGURE 13 Packing of chains in the hard segment. From Blackwell, J. and Gardner, K.H. *Polymer,* 20:13, 1979.

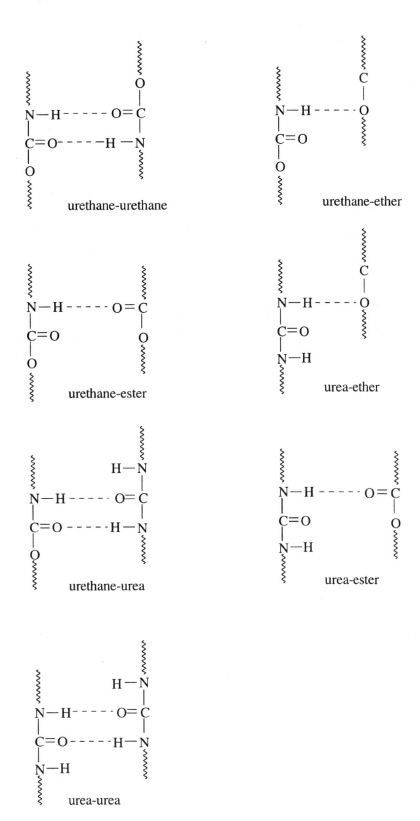

FIGURE 14 Hydrogen bonding interactions in polyurethanes.

its consequences in polyurethanes.[26,33,37-40] A comparison of IR and DSC results on samples with varying thermal history has shown that the dissociation of hydrogen bonding is insensitive to the degree of ordering present and is accelerated at temperatures above the T_g of the hard segments.[37] Several studies[26,40] have concluded the increase in the molecular mobility of the polymer chains as the temperature of the material passes through the hard segment T_g leads to the disruption of H-bonds, implying that hydrogen bonding in polyurethanes does not control the molecular mobility of the polymer chains, and thus does not contribute to the mechanical properties of the polyurethanes directly.

The effect of hard-segment diisocyanate content on the hydrogen bonding index (the ratio of bonded to free urethane carbonyl groups) is shown in Figure 15. As would be expected, at high hard-segment contents, there is a greater degree of interurethane hydrogen bonding, due to an increased extent of microphase separation. At 25°C, 80–90% of the N-H groups in the hard segment of a typical polyurethane are hydrogen bonded. As the temperature is raised, the number of free N–H groups increases, indicating a disruption of hydrogen bonding. The hard segment-soft segment hydrogen bonds are disrupted first, as interurethane hydrogen bonds formed with other hard segments are much stronger than the hydrogen bonds between the hard and soft segments. Furthermore, the hard segments are usually below their melting or glass transition temperature, which prevents disruption of these bonds. A change in the slope of the temperature dependence of hydrogen bonding at 75 to 100°C is attributed to the onset of accelerated hydrogen bond dissociation which occurs at the T_g of the hard segments. The rigidity of the hard segments below their T_g restricts hydrogen bond disruption. As the temperature is raised, and sufficient mobility is attained, secondary bond dissociation can occur more readily. It is important to note that there is still significant hydrogen bonding even at 200°C.

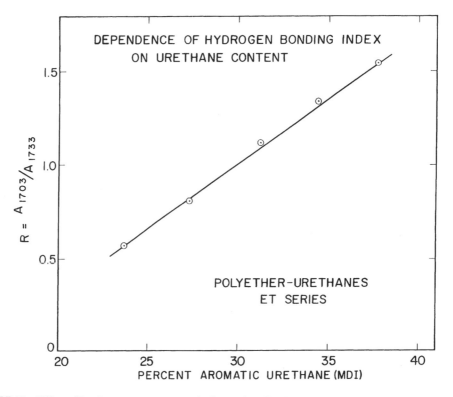

FIGURE 15 Effect of hard segment content on hydrogen bonding index. From Lelah, M.D. and Cooper, S.L. *Polyurethanes in Medicine*, CRC Press, Boca Raton, FL, 1986. With permission.

Wang and Cooper have studied hydrogen bonding in polyetherurethane ureas.[35] They deduced the presence of three-dimensional inter-urea hydrogen bonding as illustrated in Figure 16. A decrease in hard-segment content, results in some soft segments dispersed in the hard domains. This interferes with the ordering of the hard segments and also allows the polyether oxygens to compete with urea carbonyls for the urea NH groups. This results in a system with a mixed state of hydrogen bonding, containing conventional as well as three-dimensional inter-urea bonds.

Studies of ionic polyurethanes also have demonstrated the importance of phase separation as a determinant of the physical properties of polyurethanes. Grasel et al.[41] studied sulfonated polyurethanes, where the urethane hydrogens were replaced by propyl sulfonate groups up to a level of 20%. Using DSC and FTIR to examine hydrogen bonding and phase transitions, they found that as the degree of sulfonation of the urethane hydrogens increased, the degree of phase separation initially decreased. At higher levels (20% sulfonation) the phase separation increased once more, hydrogen bonding providing the driving force, and the resultant morphology was comparable to the unmodified polyurethane. IR spectroscopy showed that there were more free carbonyls in this sample, implying that the urethane groups were hydrogen bonding with the sulfonate groups rather than the urethane carbonyl groups. Studies of polyurethane ionomers by Cooper et al.[42,43] showed that the neutralizing cation may influence the mechanical properties through the structuring and ordering of the associating anions. They concluded that the local environment determines the aggregate morphology; the aggregate structure influences the overall morphology and material properties.

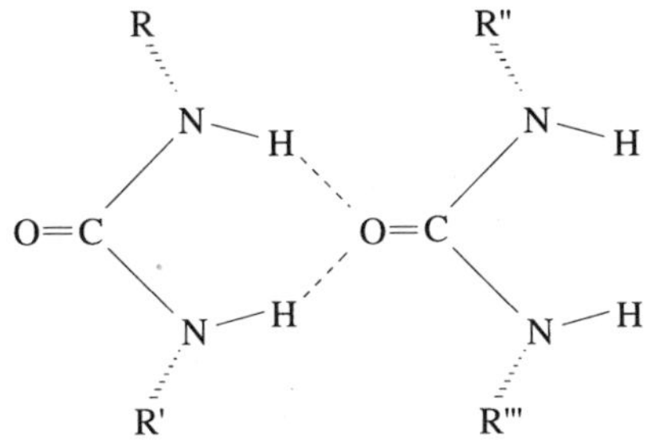

FIGURE 16 Representation of the 3-d inter-urea hydrogen bonding in polyurethaneurea.

E. CROSSLINKING

The extent of crosslinking within a polyurethane will affect its mechanical properties. Crosslinking affects the mobility of the polymer chains. If the degree of crosslinking is low in single phase elastomers, then the elastic properties of the material can be retained, with enhanced strength and creep resistance. As the degree of crosslinking increases, the modulus increases, as does the hardness. The materials no longer behave as elastomers, but start to resemble rigid thermosetting plastics. The alteration in physical properties of polyurethanes that occur via crosslinking are shown in Figure 17. In microphase separated polyurethanes, crosslinking typically occurs via use of multifunctional polyols or chain extender molecules. The use of the latter can provide an anomalous decrease in modulus due to the disruption of the domain morphology of the system.[44]

F. THE EFFECT OF POLYURETHANE CHEMISTRY ON PHYSICAL PROPERTIES

1. Isocyanate

The presence of an aromatic isocyanate in the hard segment produces a stiffer polymer chain with a higher melting point than a material synthesized from an aliphatic isocyanate. Polyurethanes containing aromatic isocyanates tend to be hard, and of low elasticity. As stated in Chapter 2, the

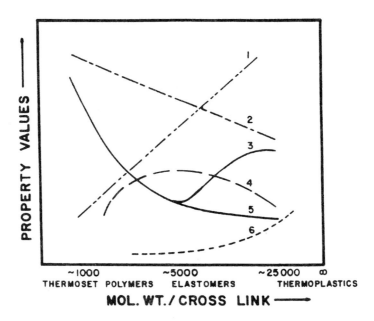

FIGURE 17 Effects of crosslinking on the properties of polyurethanes. Curve 1: solvent swelling, elongation and tear strength, Curve 2: glass transition temperature and melting point, Curve 3: modulus and hardness for polymers with high intermolecular attractions, Curve 4: elasticity, Curve 5: modulus and hardness for polymers with realtively low intermolecular attractions, Curve 6: creep and compression set. From Saunders J.H. and Frisch K.C. *Polyurethanes: Chemistry and Technology.* Copyright Interscience, New York, 1962. Reprinted by permission of John Wiley & Sons.

two most commonly used aromatic isocyanates in polyurethane synthesis are toluene diisocyanate (TDI) and 4,4'-diphenylmethane diisocyanate (MDI). Of these, MDI has superior reactivity, and polymers based on MDI may possess better physical properties. Furthermore, MDI is crystallizable whereas the mixed isomer 2,4-TDI and 2,6 TDI does not crystallize in the solid state. Aromatic diisocyanates such as naphthalene diisocyanate (NDI) and 3,3' bitoluene diisocyanate (TODI) also can produce high-performance polymers. NDI produces less extensible and harder materials than MDI. Typical aliphatic isocyanates include 1,6-hexane diisocyanate (HDI), isophorone diisocyanate (IPDI), and methylene bis (p-cyclohexyl isocyanate) (H_{12}MDI). At equivalent stoichiometry, H_{12}MDI polyurethanes possess comparable mechanical properties compared to analogous MDI based polyurethanes. H_{12}MDI-based hard segments are not particularly crystallizable due to the presence of the three H_{12}MDI isomers, whereas MDI-based hard segments will readily crystallize under favorable conditions. However, H_{12}MDI based polyurethanes possess lower high temperature properties and lower solvent resistance. The symmetry of the isocyanate also is important. Increasing symmetry favors the crystallization of the hard segment and so increases the degree of phase separation, modulus, hardness, and abrasion resistance. Methyl substituents on the aromatic ring will impede packing and crystallization of the hard segment, lowering the modulus and abrasion resistance.

2. Polyols

Polyols used in polyurethane synthesis are responsible for the flexibility of the material, particularly at low temperatures and elongation at break. As the molecular weight of the soft segment increases, the T_g of the polyurethane decreases. A higher degree of microphase separation increases the ease of backbone rotation in the soft segment component producing a lower glass-transition temperature resulting in a more extensible material. Polyurethanes synthesized from polyesters possess relatively good physical properties; however, they are susceptible to hydrolytic cleavage of the ester linkage. In applications where hydrolytic stability is required, polyether-based polyurethanes are preferred; however, polyetherurethanes typically do not possess the same degree of mechanical strength as polyesterurethanes. Polytetramethylene oxide (PTMO or PTMEG) polyurethanes show a level of mechanical strength comparable to that of polyester polyurethanes and possess relatively good hydrolytic stability.[45] As the weight fraction of the soft segment increases, the properties of the polyurethane will change from that of a hard plastic to those of flexible elastomers. High molecular weight polyethers and polyesters will have better tensile properties than low molecular weight counterparts. Polyurethanes containing high molecular weight polyols are also more likely to cold-harden, due to soft segment crystallization. Polyesterurethanes are also likely to exhibit more phase mixing, compared to polyetherurethanes.

3. Chain Extenders

The chemistry of the chain extender used in polyurethane synthesis also can affect the physical properties of the material. The use of a chain extender to increase the molecular weight of the hard segment facilitates the phase separation in the final material. The selection of a diamine or a diol determines whether urea groups or urethane groups are formed. This influences the degree of phase separation that occurs, which in turn influences the mechanical properties. However, polyurethaneureas are more difficult to melt process and have lower solubilities in common solvents than conventional polyurethanes. Generally, aliphatic chain extenders yield softer materials than aromatic chain extenders. The number of carbon atoms in the chain extender also affects the crystallizability of the hard segment. A crystalline hard domain improves the physical properties of the material. Glycol extended polyurethanes are more flexible, softer and less strong than their amine-extended analogs. Cyclic chain extenders increase the strength of the material when compared with their linear analogs.

III. CHARACTERIZATION OF POLYURETHANES

The primary focus of this section is the bulk characterization of polyurethanes. The methods used to determine the mechanical and physical properties of polyurethanes will be discussed, and examples will be given. Bulk characterization is important for a number of reasons:[46]

1. It provides assurance that the material is that which the user expects.
2. It provides an insight into the presence of fillers, plasticizers, antioxidants, low molecular weight components, unreacted monomer, solvent residues etc.
3. It can provide information about potential leachables, which may be irritant or toxic.
4. It provides a basis for interpreting the results of surface analyses.
5. It yields information on the basic mechanical properties that are important in the structural use of the material, and may provide insight into the possible mechanisms of biodegradation.

Prior to any type of bulk characterization, it is important to have some information regarding the synthetic route of the polymer. This can greatly facilitate interpretation of the data, both from bulk and surface analyses.

Methods of physical characterization of biomaterials are relatively well defined when compared with the protocols for biological evaluation. The American Society for Testing and Materials (ASTM) has developed a large number of tests for the physical characterization of materials, that are widely accepted, and reviewed on a regular basis. The advantages of test methods that are globally adopted and applied means that data obtained from different laboratories can be compared;

this is in sharp contrast to the current status of the biomedical evaluation of materials where test methods and parameter measurement are not so well defined making interpretation and comparison of data from different laboratories complicated.

A. GEL PERMEATION CHROMATOGRAPHY

As discussed in Chapter 2, the molecular weight of polymers is usually defined as a number average or a weight average. Number average molecular weights can be measured by membrane osmometry, vapor pressure depression, and end-group analysis. Weight average molecular weights can be measured by light scattering techniques. Gel Permeation Chromatography (GPC), also called size exclusion chromatography, is a separation technique that separates a complex mixture according to molecular size. A solution of the polymer is injected into a column comprised of a bed of microporous particles. Diffusion of the polymer into and out of the pores depends on the molecular size of the polymer molecules. Larger molecules will be less able to penetrate the pores and will be eluted first. Smaller molecules will pass through the pores and take longer to pass through the column. The pore size distribution of the particles determines the size range within which separation occurs. Standards of known molecular weight and narrow molecular weight distribution, such as anionically polymerized polystyrenes are used as calibration standards, to allow quantification of the relative molecular weight and molecular weight distribution of the polymer. More accurate molecular weight determination may be achieved using multi-detector methods.[47]

Belisle et al.[48] have examined the composition of Biomer using GPC through hydrolysis of the polyurethane and analysis of the fragments by GPC, mass spectrometry and infrared spectroscopy. They concluded that Biomer was composed of MDI, PTMO (1800 molecular weight), ethylene diamine, 1,3- diaminecyclohexane, poly (diisopropylaminoethylmethacrylate-co-decyl) methacrylate, and Santowhite powder. Differences in the molecular weight between two batches of Biomer also have been reported.[49] These differences were attributed to differences in the molecular weights of the batches during synthesis, and not to effects of aging. Irganox 1010, an ester, has been identified as an antioxidant present in Tecoflex.[50] GPC analysis of molecular weight distribution has been used to study the degradation of some commercially available polyurethanes.[51]

B. INFRARED SPECTROSCOPY

Infrared spectroscopy can be used to identify chemical groups within a compound. Chemical bonds within a material vibrate at characteristic frequencies, and so when infrared radiation is passed through the material, at certain frequencies, the molecule will absorb the energy and vibrate. Each group is capable of a number of different modes of vibration, such as stretching and bending, so a number of peaks can often be attributed to the presence of a particular chemical structure. Identification of these peaks and their magnitude can permit identification of the molecular structure. Some of the characteristic frequencies of functional groups found in polyurethanes are presented in Table 2. Spectra are obtained by splitting a beam of infrared radiation into two and passing one beam through the sample. The intensity of the beam after it has passed through the sample is compared with the intensity of the beam that has not passed through the sample. The intensity is compared over a range of frequencies or wavenumbers (cm^{-1}), usually from 4000 cm^{-1} to 600 cm^{-1}. Traditional methods of IR spectroscopy were based on transmission of the beam through the sample. The wavelength intensity of the emerging beam was scanned successively, meaning that several minutes were required to obtain each spectrum.

The development of Fourier Transform techniques introduced a number of advantages over the conventional methods of IR spectra collection. In Fourier Transform Infrared Spectroscopy (FTIR), the incident beam is split into two, and one is passed through the sample. The other beam is either passed through a longer distance within the sample, or passed straight to the detector. The two beams are compared and an interferogram produced. Fourier transform methods allow the conver-

TABLE 2
Characteristic frequencies of IR absorption bands for polyurethanes

Group[*]	Wavenumber (cm^{-1})	Comments[#]
ν(N–H) free N–H	3420	w, sh
ν(N–H) bonded N–H	3320	s
ν(N–H) cis-trans isomeric bonded N–H	3185	w
Overtone of 1530 cm^{-1} band	3115	w
ν(C–H) in benzene ring	3030	w
$ν_a$(CH$_2$)	2960	s, in ES only
$ν_a$(CH$_2$)	2935	s, in ET only
$ν_s$(CH$_2$)	2890	m, sh, in ES only
$ν_s$(CH$_2$)	2860	m, sh, in ES only
$ν_s$(CH$_2$)	2856	s, in ET only
$ν_s$(CH$_2$)	2795	m, in ET only
ν (C = O)	1733	vs, free C = O in ET only
ν (C = O)	1703	vs, bonded C = O in ET only
ν (C = O)	1740–1690	vs, free and bonded C = O in urethane and ester ES only.
ν (C = C) in benzene ring	1600	s
δ (N–H) + ν (C–N)	1530	vs
δ (CH$_2$)	1500–1430	w
ν (C–C) in benzene ring	1410	s
w(CH$_2$)	1360	m
δ (N–H) +ν (C–N), β (C–H)	1310	s
w(CH$_2$), ν (C–O–C) of ester	1250	s, sh.
δ (N–H) +ν (C–N),	1225	s
ν (C–O–C) of ester	1180	s, in ES only
ν (C H$_2$–O–C H$_2$) of aliphatic ether	1110	vs, in ET only
ν (C–O–C) of ester in hard segment	1080	s
β (C–H) in benzene ring	1020	w
γ (C–H) in benzene ring	820	w

[#] Relative intensity based on sample at room temperature: w = weak; m = medium; s = strong; vs. = very strong; sh = shoulder; ET = polyetherurethanes; ES = polyesterurethanes

[*] ν = stretching; δ = bending; w = wagging; β = in plane bending; γ = out of plane bending; νa = asymmetric stretching; vs = symmetric stretching.

sion of the interferogram into a plot of absorption against wavenumber. Spectra can be obtained within a few seconds, which allows some kinetic experiments to be monitored by FTIR methods. Digital software also allows smoothing of spectra, and spectral subtraction, enhancing analysis. FTIR data are typically taken using many scans, and addition of the spectra (multiplexing) means that very small samples can be analyzed. Spectra can be interpreted as conventional IR spectra. Adaptation of the technique to reflection rather than transmission mode (Attenuated Total Reflection Fourier Transform Infrared Spectroscopy — ATR–FTIR) has been used to study polymer surfaces, and to investigate protein adsorption onto different surfaces, including polyurethanes. This method of surface characterization is discussed in more detail in the next chapter.

Bond vibrations are sensitive to the environment, and so slight shifts in peak positions, or peak splits can be used to indicate changes in bonding interactions of the molecule. Such alterations can be induced by changes in the structure of neighboring chemical groups, or changes in intermolecular bonding, such as hydrogen bonding. Figure 18 shows typical IR spectra of a polyetherurethane and a polyesterurethane. Shifts in the position of peaks and their relative magnitude have been used to

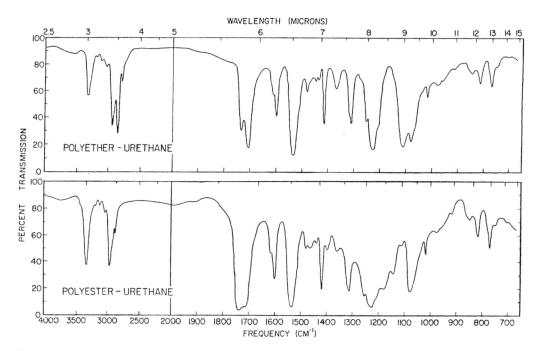

FIGURE 18 IR spectra of (a) polyetherurethane (MDI/BD/PTMO) and (b) polyesterurethane (MDI/BD/PTMA). From Seymour R.W. Ph.D. Thesis. University of Wisconsin–Madison, 1973.

assess semiquantitatively the degree of intermolecular bonding within polyurethanes. Wang and Cooper studied a series of PTMO based polyurethanes.[35] Deviations in peak position and relative peak intensity were observed in materials synthesized from identical components, but of different molar ratios. The relative ratios of absorption peaks near 1702 cm^{-1} and 1732 cm^{-1} have been interpreted as the bonded to nonbonded urethane carbonyl ratio, and used as a measure of the extent of phase separation.[52-53] Grasel and Cooper reported that for PTMO, PPO and PEO polyurethanes, the extent of urethane carbonyl hydrogen bonding increased with the hard segment content of these polyurethanes.[53] PDMS-polyurethanes, showed a very high degree of hydrogen bonding, indicating a high degree of phase separation in these systems. Other studies of polyurethanes with alkyl chains grafted to urethane nitrogen showed that as the degree of alkylation increases, the relative proportion of nonbonded hydrogens also increased, denoting a decrease in the degree of phase separation.[54]

Infrared spectroscopy also can be used to confirm the presence of functional groups within a polyurethane, identify the presence of contaminants and processing aids, and serve as a reference spectrum for surface characterization by attenuated total reflection FTIR.

C. Differential Scanning Calorimetry

Differential Scanning Calorimetry (DSC) is a thermal analysis technique. It is used to characterize the T_g and T_m of a material, the degree of crystallinity, the degree of phase separation and morphological changes that occur on annealing. A sample of the material is placed inside the calorimeter and heated at a fixed rate. The amount of energy needed to maintain a fixed rate of temperature increase is measured. Changes in the specific heat denote changes in the mobility of the polymer chains. Characterization of the thermal properties of segmented polyurethanes indicate that there are multiple thermal transitions in these materials. Each transition has been attributed to a specific phenomenon in each of the phases. DSC thermograms can be used identify the glass transition temperature (T_g) of a polymer. The glass transition temperature is identified by a change in heat capacity which appears as a baseline shift. As discussed earlier T_g is the temperature at which a large increase in the mobility of the polymer backbone occurs. An endothermal peak in the DSC thermogram denotes the melting temperature of the polymer, T_m. This denotes the temperature at which disordering of the crystalline regions of the hard segment occurs. Melting and crystallization events in the hard and soft segments also can be observed from DSC scans as corresponding endotherms or exotherms.

In a DSC scan for a polyurethane, as many as five transitions can be observed. These include the glass transition temperature (generally between –50 and –10°C), short range and long range order transitions (35 to 115°C, and 130 to 190°C respectively), and finally the melting temperature of the hard segments (200 to 225°C). An *in situ* quench followed by an additional scan may be performed in order to examine the effect of thermal history of the polymer sample. Annealing of polyurethanes has been studied by a number of investigators.[18,55-56]

The soft segment T_g can be used as a measure of the degree of phase separation of the polyurethane. The glass-transition temperature is affected by the purity of the phase, and so if the material is well phase-separated, the T_g will lie very close to the T_g of the soft segment polymer. The larger the deviation from this value, the larger the degree of phase mixing of the soft and hard segments. The degree of order within the hard segment of a polyurethane depends upon the chemistry, rigidity and degree of hydrogen bonding within the hard segment. The higher the degree of order within the hard segments, the higher the melting point of the polyurethane.

Typical DSC thermograms of segmented polyurethanes are shown in Figure 18. The samples are based on MDI–BD hard segments combined with either PTMO or polytetramethylene adipate (PTMA) as soft segments. The nomenclature has been established whereby the two numbers following the ET (MDI/BD/PTMO) or ES (MDI/BD/PTMA) designations indicate the weight-percent diisocyanate, and the soft-segment molecular weight in thousands, respectively. For example, ET-38-1 represents an MDI/BD/PTMO-based polyurethane with a diisocyanate (MDI) content of 38 weight percent and a soft-segment PTMO molecular weight of 1000. In Figure 19, the decrease in the DSC traces between –60 and –10°C corresponds to the T_g of the soft segment.

The sets of thermograms in Figure 19, and the data in Table 3 demonstrate the effects of hard segment content and soft-segment molecular weight on soft-segment T_g. Both the ES (polyester soft-segment) and ET (polyether soft-segment) series of polymers show a decrease in soft-segment T_g with increasing soft-segment molecular weight. Except for ET-38-1, the ET polyurethanes having a soft-segment molecular weight of 1000 show a constant soft-segment T_g at about –44°C. In the ES series, the soft segment T_g generally increases with increasing MDI content.

The variation of the T_g of the soft segment as a function of composition or segmental chemical structure has been used as an indicator of the degree of microphase separation. Factors influencing the phase separation process in these MDI-based polyurethanes have been summarized by Aitken and Jeffs as follows:[57]

1. Crystallization of either component
2. The steric hindrance of the hard segment unit in a hydrogen-bonding process
3. The inherent miscibility of the hard and soft components

Higher molecular weight segments increase phase separation and account for the low T_g of the 2000 molecular weight soft-segment samples. The miscibility arguments can rationalize the T_g terms in the 1000 m.w. soft-segment polyurethanes. The relatively constant T_g values observed as a function of composition exhibited by the polyetherurethane elastomers of 1000 m.w. soft segment (Figure 19 and Table 3) indicate that the penetration of isolated hard segments into the soft phase is limited. The polyesterurethane materials on the other hand, show a greater tendency for the hard segment to be trapped in the polyester rich soft segment phase, owing to the greater polarity of the polyester segment.[58] The T_g of the soft segment in the polyester-urethanes thus increases, as the hard-segment content is increased, due to phase mixing.

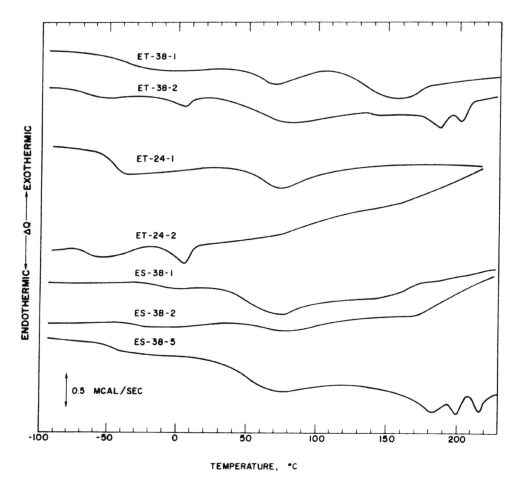

FIGURE 19 DSC curves for ET-24, ET-38 and ES-38 series of segmented polyurethanes. From Srichatrapimuk V.W. and Cooper S.L. *J. Macromol. Sci. — Phys. B,* 15:267, 1978. With permission, Marcel Dekker, Inc.

Analogous studies on two series of segmented 1000 m.w. PTMO-based polyurethanes, having either a symmetric 2,6-toluene diisocyanate (TDI) or an asymmetric 2,4-TDI-based hard segment (butanediol chain extended), show similar results.[59] The 2,6-TDI samples, having crystalline hard domains which restrict phase mixing, exhibit a soft-segment T_g which was relatively independent of hard-segment content, indicative of a pure soft segment phase. The 2,4-TDI systems, on the other hand, give soft-segment T_g values which increase with increasing hard-segment content, indicative of considerable phase mixing with the amorphous 2,4-TDI-based hard domains. In addition, Sung et al.[37] have investigated polyurethaneureas based on TDI hard segments, ethylene diamine and butanediol chain extenders, and PTMO or polybutylene adipate soft segments. They found that the extent of phase segregation improved significantly when ethylene diamine was used as the chain extender instead of butanediol.

The DSC spectra in Figure 19 exhibit several endotherms associated with disordering processes which occur in the urethane hard-segment domains. Data from early studies led to a hypothesis that these endotherms were attributable to hydrogen-bond disruption;[60-61] however, later studies have shown these transitions to strongly depend on thermal history.[18,38,62] Annealing of the sample elevated the temperature of the transition. Furthermore, endotherms still occurred in samples where hydrogen bonding was eliminated by the substitution of urethane hydrogens with alkyl chains.

TABLE 3
Effect of soft segment length on soft segment T_g for polyetherurethanes (ET) and polyesterurethanes (ES)

Sample	Soft Segment T_g (°C)
ET-24-1	−43
ET-24-2	−57
ET-24-1	−43
ET-28-1	−44
ET-31-1	−44
ET-35-1	−43
ET-38-1	−39
ET-38-2	−60
ES-24-1	−30
ES-28-1	−32
ES-31-1	−25
ES-35-1	−19
ES-38-1	−10
ES-38-1	−10
ES-38-2	−26
ES-38-5	−47

From Srichatrapimuk V.W. and Cooper S.L. *J. Macromol. Sci. — Phys. B*, 15:267, 1978.

Three characteristic endothermic transitions have been observed (Figure 20).[38] The first is an endotherm centered at approximately 70°C which is attributed to the disruption of domains with limited short-range order; the second at 120 to 190°C, which represents the dissociation of domains containing long range order; and the third, a transition above 200°C which is attributable to the melting of microcrystallites of the hard segments. The first transition can be shifted upward to merge with the second transition by annealing, the final state of order depending on the annealing history and sample composition.

Koberstein and Russell have used SAXS and DSC techniques to study the multiple endotherms in segmented polyurethanes consisting of MDI–BD hard segments and PPO soft segments.[63] Two distinct endotherms were observed in all samples. The high temperature endotherm (above 200°C) is attributed to melting of microcrystalline hard domains. A lower temperature endotherm is assigned to the onset of microdomain mixing of "noncrystalline" hard and soft segments. This accompanies the microphase separation transition (MST), which involves the disruption of microdomain structure to form a homogeneous mixed phase.[64] A representation of the morphology of segmented polyurethanes at temperatures around this region is contained in Figure 21. The MST is believed to occur in the range of 140–210°C. Further work by Koberstein's group examined the effects of thermal annealing on the morphology and properties of polyurethane elastomers. DSC studies of samples rapidly quenched from a melt at 240°C show that the melt phase is homogeneous at this temperature. The annealing of polyurethanes for a short time below the MST produces a very small increase in the molecular weight of the polymer. Annealing of polyurethanes above the MST can promote chain branching reactions, resulting in an increase in molecular weight.[65] The T_g of the soft segment

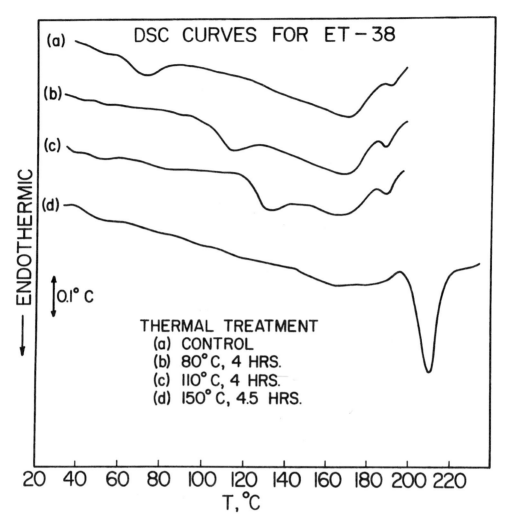

FIGURE 20 Effect of annealing on the DSC curves for ET-38-1 (a) control; (b) 80 °C, 4 hour; (c) 110°C, 4 hour; (d) 150 °C, 4.5 hour. Reprinted with permission from Seymour R.W. and Cooper S.L. *Macromolecules*, 6:48, 1973. Copyright 1973, American Chemical Society.

phase has been reported to increase after annealing, indicating that a greater proportion of the hard segments are dispersed within the soft segments.[16,18,64]

D. DYNAMIC MECHANICAL THERMAL ANALYSIS

Dynamic Mechanical Thermal Analysis (DMTA) is an important technique capable of providing considerable information on the position of transitions and the mechanical properties of polymers. DMTA measures the storage modulus (E') and the loss modulus (E'') as a function of temperature. A sinusoidal mode of deformation is applied to the sample, as the temperature is scanned from well below the glass transition temperature to the point when the sample becomes too soft to test in a given apparatus. DMTA provides information on first and second-order transitions (T_m and T_g, respectively), the degree of phase separation, crystallinity and crosslinking of the polymer, and the mechanical properties such as the glassy state and the rubbery plateau modulus.

Typical storage modulus data for several polymer systems are shown in Figure 22. Curves D and E represent thermomechanical spectra for two polyurethanes. Two distinct transitions are

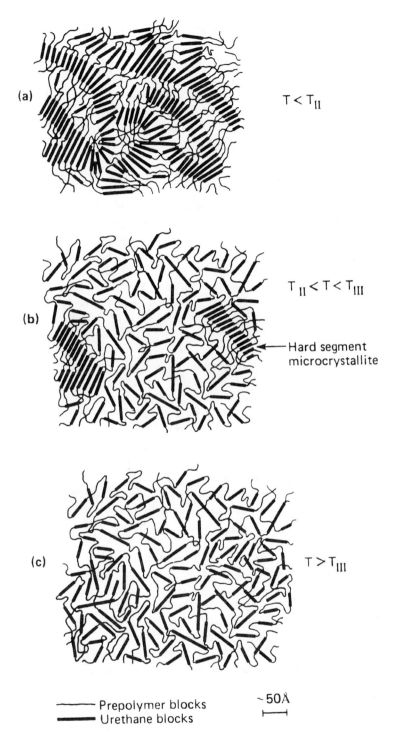

FIGURE 21 Schematic model for the morphological changes that occur during DSC scans of polyurethane elastomers: (a) below the the microphase mixing transition temperature (T^{II}) (b) between the microphase mixing transition temperature and the melting temperature (T^{III}); and (c) above the melting temperature. The microcrystalline hard-segment domains are indicated. Reprinted with permission from Koberstein J.T. and Russell T.P. *Macromolecules,* 19:714, 1986. Copyright 1986 American Chemical Society.

indicated by the dramatic drops in storage moduli. Ideally, for well phase separated block copolymers, these transitions are located at the T_g or T_m of the corresponding component homopolymers. The low temperature transition is related to the T_g of the soft-segment phase. When this soft segment phase is relatively pure, the correlation between this storage modulus transition and the T_g of the soft-segment homopolymer is very good. The high temperature transition correlates well with the temperature at which hard-segment rich domains begin to dissociate or drastically soften. Again, high purity in these domains shifts the transition to higher temperatures, approaching the softening temperature of the hard-segment homopolymer. Sample composition, segmental length, inherent inter-segment solubility, and sample preparation technique have been found to influence the degree of phase separation and thereby the shape and temperature location of the dynamic-mechanical transition points. Phase mixing between domains tends to produce a decreased slope in the storage modulus transition region and broadened loss peaks. Dynamic mechanical analysis is a sensitive tool for characterizing polymers with similar chemical structures or detecting the presence of additives which may be present in moderate quantities.

Figure 23 shows the storage modulus (E') and the dissipation factor (tan δ) as a function of temperature for a series of polyetherurethanes with the same 1000 m.w. PTMO soft segment, but different MDI contents.[66] As the hard-segment diisocyanate content is increased, the modulus, high-temperature softening point, and the T_g also increase. This is a characteristic of an incompatible system where the hard-segment domains behave as reinforcing filler particles. The dissipation factor spectra show at least two peaks: a large peak at about 0°C (α^a) which corresponds to the soft segment T_g, and a secondary transition at about –100°C (γ), which is attributed to localized methylene rotations in the polyether sequences.

Figure 24 shows dynamic mechanical spectra for a series of polyesterurethanes with different soft-segment molecular weights. In these polymers the hard to soft-segment ratio was kept constant.[66] An increase in the molecular weight of the polyol results in an increased propensity for the soft segment to crystallize. This is indicated by a rise in the modulus and a secondary peak αc, in tan δ for ES-38-5. The increase in crystallinity also results in a decrease in the T_g (the position of the αa peak). This is due to crystallization brought about by longer segment lengths, which promotes greater purity in the microphase separated soft segment phase.

The effect of cross linking a polyesterurethane Estane® 5740-070 with MDI is shown in Figure 25.[44] The crosslinking reaction in this case proceeds through reaction of the isocyanate with the urethane hydrogen, resulting in an increased content of aromatic allophanate linkages. The T_g is seen to increase with cross linking, and the increase in the plateau modulus with increasing MDI is the result of a greater percentage of bulky groups present acting as reinforcing filler. Above the MDI phase softening point, rubber-like behavior is seen in Samples 2 to 4.

Polyurethanes are sometimes plasticized in order to modify properties, to reduce cost, or to improve processability. Figure 26 shows the effect of plasticizer incorporation in Estane® 5740-070.[44] The data show that the polyesterurethane is affected as a two-component system. The soft polyester segments are preferentially plasticized by the less polar diluent Carbowax®, as shown by a shift in T_g toward lower temperatures. The plateau modulus is affected mostly by the incorporation of the highly polar DMSO diluent. These complementary results indicate that hard and soft domains can be preferentially solvated by different plasticizers.

E. Electron Microscopy

Scanning Electron Microscopy (SEM) studies have primarily been used to study the surface topography of polymeric materials. SEM techniques are used to view cross sections of polymer specimens and examine the morphological structure of the material, and assess the gross uniformity of the sample. The material is usually frozen in liquid nitrogen prior to fracture in order to inhibit molecular rearrangement at the new interface, particularly if the glass transition temperature of the polymer is below room temperature. The presence of large scale phase separation, pores, voids,

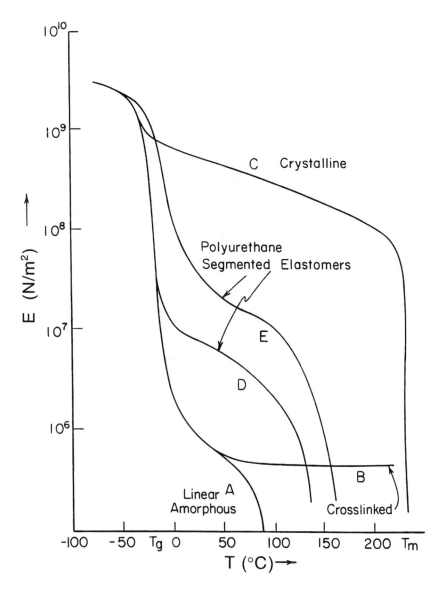

FIGURE 22 Storage modulus v temperature curves for (A) linear amorphous polymer, (B) crosslinked polymer, (C) semicrystalline polymer, (D) MDI/BD/PTMA segmented polyurethane (32% MDI by weight), (E) MDI/BD/PTMA segmented polyurethane (38% MDI by weight). From Cooper S.L. and Tobolsky A.V. *J. Appl. Polym. Sci.*, 10:1837, Copyright 1966. Reprinted with permission by John Wiley & Sons.

particulate contaminants, fillers, fatigue cracking, and environmental stress cracking all can be detected by SEM. Sample preparation of polymers for SEM is specimen-specific and usually involves coating the polymer sample with a thin conducting layer of gold. Some samples may require staining in addition to the conducting overlayer. Exposure to radiation and heat may cause the polymer to degrade. High resolution, low-voltage SEM allows study of specimens without the need of a conducting layer, and reduces radiation damage to the polymer specimen. Due to the small size of the hard segment domains (50 to 100 Å), interpretation of SEM micrographs for information regarding surface microphase separation is difficult.

Transmission Electron Microscopy (TEM) also has been carried out on polyurethane systems. TEM has a higher resolution than SEM but in general, sample preparation is more difficult. Solvent

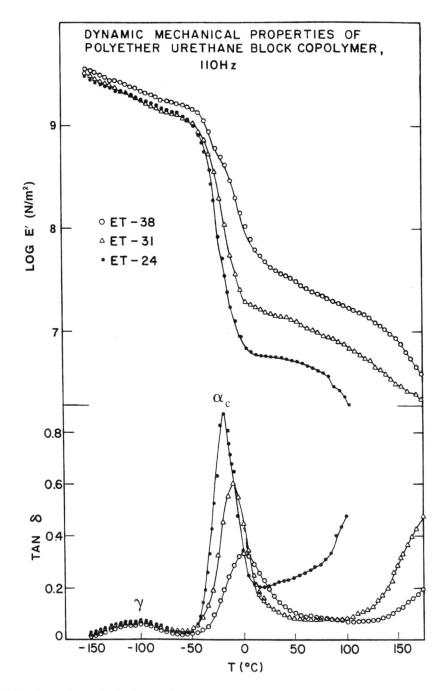

FIGURE 23 Dynamic mechanical properties of polyetherurethanes at 110Hz. From Huh D.S. and Cooper S.L. *Polym. Eng. Sci.*, 11:369, 1971. With permission.

casting techniques can be used to prepare thin films for analysis, although specimens may possess a morphology unrepresentative of the bulk.[67] Ultramicrotomy can provide thin sections, but must be performed at low temperatures (i.e., below the glass transition temperature of the soft segment) to prevent rearrangement of the soft and hard phases. Staining also is necessary; osmium tetroxide and ruthenium tetroxide are commonly used to provide contrast between hard and soft segments.

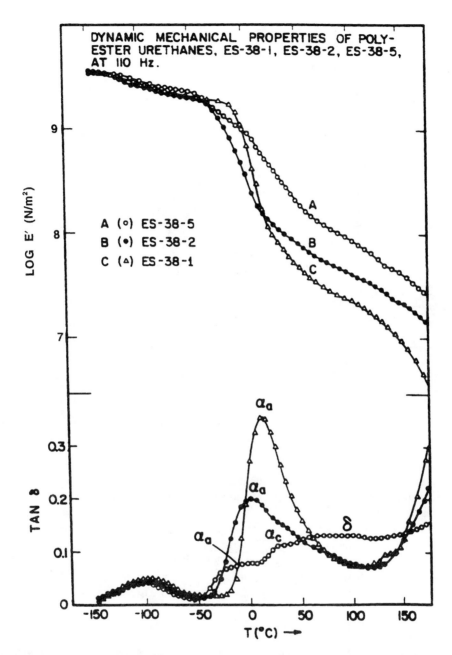

FIGURE 24 Dynamic mechanical properties of polyesterurethanes at 110 Hz. From Huh D.S. and Cooper S.L. *Polym. Eng. Sci.*, 11:369, 1971. With permission.

Microphase separation in polyurethane samples has been observed by TEM by several researchers.[7,8,23,67]

Li and Cooper have examined the morphology of osmium tetroxide stained films of polyurethane-polybutadiene systems using TEM.[67] Figure 27 is a schematic representation of the domain structure and corresponding surface morphology for a series of polybutadiene polyurethanes. These materials exhibit almost complete phase separation, due to the high degree of incompatibility between the hard and soft segments. Below a hard segment volume fraction of 32%, the morphology of the material can be described by short cylindrical hard segment microdomains within the soft

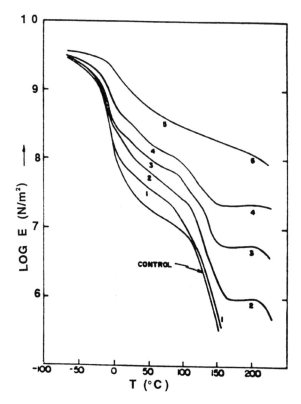

FIGURE 25 Modulus-temperature curves of Estane 5740-070 crosslinked with MDI. (1) 5.1 pph; (2) 1.6 pph; (3) 25.2 pph; (4) 99.3 pph MDI. From Cooper S.L. and Tobolsky A.V. *J. Appl. Polym. Sci.*, 11:1361, 1967.

segment phase. Between 35% and 75%, the hard segment domains have rod-like or lamellar character. Increasing the hard segment content results in an increase in the length of the lamellae, but not the width. Above 75% hard segment content, the soft segments form isolated, globular but nonspherical microdomains.

Li and Cooper also examined the morphology of polyetherurethane thin films, reporting that for polyurethane thin films containing PTMO soft segments and MDI/BD hard segments, short cylinder or lamellar morphology was adopted, depending on the sample's composition.[68] The samples with a higher hard segment content adopted the lamellar morphology. Differences in the state of order between samples that were molded and solvent cast were also observed.

F. Stress-Strain Properties and Ultimate Tensile Strength

The fracture process can be represented by three steps: initiation of microcracks or cavitation, slow crack propagation, and catastrophic failure. Dispersed phases tend to interfere with the crack propagation step, through redistribution of energy that would otherwise cause the cracks to reach catastrophic sizes. Thus, a two-phase morphology is essential to the achievement of high strength in elastomers. The presence of hard-segment domains also increases energy dissipation by hysteresis and other viscoelastic mechanisms.

Growing cracks can be deflected and bifurcated at phase boundaries. Upon deformation, triaxial stress fields are formed about hard-phase particles, tending to inhibit the growth of cavities. Cavities which do form can be limited to small sizes, stabilized by surface energy effects. The hard phase can relieve stress concentrations by undergoing deformation or internal structural reorganization.

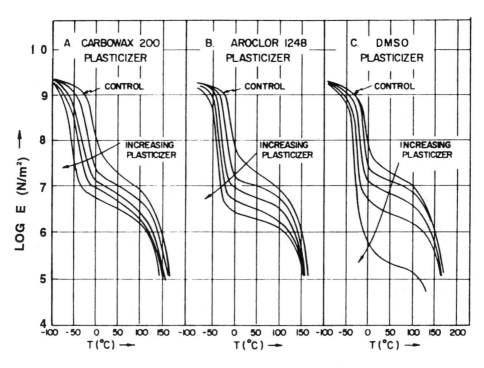

FIGURE 26 Modulus temperature curves of plasticized polyesterurethane, Estane 5740-070. (A) Carbowax 200; (B) Arclor 1248; (C) DMSO. From Cooper S.L. and Tobolsky A.V. *J. Appl. Polym. Sci.,* 11:1361, 1967.

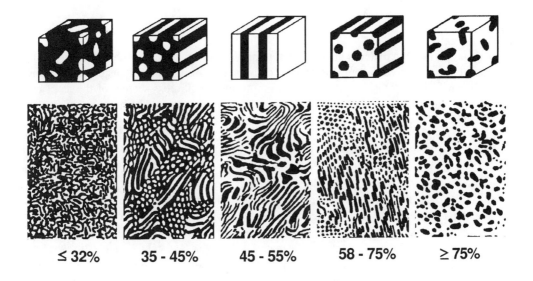

Hard Segment Weight Fraction

FIGURE 27 Morphological models of polybutadiene-polyurethanes, of increasing hard segment content. The light areas represent hard segment, dark regions, soft segment. Li, C. Ph.D. Thesis, University of Wisconsin, Madison. 1988.

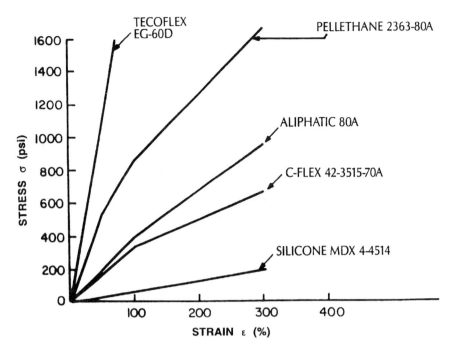

FIGURE 28 Stiffness of some biomedical polyurethanes. From Szycher M. In *Blood Compatible Materials and Devices,* Ed. Sharma C. P., Szycher M. Technomic, Lancaster, PA, 1991. With permission.

Although hydrogen bonding can contribute to domain cohesiveness, hydrogen bonding itself is not directly responsible for high physical properties.

1. Tensile Properties

The tensile properties of a material are measured to provide information on the mechanical strength of a material. Tests involve the application of a constant rate of uniaxial extension to the sample. The engineering stress, defined as the force normal to the initial cross-section of the test sample is measured as a function of extension, under a constant rate of extension. The stress-strain responses for some biomedical polyurethanes are shown in Figure 28. Young's Modulus, ultimate tensile strength (UTS) and ultimate elongation are obtained from such tests. Typical values for polyurethanes used as biomaterials are listed in Table 4. The chemistry of the hard and soft segments, the degree of phase separation of the polyurethane, and the molecular weight can affect the values obtained for Young's Modulus, UTS and ultimate elongation.

The tensile strength of a polyurethane is dependent on temperature. Below the soft segment glass transition temperature, polyurethanes are rigid and behave plastically. Above the hard segment glass transition or melting temperature, the materials behave as amorphous, noncrosslinked rubbers. Between these two transition temperatures, the materials behave as typical thermoplastic elastomers, with strength and modulus decreasing as temperature increases. The properties also decrease depending on the difference between the service temperature and the glass temperature. This can be attributed to differences in soft segment glass transition temperatures, but could also be partially determined by the degree of phase mixing in the material. The degree of phase mixing is influenced by the polarity of the soft segment. Speckhard and Cooper compared the tensile properties of polyurethane elastomers, taking into account the difference between the service temperature and the glass transition temperature of the material.[69] Their results suggested that the lack of soft segment crystallizability under strain and possibly a very high degree of phase separation limit the tensile properties of polyurethanes with nonpolar soft segments, which generally have lower tensile

TABLE 4
Mechanical properties of biomedical polyurethanes

Name	Tensile Strength (MPa)	Initial Modulus (MPa)	Ultimate Elongation (%)	Hardness (Shore Durometer)	Water absorption (%)
Biomer SolG	31–41	2.8–5.5	600–800	75A	1.2
Biomer ExtG	28–35	12.4 Flx			0.18
Cardiothane 51	43		580	72A	1.6
Cardiomat 610	27.6	8.1*	500	80A	
Corethane 80A	44.8–51.7	4.8–9.6*	400–490	80A	1.2
55D	48.2–58.6	11.7–13.8*	365–440	55D	0.9
75D	48.2–62.7	18.6–22.1*	255–320	75D	0.8
Pellethane 2363 Series	35–48	3.6–14	350–600	55D, 75D, 80A, 90A	
Tecoflex 80A	42	2.8	580–800	80A,	
60D	42	15.0	400	60D,	
72D	55	15.4		72D	
Rimplast					
PYUA 102	21	28 Flx	700	70A	
PYUA 103	10	13.8 Flx	1000	60A	1.5
BioSpan	41	8.1	850	70A	
Thoratec BPS-215	38	10.3	700	75A	
BPS-105	35	4.1	870	70A	
Texin AM, DM, M series	48	8.3	175–550	885A, 65D, 70D	
Biothane	18	12.0	136	44D	
Erythrothane	43	4.8	520	83A	

Flx = flexural modulus* modulus at 300%

TABLE 5
Tensile properties of MDI/ED/PTMO polyetherurethaneureas

Hard Segment (wt%)	Soft segment (m.w.)	Young's Modulus (10^6 Pa)	Elongation at failure (%)	UTS (10^6 Pa)
46	1000	69.2	600	43.0
46	2000	188.5	570	388.8
36	1000	9.3	850	34.6
36	2000	42.6	770	40.1
25	1000	3.3	1550	7.1
25	2000	4.3	1160	18.6

From Wang C.B. and Cooper S.L. *Macromolecules,* 16:775, 1983.

properties. Polyurethanes with ionic groups show enhanced mechanical properties in the dry state. These properties are compromized when the materials are hydrated.

Table 5 lists the tensile properties of a series of polyetherurethane ureas based on MDI/ED/PTMO.[35] These data show that an increase in either the hard-segment content (at constant soft-segment molecular weight) or the block length (at constant hard-segment content) leads to a higher Young's modulus and lower elongation at failure. The higher moduli arise from the introduction of higher volume fractions, as well as greater order in the hard-segment domains. The higher moduli and tensile strengths of the high soft-segment (2000) series is consistent with their higher urea content, which results in more cohesive hard domains.

2. Tensile Stress Hysteresis

Stress hysteresis of polyurethanes can limit the applications of polyurethanes. Repeated application of stress to a polyurethane leads to a decrease in the stress-strain properties, which is attributed to disruption of hard segments. Figure 29 shows an example of stress hysteresis for ET-38-1 polyetherurethane.[70] Unlike the low-strain Young's Modulus which depends on the rigidity and morphology of the hard-segment domains, stress hysteresis is a function of domain ductility and restructuring, and the nature of the mixed hard and soft-segment interfacial regions.[27] In the polyurethanes, hard-segment crystallization has been found to increase stress hysteresis, permanent set, and tensile strength. Heat build-up in polyurethanes attributable to their high hysteresis losses has limited their suitability in applications such as high-speed automobile tires.

3. Fatigue Testing

Many polymers used in biomedical applications must endure large cyclical deformations through their lifetime, which can be expected to be a number of years depending on the type of implanted device. Materials used under cyclical conditions may fail due to fatigue. This is most relevant for cardiovascular devices such as left ventricular assist devices (LVADs), heart valves and vascular grafts. Polyurethanes are also candidate materials for the outer housing of total artificial hearts. Fatigue failure can be defined as complete failure, or significant reduction in the physical properties such as the compliance or the modulus, that would prevent the device performing its intended function. Properties such as the modulus and strength also may start to deteriorate long before final failure occurs, even if the maximum stress level in the fatigue test is significantly lower than the ultimate static strength of the material.

The actual mechanical performance of a material also is influenced by the final geometry of the device or component, and by the environment. Two levels of tensile tests are recommended as

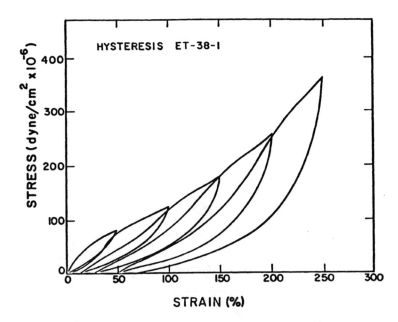

FIGURE 29 Tensile stress hysteresis. From Lelah, M.D. and Cooper, S.L. *Polyurethanes in Medicine*, CRC Press, Boca Raton, FL, 1986. With permission.

part of a biomaterials characterization program.[46] Initially, uniaxial tests should be performed, in order to rank materials, using materials in a standard geometry and under standard conditions. Second level biaxial tests are recommended on candidate materials, as it must be remembered that most biomaterials are employed under conditions where they are required to withstand biaxial, rather than uniaxial, deformation. The test environment, loading and environmental conditions and the sample preparation and geometry can affect the fatigue characteristics.[71,72]

The fatigue behavior of polyurethanes for biomedical applications has been investigated by a number of researchers, and factors including the test environment and absorption of blood components have been suggested as contributors to the fatigue response of polyurethanes. Differences in the fatigue strength of polyurethanes have been observed with differences in media, e.g., between tests performed in air, saline and lipid solutions or blood. McMillin reported that the fatigue resistance of polyurethanes was greater in blood than in air or physiological solution.[71] The dependence of the fatigue strength on the test conditions puts further limitations on the interpretation of reports in the literature, many of which have been conducted in air. Takahara *et al.* have concluded that the absorption of lipids by polyurethanes can affect the fatigue resistance of polyurethanes, and that the state of aggregation of the polyurethane hard segments determines the fatigue resistance of polyurethanes when immersed in biological fluids.[73,74] It is possible that absorbed lipids may act as plasticizers and promote hard segment domain disruption. Lipid absorption by biomaterials also is believed to be associated with calcification of implanted materials which can lead to material hardening and failure. Liu *et al.*[75] found that after 10^5–10^6 loading cycles, the degree of phase mixing of the soft and hard segments increased. The interfacial regions between the hard and soft segments were the first to be disrupted. Cyclic loading of materials also may result in surface defects that may affect the hemocompatibility. Sevestianov and Parveev,[76] studied platelet adhesion to polyurethanes before and after cyclic loading and found that the number of adherent platelets increased after cyclic loading, although the morphology of adherent cells was unchanged. The increase in adhesion was believed to be due to an increase in surface defects, although there was no drastic change in the bulk properties of the materials.

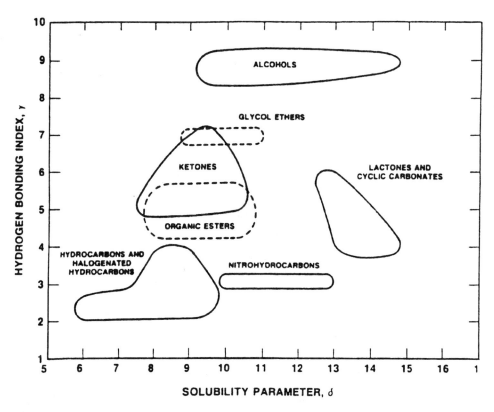

FIGURE 30 Parameter locations for major solvent groups. From Szycher M. In *Blood Compatible Materials and Devices,* Ed. Sharma C. P., Szycher M. Technomic, Lancaster, PA, 1991. With permission.

G. Solubility Tests

Polyurethanes are polar materials and offer resistance to nonpolar solvents such as hydrocarbons and fuel oil. Polyurethanes are also more resistant to ozone and oxidative aging compared with unsaturated rubbers such as the dienes. Their polarity, however, means that polyurethanes will swell or dissolve in polar organic solvents. Water absorption and swelling can cause problems in hydrous environments, including the biological one. Szycher has developed a solubility map of various solvents for the polyurethanes (Figure 30).[77] Preferential solubility of a particular compound into either the hard or soft segment component of a polyurethane also may occur.[44] Knowledge of the solubility characteristics of a polymer can aid in the selection of correct fabrication and cleansing techniques.

Knowledge of the solubility characteristics of a polymer also is useful in the evaluation of polymeric biomaterials. High absorption of physiological fluid into a biomaterial may compromise the mechanical properties through plasticization, induced crystallization, or alterations in phase relationships. Understanding of the solubility and swelling characteristics of polymers will facilitate prediction of the useful life of biomedical devices. Generally, polymer solubility characteristics can be predicted using a solubility parameter, δ. The Hansen solubility parameters considers three components to δ that reflect hydrogen bonding interactions, permanent dipole-dipole interactions and nonpolar interactions between the polymer and the solvent. The solubility parameters for various polyurethanes, polyurethane components and biological species are presented in Table 6 below.[77]

H. Permeability and Extractability

The extraction of nonpolymers from a polymeric material, including oligomers and manufacturing and processing additives can have implications for the final physical and biological performance

TABLE 6
Solubility parameters of blood components and biomaterials

Polymer or blood component	Solubility Parameter, δ $(cal/cm^3)^{1/2}$
Segmented polyurethane (Biomer)	
Soft segment	10.5
Hard segment	13.0
Aliphatic Polyurethane	
Soft grades (80A–85A)	9.0–12.0
Hard grades (60D–72D)	10.0–13.0
PTMEG	8.0–9.5
Silicone Oil	6.2
Polydimethylsiloxane (silicone rubber)	7.3–7.6
Polyethylene terephthalate	9.7–10.7
Cholesterol and esters	8.4–8.9
Triglycerides	8.0–8.3
Lipid-soluble vitamins	8.6–10.9
Phospholipids	>16
Proteins	>18
Water	23.2

From Szycher M. In *Blood Compatible Materials and Devices,* Ed. Sharma C. P, Szycher M. Technomic, Lancaster, PA, 1991. Reproduced with permission.

of a given material. Low mobility of solvents can result in the slow release of components over time, with potential toxic or other biological effects. Removal of these components also may lead to alterations in the physical properties of the material. The extraction of processing additives from polyurethanes also has been carried out as part of the determination of the composition of medical grade polyurethanes.[78-81]

Assessment of the permeability characteristics of a material is important for membrane applications of polyurethanes.[82-85] Oxygen and carbon dioxide permeability are critical in applications such as membrane oxygenators. Water and oxygen permeability are of importance in wound dressings. The phase separated nature of polyurethanes means that gas transport cannot be modeled as for homogenous polymers. Diffusion of species through amorphous regions will be higher than through the glassy or semicrystalline regions. Hence, the degree of phase separation in the material must also be considered in addition to the chemistry of the phases.

I. ELECTRICAL PROPERTIES

The electrical properties of polyurethanes are important in certain medical applications, such as pacemaker lead insulation, where low electrical conductivity or high resistivity are required. Conductivity may be measured directly, or it may be characterized by the low-frequency loss component of the complex dielectric constant. Polyurethanes are considered to be polar macromolecules, as they contain groups with hydrophilic character. These polar groups can reorient in an electric field, giving rise to high dielectric constants. The dielectric constant of polyurethanes may be lowered by improving microphase separation and reducing ionic mobility.

The water absorption characteristics of a polyurethane can affect the electrical conductivity of the material. The presence of hydrophilic groups results in water absorption from the environment, which can reduce the insulating properties. Similarly, the chemical composition of the polyol can affect the electrical properties, through differences in water absorption. Table 7 shows data on the effect of polyurethane chemistry, water absorption and electrical properties.[86]

TABLE 7
Water absorption effects on polyurethane elastomer chemical structure and electrical properties

Property	Polyurethane based on adipic acid-diethylene glycol polyester	Polyurethane based on adipic acid-hexane diol polyester
Volume resistivity, (Ω cm^{-1}) dry	$4 * 10^{11}$	$3 * 10^{12}$
Volume resistivity, (Ω cm^{-1}) wet	$1 * 10^{9}$	$8 * 10^{11}$
Swelling (wt %)	2.1	0.9

From Wright P. and Cumming A.P.C. *Solid Polyurethane Elastomers*. Maclaren & Sons, London, 1969. With permission.

SUMMARY

In this chapter, we have provided an overview of polymer structure-property relationships, focussing on polyurethane elastomers. The microphase structure of polyurethanes contributes to their mechanical properties; the phase separated structure is believed to account for their good biocompatibility as well. Researchers are continuing to study polyurethane structure, in order to understand how synthesis and processing treatments ultimately affect the properties of the material.

Bulk characterization of biomaterials is a critical feature of any evaluation program. It is necessary to ensure that, among other things, the material possesses adequate mechanical properties for its intended application. A number of the tests commonly used to characterize polyurethane biomaterials have been described here. Studies of polyurethane elastomers in the literature have been discussed to demonstrate both the application of each technique, and the factors that influence the mechanical and physical properties of the polyurethanes, such as chemical modification, incorporation of additives and thermal treatment.

REFERENCES

1. Rodriguez F. *Principles of Polymer Systems*. (4th Ed.): Hemisphere Pub. Corp., New York, 1996.
2. Cowie J. M. G. *Polymers: The Chemistry and Physics of Modern Materials*. International Textbook, Aylesbury, UK, 1973.
3. Blackwell J. and Gardner K. H. "Structure of hard segments in polyurethane elastomers." *Polymer*, 20:13, 1979.
4. Harrell L. L. "Segmented polyurethanes. Properties as a function of segment size and distribution." *Macromolecules*, 2:607, 1969.
5. Schollenberger C. S. and Dinsberg K. "Thermoplastic urethane molecular weight property relations." *J. Elast. Plast.*, 5:222, 1973.
6. Cooper S. L. and Tobolsky A. V. "Properties of linear elastomeric polyurethanes." *J. Appl. Polym. Sci.*, 10:1837, 1966.
7. Koustky J. A., Hien N. V. and Cooper S. L. "Some results on electron microscopic investigations of polyether-urethane block copolymers." *J. Appl. Polym. Sci.*, B8:353, 1970.
8. Fridman I. D. and Thomas E. L. "Morphology of crystalline polyurethane hard segment domains and spherulites." *Polymer*, 21:388, 1980.
9. Grady B. P. and Cooper S. L. "Thermoplastic Elastomers." In *Science and Technology of Rubber*, Ed. Mark J. E. Academic Press, 1994: 601.
10. Krause S. "Microphase separation in block copolymers. Zeroth approximation." *J. Polym. Sci. Part A*, A2, 7:249, 1969.
11. Krause S. and Reismiller P. A. "Micelle formation in butanone solutions of styrene-butadiene-styrene triblock copolymers." *J. Polym. Sci. Part A*, A2, 13:663, 1975.

12. Meier D. J. "Statistical thermodynamics of block copolymers: network statistics." *J. Macromol. Sci. Phys.,* 17:181, 1980.
13. Helfand E. and Tagami Y. "Theory of the interface between immiscible polymers." *J. Polymer Sci., Part B,* B9:741, 1971.
14. Helfand E. and Wasserman Z. R. "Proposed experiment to estimate the mixing free energy of polymers." *Macromolecules,* 11:683, 1978.
15. Grand A. D. L., Vitale G. G., and Grand D. G. L. "Small angle X-ray scattering from block polymers. II the Bulk state." *Polym. Eng. Sci.,* 17:598, 1977.
16. Wilkes G. L. and Emerson J. A. "Time dependence of small angle X-ray measurements segmented polyurethanes following thermal treatment." *J. Appl. Phys.,* 47:4261, 1976.
17. Ophir Z. H. and Wilkes G. L. "Time dependence of mechanical propertes and domain morphology of linear and crosslinked segmented polyetherurethanes." *Polym. Prepr. Am. Soc. Div. Polym. Chem.,* 19:26, 1978.
18. Hesketh T. R., Bogart J. W. C. v. and Cooper S. L. "Differential Scanning Calorimetry analysis of morphological changes in segmented elastomers." *Polym. Eng. Sci.,* 20:190, 1980.
19. Kwei T. K. "Phase separation in segmented polyurethanes." *J. Appl. Polym. Sci.,* 27:2981, 1982.
20. Chu B., Gao T., Li Y., Wang L., Desper C. R., and Byrne C. A. "Microphase separation kinetics in segmented polyurethanes: effects of soft segment length and structure." *Macromolecules,* 25:5724, 1992.
21. Tao H.-J., Meuse C. W., Yang X., MacKnight W. J., and Hsu S. L. "A spectroscopic analysis of phase separation behavior of polyurethane in restricted geometry: chain rigidity effects." *Macromolecules,* 27:7146, 1994.
22. Lee H. S. and Hsu S. L. "An analysis of phase separation kinetics of model polyurethanes." *Macromolecules,* 22:1100, 1989.
23. Russo R. and Thomas E. L. "Phase separation in linear and crosslinked polyurethanes." *J. Macromol. Sci. — Phys. B,* 22:553, 1983.
24. Clough S. B., Schneider N. S., and King A. O. "Small angle X-ray scattering from polyurethane elastomers." *J. Macromol. Sci. Phys.,* B2:641, 1968.
25. Estes G. M., Seymour R. W., and Cooper S. L. "Infrared studies of segmented polyurethane elastomers. II. Infrared dichroism." *Macromolecules,* 4:452, 1971.
26. Tanaka T., Yokoyama T., and Yamaguchi Y. "Quantitative study on hydrogen bonding between urethane compound and ethers by infrared spectroscopy." *J. Polym. Sci. Part A,* A1, 6:2137, 1968.
27. Bonart R. "X-ray investigations concerning the physical structure of crosslinking in segmented elastomers." *J. Macromol. Sci. Phys.,* B2:115, 1968.
28. Wilkes C. E. and Yusek C. S. "Investigation of domain structure in urethane elastomers by X-ray and thermal methods." *J. Macromol. Sci. — Phys. B,* B7:157, 1973.
29. Blackwell J. and Lee C. D. "Hard segment domain sizes in MDI/diol polyurethane elastomers." *J. Polym. Sci. Polym. Phys. Ed.,* 21:2169, 1983.
30. North A. M. "Dielectric relaxation in polymers with particular reference to two-phase systems." *J. Polym. Sci., C.,* 50:345, 1975.
31. North A. M., Reid J. C., and Shortall J. B. *Eur. Polym. J.,* 8:1129, 1969.
32. Bonart R., Morbitzer L., and Hentze G. "X-ray investigation concerning the physical structure of crosslinking in urethane elastomers. II. Butanediol as chain extender." *J. Macromol. Sci. Phys.,* 3:337, 1969.
33. Seymour R. W. and Cooper S. L. "Segmental orientation studies of block polymers. I. Hydrogen-bonded polyurethanes." *Macromolecules,* 6:896, 1973.
34. Allegrezza A. E., Seymour R. W., Ng H. H., and Cooper S. L. "Segmental orientation studies of block copolymers. II. Non-hydrogen bonded polyurethanes." *Polymer,* 15:433, 1974.
35. Wang C. B. and Cooper S. L. "Morphology and properties of segmented polyether polyurethane ureas." *Macromolecules,* 16:775, 1983.
36. Seymour R. W. and Cooper S. L. "Viscoelastic properties of polyurethane block copolymers." *Rubber Chem. Technol.,* 47:19, 1974.
37. Sung P. C. S., Hu C. B., and Wu C. S. "Properties of segmented poly(urethaneureas) based on 2,4 toluene diisocyanate. I. Thermal transitions, X-ray studies and comparison with segmented poly(urethanes)." *Macromolecules,* 13:111, 1980.

38. Seymour R. W. and Cooper S. L. "Thermal analysis of polyurethane block copolymers." *Macromolecules,* 6:48, 1973.
39. Srichatrapimuk V. W. and Cooper S. L. "Infrared thermal analysis of polyurethane block copolymers." *J. Macromol. Sci. — Phys. B,* 15:267, 1978.
40. Brunette C. M., Hsu S. L., and MacKnight W. J. "Structural and mechanical properties of polybutadiene-containing polyurethanes." *Polym. Eng. Sci.,* 21:163, 1981.
41. Grasel T. G. and Cooper S. L. "Properties and biological interactions of polyurethane anionomers: effect of sulfonate incorporation." *J. Biomed. Mater. Res.,* 23:311, 1989.
42. Yang C. Z., Grasel T. G., Bell J. L., Register R. A., and Cooper S. L. "Carboxylate containing chain-extended polyurethanes." *J. Polym. Sci. Polym. Phys. Ed.,* 29:581, 1991.
43. Visser S. A. and Cooper S. L. "Effect of neutralizing cation type on the morphology and properties of model polyurethane ionomers." *Polymer,* 33:920, 1992.
44. Cooper S. L. and Tobolsky A. V. "Anomalous depression of rubbery modulus through crosslinking." *J. Appl. Polym. Sci.,* 11:1361, 1967.
45. Frisch K. C. "Recent advances in the chemistry of polyurethanes." *Rubber Chem. Technol.,* 45:1442, 1972.
46. Hergenrother R. W., Silver F. H., Kardos J. L., and Cooper S. L. "Bulk Characterization." *Cardiovasc. Pathol.,* 2:73S, 1993.
47. Lee D., Speckhard T. A., Sorensen A. D., and Cooper S. L. "Methods for determining the molecular weight and solution properties of polyurethane block copolymers." *Macromolecules,* 19:2383, 1986.
48. Belisle J., Maier S. K., and Tucker J. A. Compositional analysis of Biomer. *J. Biomed. Mater. Res.,* 24:1585, 1990.
49. Tyler B. J., Ratner B. D., Castner D. G., and Briggs D. "Variations between Biomer™ lots. 1. Significant differences in the surface chemistry of two lots of a commercial poly(ether urethane)." *J. Biomed. Mater. Res.,* 26:273, 1992.
50. Sreenivasan K. "A combined chromatographic and IR spectroscopic method to identify antioxidant in biomedical polyurethane." *Chromatographia,* 32:285, 1991.
51. Ratner B. D., Gladhill K. W., and Horbett T. A. "Analysis of *in vitro* enzymatic and oxidative degradation of polyurethanes." *J. Biomed. Mater. Res.,* 22:509, 1988.
52. Ishihara H., Kimura I., Saito K., and Ono H. "Infrared studies on segmented polyurethane-urea elastomers." *J. Macromol. Sci. Phys.,* B10:591, 1974.
53. Grasel T. G. and Cooper S. L. "Surface properties and blood compatibility of polyurethaneureas." *Biomaterials,* 7:315, 1986.
54. Pitt W. G., Grasel T. G., and Cooper S. L. "Albumin adsorption on alkyl chain derivatized polyurethanes: II. The effect of alkyl chain length." *Biomaterials,* 9:36, 1988.
55. Jacques C. H. M. "Effect of annealing on the morphology and properties of thermoplastic polyurethanes." In *Polymer Alloys,* Ed. Klempner D, Frisch K. Plenum Press, New York, 1977: 287.
56. Bogart J. W. C. v., Bluemke D. A., and Cooper S. L. "Annealing-induced morphological changes in segmented elastomers." *Polymer,* 22:1428, 1981.
57. Aitken R. R. and Jeffs G. M. F. "Thermoplastic polyurethane elastomers based on aliphatic diisocyanates: thermal transitions." *Polymer,* 18:197, 1977.
58. Seymour R. W., Estes G. M., and Cooper S. L. "Infrared studies of segmented polyurethane elastomers I. Hydrogen bonding." *Macromolecules,* 3:579, 1970.
59. Schneider N. S., Sung P. C. S., Matton R. W., and Illinger J. L. "Thermal transitions behavior of polyurethanes based on toluene diisocyanate." *Macromolecules,* 13:111, 1975.
60. Clough S. B. and Cooper S. L. "Structural studies on urethane elastomers." *J. Macromol. Sci. — Phys. B,* 2:553, 1968.
61. Miller G. W. and Saunders J. H. "Thermal analysis of polymers. III. Influence of isocyanate structures on the molecular interactions in segmented polyurethanes." *J. Polym. Sci. Part A,* 1:1923, 1970.
62. Schollenberger C. S. and Hewitt L. E. "Thermoplastic polyurethane elastomer structure-thermal transition relation." *Polym. Prepr. Am. Soc. Div. Polym. Chem.,* 19:17, 1978.
63. Koberstein J. T. and Russell T. P. "Simultaneous SAXS-DSC study of multiple endothermic behavior in polyether-based polyurethane block copolymers." *Macromolecules,* 19:714, 1986.
64. Leung L. M. and Koberstein J. T. "DSC annealing study of microphase separation and multiple endothermic behavior in polyether-based polyurethane block copolymers." *Macromolecules,* 19:706, 1986.

65. Hu W. and Koberstein J. T. "The effect of thermal annealing on the thermal properties and molecular weight of a segmented polyurethane copolymer." *J. Polymer Sci., Part B,* 32:437, 1994.
66. Huh D. S. and Cooper S. L. "Dynamic mechanical properties of polyurethane block copolymers." *Polym. Eng. Sci.,* 11:369, 1971.
67. Li C., Goodman S. L., Albrecht R. M., and Cooper S. L. "Morphology of segmented polybutadiene-polyurethane elastomers." *Macromolecules,* 21:2367, 1988.
68. Li C. and Cooper S. L. "Direct observation of the micromorphology of polyether polyurethanes using high voltage electron microscopy." *Polymer,* 31:3, 1990.
69. Speckhard T. A. and Cooper S. L. "Ultimate tensile strength properties of segmented polyurethane elastomers: factors leading to reduced properties for polyurethanes based on nonpolar soft segments." *Rubber Chem. Technol.,* 59:405, 1986.
70. Estes G. M. *A study of orientation in segmented polyurethane elastomers* [Ph.D.]. University of Wisconsin–Madison, 1971.
71. McMillin C. R. "Physical testing of materials for cardiovascular applications." *Artif. Organs,* 7:78, 1983.
72. Myers C. W. S. *Morphology and fatigue properties of polyurethane elastomers* [Ph.D.]. University of Wisconsin–Madison, 1993.
73. Takahara A., Murakani A., Tashita J., Kajiyama T., and Takayanagi M. "Influence of lipid absorption on fatigue strength of poly(urethaneureas)." *Rep. Progr. Polym. Phys. Japan,* 25:849, 1982.
74. Takahara A., Tashita J., Kajiyama T., and Takanagi M. "Effect of aggregation state of hard segment in segmented poly(urethaneureas) on their fatigue behavior after interaction with blood components." *J. Biomed. Mater. Res.,* 19:13, 1985.
75. Liu L. M., Sumita M., and Miyasaka K. "Characterization of fatigue by segmented polyurethanes by using thermoluminescence and pulse NMR." *J. Macromolecular Sci.; Physics,* B28:309, 1989.
76. Sevestianov V. I. and Parveev V. M. "Fatigue and hemocompatibility of polymer materials." *Artif. Organs,* 11:20, 1987.
77. Szycher M. "Biostability of polyurethane elastomers: a critical review." In *Blood Compatible Materials and Devices,* Ed. Sharma C. P., Szycher M. Technomic, Lancaster, PA, 1991: 33.
78. Marchant R. E., Anderson J. M., Hiltner A., Castillo E. J., Gleit J., and Ratner B. D. "The biocompatibility of solution cast and acetone-extracted Biomer." *J. Biomed. Mater. Res.,* 20:799, 1986.
79. Grobe G. L., Gardella J. A., Chin R. L., and Salvati L. "Characterization of solution-cast extracts from Biomer by FT-IR and ESCA." *Appl. Spectr.,* 42:989, 1988.
80. Grobe G. L., Nagel A. S., Gardella J. A., Chin R. L., and Salvati L. "Characterization of solution-cast extracts from Cardiothane-51 by FT-IR and ESCA." *Appl. Spectr.,* 42:980, 1988.
81. Renier M., Wu Y. K., Anderson J. M., Hiltner A., Lodoen G. A., and Payet C. R. "Characterization of extractable species from poly(etherurethane urea) (PEUU) elastomers." *J. Biomater. Sci., Polym. Ed.,* 5:511, 1994.
82. Knight P. M. and Lyman D. J. "Evaluation of the gas transfer characteristics of porous copolyurethane oxygenator membranes." *Ann. Biomed. Eng.,* 13:25, 1985.
83. Behar D., Juszynski M., Ben Hur N., and Rudensky B. "Omiderm, a new synthetic wound covering: Physical properties and drug permeability studies." *J. Biomed. Mater. Res.,* 20:731, 1986.
84. Jayasree G. and Sharma C. P. "Permeability of PEUU membranes: their modification towards blood compatibility." *J. Biomater. Appl.,* 3:405, 1989.
85. Wu P., Fisher A. C., Foo P. P., Queen D., and Gaylor J. D. S. "*In vitro* assessment of water vapour transmission of synthetic wound dressings." *Biomaterials,* 16:171, 1995.
86. Wright P. and Cumming A. P. C. *Solid Polyurethane Elastomers.* Maclaren & Sons, London, 1969.

5 Surface Characterization of Polyurethanes

I. INTRODUCTION

The interactions between biological systems and artificial surfaces occur at the tissue-biomaterial interface, and it is reasonable to expect that the nature of this surface influences these interactions. Therefore, the biological response to a biomaterial must be at least partly mediated by the surface properties of the material. Realization of the importance of surface structure in determining the biocompatibility of a material has promoted research activity into understanding surface structure-property relationships to enable the design of improved biomaterials. Characterization of surfaces is an important factor in defining these relationships, providing information on the chemical structure, orientation and mobility of groups within the topmost atomic layers at the interface. The composition of a surface often differs significantly from the composition of the bulk.

There are many different surface and interfacial parameters that may play a role in biocompatibility aside from surface chemistry. The physicochemical properties of a surface also may influence interfacial reactions, through parameters such as the hydrophilic/hydrophobic ratio, surface electric charge, hydrogel character, the presence of receptor sites, and roughness. A number of techniques have been developed in order to study surfaces, some of which have been used to study biomaterials. Ratner has proposed a scheme for biomaterial characterization, which is shown in Figure 1.[1] At present there is no single technique that can provide all the relevant information about a surface, if one includes factors such as conformation and mobility in addition to chemistry. Therefore, as far as possible, more than one technique should be employed in order to gain as much information as possible about a particular surface. The most commonly used surface characterization techniques for polymers are contact angle measurements, attenuated fourier transform infrared spectroscopy (ATR–FTIR) and surface spectroscopic and spectrometric techniques such as ESCA and SIMS. Other techniques such as scanning electron microscopy (SEM) often are employed to study the surface morphology of polymeric materials, as well as the morphology of adherent cells after exposure to biological media. A comparison of the surface depth that each method can analyze is shown in Figure 2 and Table 1.[1] Surface electrical properties may be investigated using zeta potential measurement techniques.

One of the major problems with surface analysis and characterization studies is that of surface contamination. Surfaces pose a very reactive environment and are readily contaminated. There are many sources of contamination, from fingerprints, transfer of species from packaging, the laboratory environment, and from surface characterization equipment. Silicones will readily migrate to or transfer between surfaces, and silicone contamination of laboratory-synthesized polyurethanes is not uncommon. This must be remembered when handling samples and interpreting data.

II. SURFACE ENERGY AND SURFACE TENSION

Excess surface energy results from the different atomic or molecular environment encountered by atoms and molecules at the surface or interface when compared with the environment of the molecules contained within the bulk of the material. These differences arise from the reduction in the number of nearest neighbors of the atoms or molecules with which they would associate in the bulk, which in turn reduces the magnitude of stabilizing interactions with their nearest neighbors.

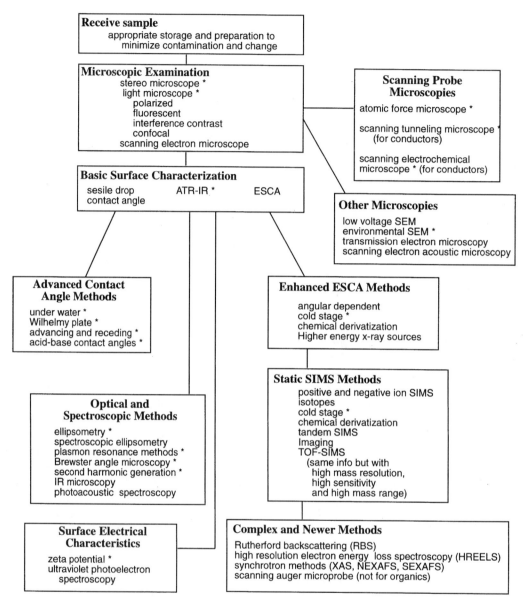

FIGURE 1 Scheme for Biomaterial characterization. Reproduced by permission of the publisher from Ratner B.D. *Cardiovasc. Pathol.*, 2(3 Suppl):87S. Copyright 1993 by Elsevier Science.

This means that the molecules at the surface possess excess energy when compared with molecules in the bulk. This leads to a difference in forces acting parallel to the surface. Surface tension is equal to the change in the Helmholtz free energy of the whole system, associated with a change in area, whereas the surface free energy is equal to the change in the Helmholtz free energy of the surface, associated with a change in surface area. Surface tension is equal to the force per unit length and is usually given the symbol γ. Surface energy is measured as the energy per unit area. Surface energy is often used interchangeably with surface tension. For certain systems, including polymers, the differences in surface energy and surface tension are assumed to be close to zero.

Surface Characterization of Polyurethanes

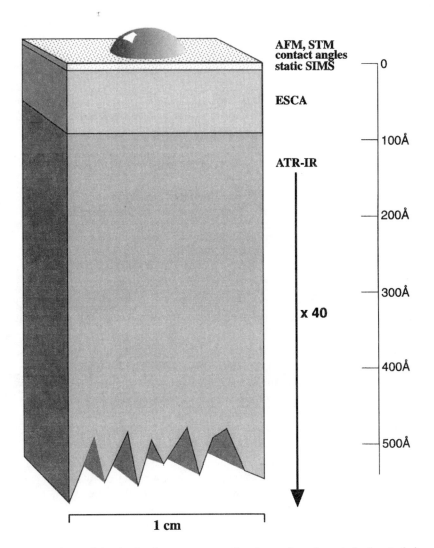

FIGURE 2 Comparison of the depth of measurement of major surface characterization techniques. Reproduced by permission of the publisher from Ratner B.D. *Cardiovasc. Pathol.*, 2(3 Suppl):87S. Copyright 1993 by Elsevier Science.

TABLE 1
Depth of analysis of surface characterization techniques

Technique	Depth of Analysis	Lateral Resolution
Contact Angles	3–20Å	1 mm
XPS (ESCA)	10–250Å	10–150 μm
SIMS	10 Å (static) to 1 μm (dynamic)	500 Å
ATR–FTIR	1–5 μm	10 μm
SEM	5 Å	1 μm

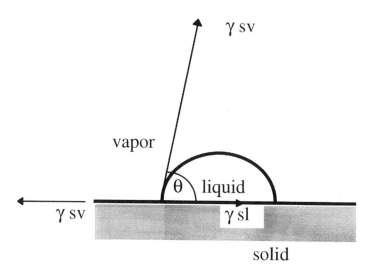

FIGURE 3 A drop of liquid on a solid surface in a vapor environment.

An interface is formed when two different phases come into contact. The interfacial tension is a measure of the degree of interaction between two phases at their common boundary. Interfacial tension measurements have been pursued in biomedical engineering as a means of measuring and perhaps correlating the surface energies of the two phases, such as the interactions between blood or other solutions containing proteins and synthetic materials. It was hoped that surface free energy measurements of materials could be used as a predictor of blood compatibility; however, most studies have used water as the model fluid, on the basis that biomaterials are employed in an aqueous environment. However, it is possible that the presence of proteins in plasma and the blood alters the surface energetics of the blood. Furthermore, tensiometric methods are best interpreted within a thermodynamic framework whereas biological processes are usually considered in physicochemical terms.[2] These interpretative differences also may hinder correlation of surface energy with the biological response and its use to predict the biological response. Vogler has recently published an excellent review and discussion of tensiometric measurements, pertaining to biomaterials evaluation.[2]

A. Contact Angles

Contact angle goniometry is the most widely used method of tensiometric characterization of biomaterial surfaces. A surfaces' contact angle is one of the few parameters in surface science that can be measured readily. The contact angle is that angle at the junction of three phases, e.g., a drop of liquid on a solid surface, in an air environment (Figure 3). The contact angle reflects the tendency of a liquid to wet a surface. It can be considered to reflect the competing tendencies of the drop to spread over the surface, as to wet it, or bead up, in order to minimize the contact area with the solid. Contact angle equilibria also balance the reduction of the interface and contact area with the surface and the contact area with the third phase, e.g., air. As the magnitude of the contact angle increases, the material is considered to be less wettable by the liquid. As the contact angle approaches zero, the liquid spreads over the solid, increasing the contact area between the liquid and the solid, and the liquid is said to wet the surface.

The Young Equation (5.1) relates the equilibrium contact angle, θ, at the solid-liquid-vapor or solid-liquid-liquid boundary to the interfacial tensions between the phases:

$$\gamma_{LV} \cos\theta = \gamma_{SV} - \gamma_{SL} \tag{5.1}$$

where γ_{LV} is the liquid-vapor interfacial tension
 γ_{SV} is the solid-saturated vapor interfacial tension
 γ_{SL} is the solid-liquid interfacial tension.

Measurements of γ_{LV} can be made, but determination of γ_{SV} and γ_{SL} is more difficult. Fowkes postulated that the interfacial tension between two surfaces could be considered to consist of a variety of different energy components, depending on the type of interaction:

$$\gamma = \gamma_{dispersion} + \gamma_{polar} + \gamma_{metallic} + \gamma_{hydrogen\ bond} + \cdots \qquad (5.2)$$

Many other researchers have proposed different interrelationships between the individual surface free energy components and the interfacial tension. None is considered sufficient for characterizing the surface free energy of biomaterials. In the past, contact angle measurements have been taken, and the polar, dispersive and other components of the surface free energy have been calculated. There has been debate as to whether the angle described in the Young Equation is the same as the measured contact angle, and this raises questions regarding the validity of surface energy measurements obtained through the measurement of contact angles. Arguments against the calculation of such parameters from measurements of contact angles revolve around the assumptions that the system is in equilibrium, which is required for thermodynamic interpretation of measurements, and that there is no permeation of the liquid into the perfectly smooth surface.[3] Additional factors that limit the interpretation of contact angle measurements include the physical properties of a surface that may influence the formed angle, such as roughness, and adsorption of solute molecules onto the surface.

The concept of a critical surface energy, γ_c, has been developed by Zisman *et al.* as an alternative approach to calculation of surface energy. The critical surface tension can be obtained through measurements of the advancing contact angles for a series of homologous liquids and extrapolation of the data to $\cos\theta = 1$.[4] This gives the value of the surface tension of a liquid that would just wet the surface, i.e., have a contact angle of zero when placed on the surface. Simple hydrocarbons work best for these studies, and have been used by Baier and coworkers to characterize a large number of biomaterials. They have proposed that a zone of biocompatibility may exist when γ_c lies between 20–30 dynes per cm. Within this zone, minimum bioadhesion and thrombus formation would occur. However, the relevance of calculations of the critical surface tension for biomaterials has been questioned, as measurements are made using fluids that do not contain proteins.[2] Thus, determination of the critical surface energy of a material cannot be expected to provide a direct correlation to the biological response.

B. Contact Angle Measurement

A number of different techniques exist for measuring contact angles and interfacial tension, as the configuration of materials can vary from flat solid surfaces to tubes, capillaries, fibers, beads and powders. Measurements of contact angles often are taken in air or underwater, using water or air as the medium for droplet or bubble formation. Measurement of contact angles in an aqueous environment is particularly useful for biomedical materials, as they are employed in an environment that is predominantly water; however, the presence of proteins within the plasma and blood does limit the relevance of measurements made using water. A review of methods is given by Neumann and Good.[5] Figure 4 is a schematic showing the various different methods of contact angle measurement.[1] The methods that are most frequently encountered in the biomaterials literature are contact angle goniometers, the Hamilton technique, and the Wilhemy plate balance. It must be remembered that contact angles are very sensitive to contamination and roughness. Differences in contact angles can be observed between freshly cleaved materials and surfaces that have been allowed to equilibrate with the environment.

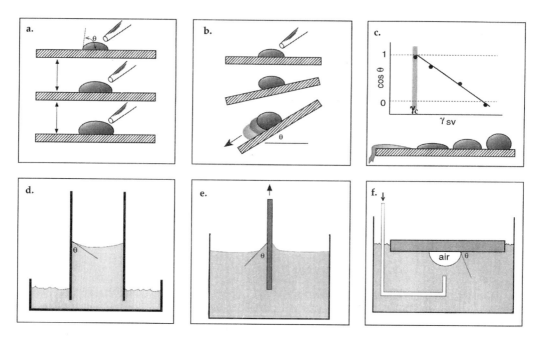

FIGURE 4 Different methods of contact angle measurement: (a) sessile drop technique to measure advancing and receding contact angles. (b) drop stability on a tilting substrate. (c) critical surface tension measurement using the Zisman method. (d) capillary rise method. (e) Wilhemy balance determination of contact angle. (f) underwater contact angles. Reproduced by permission of the publisher from Ratner B.D. *Cardiovasc. Pathol.*, 2(3 Suppl):87S. Copyright 1993 by Elsevier Science.

Contact angle goniometry utilizes a horizontal microscope with a reticular eyepiece for observation and measurement of the contact angle. The apparatus can be equipped with a tilting stage, in order to allow the measurement of receding and advancing contact angles. This method is suitable for the measurement of contact angles on planar surfaces. Numerous measurements are usually taken for each sample.

The Wilhemy plate balance measures the interfacial tension and can be used to measure contact angles. The techniques involves weighing a fluid meniscus that adheres to a rigid material as it is immersed or withdrawn from a liquid. The forces are monitored as a function of the immersion depth of the sample in the fluid. Contact angle hysteresis can be evaluated from comparison of the advancing and receding angles that are formed at the junction of the three phases; the advancing angle is observed when the material is immersed in the solution and the receding angle is formed when the material is pulled out of the liquid. If the speed of the plate is zero or very low, then static contact angles can be estimated. Numerous immersion cycles can be performed, so the reproducibility or drift of the response can be examined. With respect to sample geometry, the Wilhemy plate balance is the most versatile technique. Flat sheet materials work best, but measurements also can be made on cylindrical rods and fibers.

The Hamilton technique also has been used to measure underwater contact angles.[6] The flat sample of interest is placed face down in a glass cell containing water. Air or octane bubbles are released which rise and adhere to the surface of interest. The contact angle is then measured. This is a particularly useful technique for biomaterials evaluation as materials are usually used in a hydrous environment. Originally developed for flat sheet measurements, Lelah *et al.* have used this method for tubular materials, adapting the calculations to account for the curved geometry.[7]

Contact angles are very difficult to measure consistently. Variations in measurements obtained on similar materials within the same laboratory are not uncommon, although with practice the

TABLE 2
Surface tensions and critical surface tensions of commercial biomedical polyurethanes

Material	Surface Tension (dyne/cm)	Critical Surface Tension γ_c (dyne/cm)	Source
Extruded grade Biomer	70		7
Solution cast extruded grade Biomer	63		7
Solution grade Biomer	52		7
Extruded Grade Biomer	24.5		9
Extruded Grade Biomer (solvent extracted)	8.8		9
Solution grade Biomer (high soft segment content)	10.6		9
Solution grade Biomer (high soft segment content — solvent extracted)	7.0		9
Solution Grade Biomer		27	10
Biomer — autoclaved	31.8		11
Cast Biomer	33.4		12
Extracted Biomer	31.4		12
Biomer	59.0		13
Avcothane-51	19.5	22	14
Avcothane balloon (outer surface)	21.6		11
MDI/MDEA/PTMO1000 3/2/1	50.6		15
MDI/PTMO 1000 1/1	50.8		15
Vialon 510X-45		45	16
Vialon 510X-55		46	16
Vialon 510X-65		45	16
Vialon 510X-75		46	16

magnitude of these differences may be reduced. The surface tensions and critical surface tensions of various commercial polyurethanes, as calculated from contact angle measurements, are presented in Table 2. The contact angle that a polyurethane surface forms underwater can change with time due to hydration effects and, in the longer term, surface rearrangement, possibly due to the migration of hard segments to the surface in order to reduce the interfacial tension.[8] Contact angles remain one of the most common methods of surface characterization, as they do not require very expensive, specialized equipment. They can therefore be performed in most laboratories.

C. CONTACT ANGLE HYSTERESIS

Contact angle hysteresis is the term used to denote differences in the measured contact angles of a drop of fluid when it is spreading over the surface (the advancing contact angle), and when the droplet is receding (receding contact angle). Contact angle hysteresis can be observed on most surfaces and is thought to arise from surface heterogeneity or surface roughness. Hysteresis can be observed on molecularly smooth surfaces and hence, hysteresis also may arise from differing surface energies at a microscopic level. Surface roughness also can influence the degree of hysteresis, and a rough surface can increase the advancing angle and decrease the receding angle. Researchers also have attributed contact angle hysteresis to molecular rearrangement at the surface which can occur in order to reduce the interfacial tension. The advancing contact angle has been attributed to the nonwetting component of the surface energy, and the receding angle has been attributed to the wetting component. The receding contact angle also may be a function of ion concentration.

TABLE 3
Static and Dynamic contact angle measurements of commercial biomedical polyurethanes

Material	Static Contact Angle		Dynamic Contact Angles		Source
	Water–air	Octane–air	Advancing θ_A	Receding θ_R	
Cast Biomer			70 ± 2	46 ± 7	12
Extruded Biomer			72 ± 2	50 ± 11	12
Biomer			86 ± 3	44 ± 4	17
Spin coated Biomer	38.5 ± 4.3	45.6 ± 7.5			13
Extruded Grade Biomer	47	77			7
Extruded Grade Biomer-solvent cast	55	86			7
Solution grade Biomer	56	76			7
Pellethane			85 ± 3	47 ± 1	18
MDI/BD/PTMO 1000 3/2/1	61 ± 3	92 ± 3	75	41	19
MDI/BD/PEO 3/2/1	41 ± 3	62 ± 5	56	0	19

The maximum contact angle that can be observed on a surface is called the advancing contact angle, θ_A. Measurements of θ_A involve adding very small quantities of liquid to the droplet on the surface. θ_A is the maximum angle observed before the contact area between the droplet and the surface increases. The receding contact angle, θ_R, is the smallest angle formed between the three phases. Measurements are taken when small quantities of liquid are removed from the droplet, causing a reduction in the contact angle, just before a reduction in the contact area between the droplet and the solid surface occurs. The difference between θ_A and θ_R may be as large as the advancing contact angle, i.e., the contact area between the droplet and the surface remains the same, but when receding, the contact angle reduces to zero. Time dependent effects may be observed if the solid is slightly soluble, or if the material swells in the liquid. Reported measurements of contact angles may be of the advancing angle only, or of advancing and receding angles. Table 3 shows some of the static and dynamic contact angle measurements of some biomedical polyurethanes reported in the literature.

Two classes of hysteresis, thermodynamic and kinetic, have been assigned. Thermodynamic, or true, hysteresis is observed when the hysteresis curves can be reproduced over a number of cycles in quick succession. The curves are independent of time and frequency. This has been ascribed to microscopic domains undergoing cooperative nonequilibrium transitions. Kinetic hysteresis is indicated by the dependence of hysteresis curves on time of immersion and frequency of consecutive immersion and emersion cycles. The underlying contributors to this manifestation are believed to be slow equilibrium times, e.g., if swelling of the solid surface occurs. Thus, dynamic contact angle measurements have been used to provide information regarding the heterogeneity of surfaces, molecular mobility, roughness and swelling at the water-air-solid junction. Polymer surfaces may rearrange over long periods of time, and so long-term changes in hysteresis curves and force-immersion curves can be observed.[8]

III. ATTENUATED FOURIER TRANSFORM INFRARED SPECTROSCOPY (ATR–FTIR)

Multiple Attenuated Fourier Transform Infrared Spectroscopy (ATR–FTIR) refers to the partial absorption and attenuated reflection of an evanescent infrared wave that travels parallel to the interface through two media with different refractive indices. In this technique, the sample surface is contacted with a crystal surface, such as germanium. Infrared radiation is then reflected internally along the interface. The penetration depth of the evanescent wave is 1,000 to 10,000Å, which is much greater than the depth probed by contact angle, SIMS and ESCA methods, and hence the surface-sensitivity of the technique is regarded to be much lower. The depth of analysis can be reduced by increasing the angle of incident radiation, or by increasing the refractive index of the crystal. It should be noted that the sampling depth is unlikely to be consistent throughout one spectrum, as the depth of penetration is influenced by the wavelength of the incident radiation. The lack of surface sensitivity of ATR–FTIR compared to other techniques that are discussed in this chapter, such as ESCA and SIMS, means that much of the structural information may refer to the bulk composition rather than the topmost layers. In some cases, researchers using ATR–FTIR to characterize surfaces have reported no observable differences between the bulk and surface structure on the basis of infrared spectra, although data from other surface techniques such as ESCA and contact angle measurements showed otherwise. Sung and Hu have reduced the depth of penetration by interposing a barrier film between the polymer of interest and the crystal.[20] The barrier film must be selected so that it does not produce spectral bands in the same wavenumber region as the material of interest.

ATR–FTIR is a very versatile technique. Sample geometry is not as limited as with conventional transmission spectroscopy, and tubes, fibers, liquids, powders or gases can be examined. The use of multiple scans means that even very small quantities of a sample can be studied. Another feature of FTIR that enhances the usefulness of this technique is that subtraction of FTIR spectra is possible. This has been used to some effect in studies of protein adsorption to surfaces, including polyurethanes,[13,21-23] and in the identification of other compounds in biomedical polyurethanes.[24] One of the problems with IR spectroscopy is the deconvolution of overlapping bands. Small spectral shifts that may result from changes in the molecular environment of an atom may be difficult to distinguish from other bands in the same region. In regions where larger shifts are observed, and the region does not contain peaks from other chemical groups, peak ratios can be used to perform a semi-quantitative analysis of the states of bonding within a material. For example, carbonyl groups, in particular, are sensitive to environment and changes in peak position can be quite noticeable. Spectral shifts that are produced upon changes in the molecular environment of the urethane carbonyl within a polyetherurethane have been utilized to calculate the degree of phase separation within the material. This involves taking the ratio of hydrogen-bonded to nonhydrogen carbonyl peak areas in the sample and making some assumptions about extinction coefficients of the absorption bands being studied.[25]

A. ATR–FTIR ANALYSIS OF POLYURETHANES

Lyman and coworkers have shown that the composition of polyurethane block co-polymers varies with depth by altering the angle of incident radiation and by using different internal reflection elements.[26-28] They reported that there is less mixing of the urethane groups and polyether segments within the interfacial regions when compared to the bulk. Grasel and Cooper examined sulfonated polyurethanes and showed that as the degree of sulfonation of the bulk polymer increased the ratio of bonded to nonbonded hydrogen atoms passed through a maximum in the bulk, but not in the surface spectra. This may indicate that at low sulfonation levels there may be preferential aggregation of sulfonate groups at the surface.[29]

ATR–FTIR techniques also have been used to study biomedical polyurethanes. Many of the studies also used other characterization techiques to complement these investigations. Studies of Biomer have shown that there is some enrichment of polyether at the surface when compared with the bulk.[13] Grobe et al.[30] using FTIR and ESCA, concluded that Biomer is not really a copolymer but a blend of copolymer segments, after studying Biomer before and after extraction. Iwamoto et al. used spectral subtraction techniques to investigate the composition and surface chemistry of Cardiothane-51.[24] Both sides of six balloon pumps were examined, and the spectrum of Avcomat 610, a component of Cardiothane-51, was used as a reference spectrum. The researchers determined

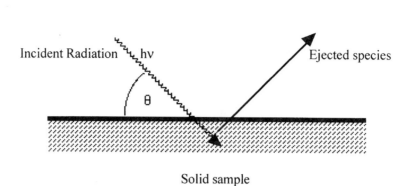

θ = take off angle

FIGURE 5 The principle of surface spectroscopy techniques.

Cardiothane-51 to consist of 90% polyurethane and 10% PDMS. Silicone was found at the surface, although in all 6 balloon pumps differences in the amount of silicone varied. Most of the balloon pumps also had more silicone on the mold-side rather than the air facing side, although two pumps showed the opposite. Fluorocarbons were also detected on some samples and were thought to derive from mold release agents used in manufacture. ATR–FTIR also has been used to study other processes. Studies of polyurethane degradation using IR spectroscopy have been performed by Takahara, and Marchant and coworkers.[12,31,32]

IV. SURFACE SPECTROSCOPIC TECHNIQUES

There exists a whole range of spectroscopic techniques that have been developed in order to probe surface chemistry and structure. Examples include X-ray photoelectron spectroscopy (XPS), Secondary Ion Mass Spectrometry (SIMS), Auger electron spectroscopy, Ion Scattering Spectroscopy (ISS), X-ray Fluorescence Spectroscopy (XRF), Rutherford Back Scattering Spectroscopy (RBS) and Conversion Electron Mössbauer Spectroscopy (CEMS). All of these surface specific techniques must be performed under ultra high vacuum conditions (UHV, $10^{-7} - 10^{-10}$ torr), or else the ejected species are lost. The techniques differ with respect to the incident beam of radiation and the measured species that are ejected from the surface. Primary sources of radiation that are used to bombard surfaces can consist of X-rays, electron beams, or ion beams. The secondary radiation may consist of ejected photons, electrons or ions, which are then detected. The techniques also differ with respect to the amount of destruction that each causes; those that bombard the surfaces with ions can simultaneously destroy and contaminate the surface. These techniques are regarded to be surface-specific, as they are capable of providing information on the top few atomic layers of a solid surface. A scheme showing the principle of surface spectroscopy is shown in Figure 5.

A. X-RAY PHOTO-ELECTRON SPECTROSCOPY (XPS)

X-ray photo-electron spectroscopy (XPS) or, to use its more common name, Electron Spectroscopy for Chemical Analysis (ESCA), is considered to be a very powerful tool for surface analysis. XPS employs the photoelectric effect and involves irradiation of a surface with a mono-energetic beam of low energy X-rays, causing excitation of the electrons within the sample, and ejection of core-level, nonvalence electrons. An XPS spectrum is a plot of the photoelectron intensity against the kinetic energy (or binding energy) of the ejected electrons. Since no two elements have the same set of binding energies, the energy distribution of the ejected electrons is characteristic of the atomic orbital, and the valence state and electron distribution within the material. Thus spectral peaks can be assigned to specific atomic and molecular orbitals and provide information on the bonding within the compound. XPS peaks are usually named according to the level from which the electron was emitted. Since there is no distinction between core and valence electrons for hydrogen and helium, these elements cannot be detected using XPS.

ESCA measurements are limited by the escape depth of the electrons, which are subject to absorption by the material, and generally ESCA can be used to analyze the upper 30–100Å of a surface. Angular dependent ESCA methods can be applied, where the incident radiation is fired at an angle to the surface altering the depth of penetration. As the take-off angle (θ in Figure 5) is reduced, the depth of penetration normal to the surface decreases, and thus the depth of analysis is reduced. The limit of detection of variable angle studies is about 10Å. Data collected in this mode suffer from reduced signal-to noise ratio, reducing the sensitivity of the technique, and the surfaces need to be very smooth. Depth-composition studies have been performed by systematically varying the angle in order to alter the depth of analysis.

ESCA is essentially a nondestructive technique, as the primary X-ray flux is quite small. This nondestructive quality compares favorably with some of the other spectroscopic techniques. As with other surface spectroscopic techniques, ESCA studies must be carried out in ultra high vacuum conditions. One of the problems associated with these conditions, particularly for polymeric samples, is that reorientation of the molecules may occur, which imposes a limit on applicability of data from ESCA studies of materials with mobile interfaces. Vacuum and air media are considered to be hydrophobic, whereas water, the main component of biological fluids, is hydrophilic. Thus, reorientation of a block copolymer comprised of segments with different hydrophilicities is likely to occur when the nature of the interface changes, in order to reduce the interfacial tension. This has been one of the strongest arguments against the use of UHV techniques for characterizing biomedical materials that are not only used at much higher pressure, but also in a predominantly aqueous environment. A number of researchers have attempted to characterize the surface of hydrated polyurethanes by freeze drying materials prior to analysis. ESCA studies on polyurethane surfaces, both hydrated and dehydrated, have been reported in the literature, and are discussed later in this chapter.

B. Secondary Ion Mass Spectrometry (SIMS)

Secondary Ion Mass Spectrometry, referred to as SIMS, is another UHV technique that has been used to investigate polyurethane biomaterial surfaces. SIMS involves the bombardment of a surface with a stream of primary ions, most commonly argon, xenon or cesium, which sputter secondary ions from the surface. Secondary ions are ejected from the surface and directed towards a quadrupole analyzer, which measures the intensity of the ions according to their mass/charge (m/z) ratio. SIMS techniques offer many advantages over XPS, including molecular specificity of the spectra, by virtue of the fact that ion fragments are measured, rather than the radiation intensity. Thus fragment weights can readily identify ions and can be used to deduce the molecular structure of the species. SIMS also is able to detect hydrogen, as well as high mass fragments, for example from proteins. Data and reference spectra from other mass spectrometric techniques have been successfully applied to interpretation of SIMS spectra, facilitating analysis. SIMS studies can be performed in a number of ways including static, dynamic, and imaging modes.

Static SIMS focuses the primary beam at one site on the surface and uses a low sputter rate, i.e., a very low primary current beam intensity. Although ions are removed from the surface, the rate of erosion of the surface is very low, so that with sensitive detection equipment, a spectrum can be obtained well within the lifetime of the surface. For this reason, static SIMS methods are considered to be nondestructive. The depth of analysis is about 10Å, and SIMS is thus regarded to be a truly surface-specific technique.

Dynamic SIMS has, at best, a lateral resolution of 10μm and can used to gain depth profiles of the chemical composition. Primary ion beams of high current density are employed, eroding the surface, while the ejected ions are simultaneously analyzed. Owing to the fast rate at which erosion occurs, dynamic SIMS cannot be considered as a nondestructive technique like static SIMS, which uses much lower primary current beam densities.

Imaging SIMS employs a highly collimated primary ion beam that is raster scanned across the surface. The mass analyzer is tuned in sequence to a particular mass. Surface maps of high resolution can be obtained by overlapping the maps of single elements. Maps of progressively deeper layers provide maps of the depth profile of the surface composition. Like dynamic SIMS, the use of high current density beams of the primary ion are required, and so destruction of the sample is likely.

Generally, SIMS is regarded to be more surface-sensitive than ESCA, and it also has a higher detection sensitivity. Through the generation and analysis of ions rather than electrons, SIMS also may be able to provide more structural information.[33] Depth profiling with SIMS destroys the surface, whereas depth profiling using variable angle ESCA methods does not, although the sensitivity is not as high. A more refined analysis of a surface can be achieved, by using both ESCA and SIMS techniques.

C. Surface Spectroscopic Studies of Polyurethanes

ESCA studies of polyurethanes have been conducted by a number of researchers in order to ascertain the precise structure at polyurethane interfaces. Several studies on laboratory synthesized polyurethanes have shown evidence of enrichment of polyether soft segments at the interface.[19] Some urethane groups, indicated by the presence of nitrogen in ESCA spectra, also can be detected, although the strength of these signals decreases as the take-off angle is increased. The ratio of hard segment to soft segments at the surface of polyurethane block-copolymers appears to be influenced by the size and chemical structure of the soft segment, as well as the bulk concentration of the hard segment.[19] Afrossman et al. synthesized a series of copolymers prepared from MDI, ethylene glycol (EG) and soft segments of polyethylene glycol (PEG) or polytetramethylene oxide (PTMO), of increasing molecular weight.[34] XPS analysis of the surfaces revealed that surfaces of polyurethanes containing PEG showed no significant segregation of the soft segment at the surface, as the surface composition of the polymer resembled that of the bulk. This was observed throughout the series of polymers as the molecular weight of the PEG soft segment increased from 200 to 3400. The polyurethane synthesized with PTMO as the soft segment showed significant segregation of the soft segment as the surface was approached. Complementary SIMS studies on these model polyurethanes showed the presence of peaks that were ascribed to CN⁻ ions, suggesting that even in polymers that show surface enrichment of the soft segment, such as the polyurethanes with a 3400 molecular weight PTMO soft segment, complete coverage cannot be assumed, and that some hard segment components may be present.

Other studies have shown that as the molecular weight of the polyether increases, the ether O1s and C1s peaks also increase.[33] An increase in the molecular weight of the polyether may enhance the ability of the soft segment to reorient, even though the ends of the molecule are tethered. Studies by Hearn and colleagues combined ESCA and SIMS techniques to examine the nature of polyurethane surfaces. ESCA studies showed enrichment of the polyether at the surface, and angular dependent studies implied that little or no hard segments were present in the topmost 20Å. However, SIMS spectra contained peaks that were associated with hard segments, implying that hard segments were indeed present within the top 10–15Å.[33] This reported increase in the segregation of the soft segment towards the surface may be a manifestation of the degree of microphase separation within the polyurethane bulk; polyurethanes containing PEG or PPG as the soft segment may not achieve the same degree of phase separation in the bulk as polyurethanes containing PTMO. The lower degree of phase separation also may provide an explanation for the higher nitrogen content detected at the surfaces of the former materials. Studies of polyurethanes containing PDMS macroglycol soft segments revealed that the PDMS molecules oriented towards the surface, and that the degree of segregation increased with an increase in bulk siloxane content; no measurable differences in blood compatibility were reported for this series of materials.[35]

As discussed earlier, electron and ionic spectroscopic techniques require ultra high vacuum environments. This raises questions concerning the applicability of such techniques to biomaterial surface characterization, as biomaterials are employed in aqueous conditions. In order to address this shortcoming, efforts have been made to perform ESCA analysis on polyurethane samples that have been freeze-dried, so that the molecular orientation at the hydrated polymer surface is preserved. Such experiments involve the hydration and freeze-drying of the material. The water is then sublimed, taking care that the temperature remains below the glass transition temperature of the soft segment to avoid any large-scale molecular restructuring. Takahara et al.[36] synthesized polyurethanes from MDI, ED, and either PEG or PPG as the soft segment. Surfaces that had been hydrated, and freeze-dried were analyzed at −30°C, and compared with the same surfaces that were dehydrated by increasing the temperature of the system to room temperature. Surface enhancement of the PPG 700 segment was observed in the dehydrated state. The strength of the ether carbon signal increased with molecular weight of the PPG segment, indicating enhancement of the polyether component at the surface, which could also be attributed to improved phase separation of the block copolymer. When hydrated, the magnitude of the N/C ratio increased. In this material, the surface free energy of the hard segment is larger than that of PPG, and so to reduce the interfacial energy, the hard segment tries to reorient to the surface. For the polyurethane samples with PEG soft segments, where the surface free energy of the soft segment is greater than that of the hard segment, ESCA analysis of freeze-dried samples showed enrichment of the soft segment at the surface. PEG also is known to swell in water which may enhance the molecular motion of PEG, promoting surface coverage. For the PPG(3000) polyurethanes, N/C ratios were larger in the hydrated polyurethane. Angular dependent studies showed that, within the limitations of ESCA spectroscopy, the PPG soft segment provides a complete over-layer at a molecular weight of 3000. Below 3000, the signal of the ether carbon was weaker, implying that the hard segment constituted some of the surface. This is in agreement with other reports indicating that the length of the soft segment component can influence the surface chemistry. Proposed surface structures are presented in Figure 6.[36]

The researchers concluded that the hydrophilic urethane/urea segments are present in higher concentrations at hydrated polyurethane surfaces. The presence of a microphase-separated structure may therefore exist at the surfaces of hydrophilic segmented polyurethanes in water, and it has been proposed that this could contribute to their good blood compatibility. Lin et al. also have employed cold-stage ESCA techniques in order to investigate polyurethane surface structure, and concluded that the more hydrophilic hard segments orient towards the surface when wet, and that the presence of the hard segment at the surface increases in the freeze-dried sample.[37]

Further studies examining the surface composition of commercially available biomedical polyurethanes have been performed. Such studies are proving to have important implications in the field of biocompatibility testing, through reports of variations in surface chemistry, identification of surface contamination, and batch to batch variation. Sung and Hu examined surfaces of Biomer and Avcothane, and reported differences in the ratios of hard to soft segment ratios on substrate and air-facing surfaces, confirming reports from Lyman et al.[26] The Biomer-air surface showed enrichment of the polyether phase.[38] Lelah et al. compared the surface and blood contacting properties of two different materials, both obtained under the trade name Biomer.[7] One material, solution grade Biomer (SB), was obtained as a 30% solution of N,N dimethylacetamide (DMA).

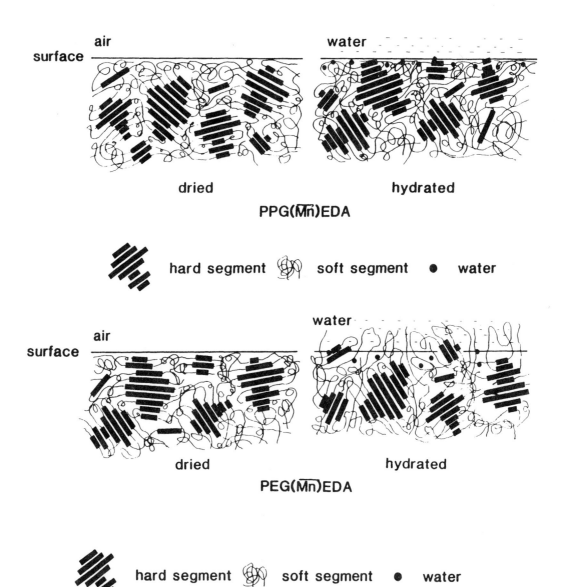

FIGURE 6 Schematic representation of the surface structure of (a) hydrophobic soft segment and (b) hydrophilic soft segment containing segmented polyurethaneureas in the hydrated and dehydrated state. From Takahara A., Jo N. J. and Kajiyama T. *J. Biomater. Sci., Polym. Ed.*, 1:17, 1989. Reproduced with permission.

This material was found to be synthesized mostly from ED, PTMO, and MDI. The second form of Biomer was extrusion grade Biomer (EB) and was believed to differ from the solution grade material in that water was used as the chain extender, rather than ED. Solution Grade Biomer had an 1800 m.w. PTMO soft segment, while Extrusion Grade Biomer had a 650 m.w. PTMO segment. Some of the Extrusion Grade Biomer was dissolved in DMA and cast (CB); the surfaces of the three samples were then compared. Bulk analysis of SB and CB by FTIR showed differences in composition. Higher soft segment concentrations were reported for the extruded material when compared with both samples prepared from solution. Washing of the surfaces led to a reduction in oxygen and an increase in the N/C ratio. More silicon contamination was detected on the extruded

Surface Characterization of Polyurethanes

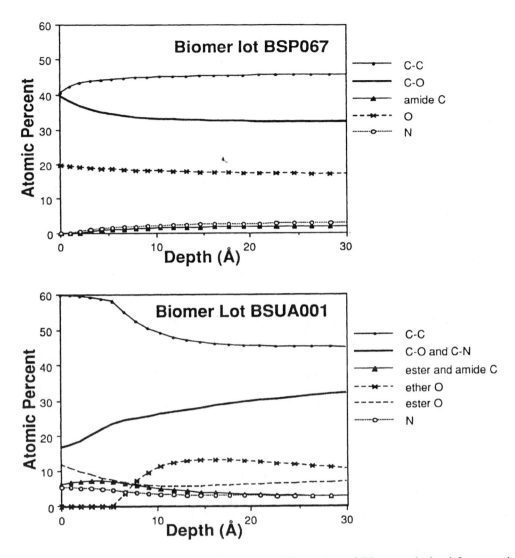

FIGURE 7 ESCA concentration-depth profiles of two different lots of Biomer, calculated from angular dependent studies. From Tyler B. J., Ratner B. D., Castner D. G. and Briggs D. J. *Biomed. Mater. Res.,* 26:273, Copyright 1992. Reprinted with permission by John Wiley & Sons.

material, which was attributed to the presence of a polydimethylsiloxane processing aid. Contamination of Biomer by polydimethylsiloxanes also has been identified and reported by Graham and Hercules,[39] who investigated the nature of the contaminant using SIMS analysis, and by Grobe *et al.*[30], although some researchers were unable to detect silicone on a Biomer surface.[40] Differences in the composition of batches of Biomer also have been reported, on the basis of spectral analyses.[41,42] Tyler and Ratner performed ESCA, SIMS and ATR–FTIR studies on two different batches of Biomer, obtained five years apart.[42-43] ESCA, SIMS and FTIR spectra are shown in Figures 7, 8 and 9. Differences between the two batches were observed in ESCA and SIMS spectra, but not in ATR–FTIR spectra. ESCA analysis showed enrichment of the polyether segment at the surface of the earlier batch of Biomer.

However, the more recent batch showed the presence of nitrogen, hydrocarbons and ester groups at the surface, accompanied by the disappearance of a signal associated with ether oxygen. Differences

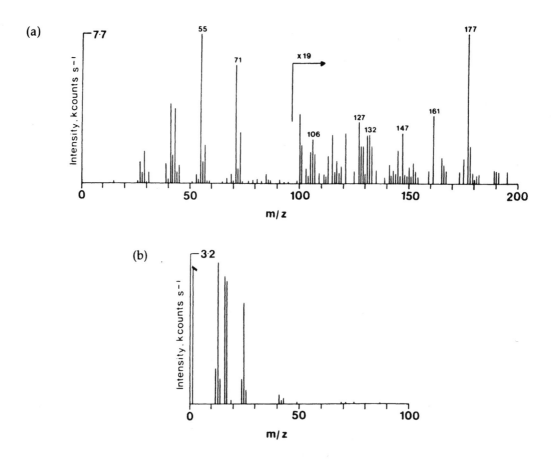

FIGURE 8 SIMS spectra of two different lots of Biomer. (a) positive ion SIMS spectrum and (b) negative ion SIMS spectrum for Biomer, lot BSP. (c) positive ion SIMS spectrum and (d) negative ion SIMS spectrum for Biomer, lot BSUA. From Tyler B. J., Ratner B. D., Castner D. G. and Briggs D. J. *Biomed. Mater. Res.*, 26:273, Copyright 1992. Reprinted with permission by John Wiley & Sons.

in the mechanisms and extent of degradation of the two materials were also detected.[42] SIMS studies confirmed the dominance of the polyether at the surface of the older batch. In the more recent batch, a number of large ions were detected from the surface that did not originate from the polyether or polyurethane components of the polymer. Comparison with other spectra suggested that the surface of the newer batch was dominated by a methacrylate polymer, possibly diisopropylamino-ethyl methacrylate (DPA–EMA). Belisle *et al.*[44] also have detected fragments of an amino compound on Biomer using SIMS analysis. Such a material may have been added to the polymer to enhance polymer stability during processing. This compound could not be removed by extraction with 12 common solvents. Similar methacrylate additives in laboratory synthesized polyurethanes have been reported to migrate to the surface of polymers, and have the capacity to influence adsorption of plasma proteins.[45] Quaternary alkyl ammonium compounds and tertiary amino compounds also have been detected on Biomer.[44,46]

Investigations of other biomedical polyurethanes also have revealed that nonpolyurethane components may be present at the surfaces of commercially available materials. Polyurethane catheters were compared with model polyurethanes of increasing hardness. Few differences in surface composition with respect to hard to soft segment ratios were observed between the model polyurethanes. The catheters were shown to contain polydimethylsiloxanes (PDMS) at the surface;

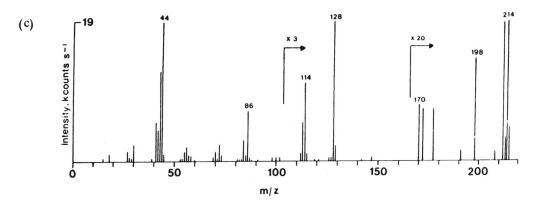

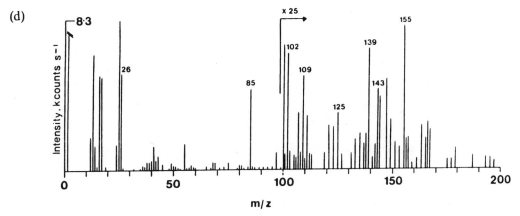

FIGURE 8 (continued)

this could have been introduced during manufacture to act as a lubricant and ease insertion of the catheter.[16] Larsson et al.[47] also examined a Pellethane catheter and found evidence of a *bis* - stearamide wax coating on the surface. Subsequent extraction of the catheter with toluene reduced the amount of amide that could be detected on the surface. The removal of this wax coating was shown to decrease *in vitro* platelet adhesion.

Avcothane and its descendant Cardiothane-51 also have been studied by surface spectroscopic techniques. Avcothane is a polyether-urethane-polydimethylsiloxane copolymer, which has been used in the manufacture of intraaortic balloon pumps. Both surfaces, mold-facing and air-facing, were examined by Sung and Hu,[38] and Graham and Hercules.[48] Sung and Hu reported differences in the polymer-substrate and polymer-air surfaces; the polymer-air surface, which is the blood-contacting surface, contained very large amounts of silicone. The investigation conducted by Graham and Hercules found that fluoride peaks were present on the spectrum of the mold-facing surface, as were peaks associated with polyether and polydimethylsiloxane. Graham and Hercules also performed SIMS studies in order to identify the contaminant, and the presence of fluorine was thought to originate from a Teflon-like mold-release agent. The air-facing surface, which is the blood-contacting surface in use, produced more peaks associated with urethane groups, and no fluorine-derived peaks. Differences in air and mold-facing surfaces also have been observed for Biomer accompanied by the detection of silicon-contamination, probably a polydimethylsiloxane.[39] Angular dependent ESCA studies of Avcothane showed that as the surface is approached, the polyether signal decreases and the signal from PDMS dominates.[46] Another study by the same researchers showed that the surface of the Cardiothane-51 was predominantly PDMS in character,

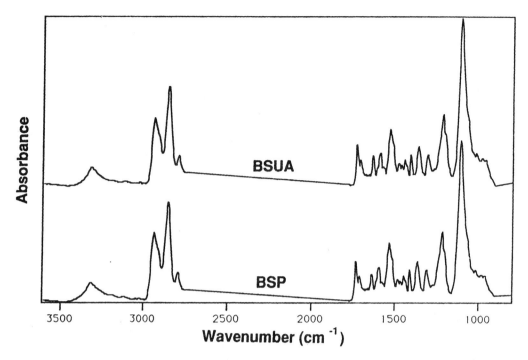

FIGURE 9 Transmission FTIR spectra for two different lots (BSUA and BSP) of Biomer. From Tyler B.J., Ratner B.D., Castner D.G.and Briggs D. J. *Biomed. Mater. Res.,* 26:273, Copyright 1992. Reprinted with permission by John Wiley & Sons.

more so than Avcothane, although some polyether could be detected. The polyether concentration was shown to decrease as the surface was approached.

ESCA studies also have demonstrated that methods of fabrication and sample treatments may alter the surface chemistry. Lelah et al.[9] demonstrated that the solvent from which the material was cast could also influence the nature of the surface. A polyurethane containing MDI, PTMO and N-methyldiethanolamine cast from THF had a lower surface hard to soft segment ratio than the same material cast from DMA. Solvent extraction of polymer samples also may produce differences in surface composition. Differences in the surface composition of Biomer also have been observed between samples cast from DMA, acetoitrile and methanol due to the differences in solvation of the components of Biomer.[30] However, Tyler et al.[43] have reported no differences in surface composition between Biomer samples cast from DMA and hexafluroroisopropane (HFIP). ESCA also has been used as a tool to investigate the effect of bulk modification on surface composition, and to study the extent and modes of degradation of polyurethanes.[12]

V. SURFACE MORPHOLOGY

The physical characteristics or morphology of surfaces can be classified according to roughness, porosity and texture. Differences in the surface structure can result from differences in the bulk chemistry, but also the physical and chemical treatments to which the material is subjected, in addition to sample handling. For example, the crystallinity of a polymer may influence the surface morphology, and fabrication methods can influence both the chemical and physical characteristics of the polymer. Morphological variations can be observed on a number of scales, from microns down to an atomic level. Surface characterization of polymer morphology can be difficult and time consuming. It must be realized that surfaces are in fact three-dimensional, but many methods are unable to study or characterize surfaces in more than two dimensions.

The roughness of a material can be described at three levels:[49] primary roughness, secondary waviness and errors of form. Other important features of the periodicity of surface morphology are the skewness and kurtosis. Skewness is a measure of the lack of symmetry about the mean distribution of heights, and kurtosis is an indication of the peakedness of a distribution.

Reports of quantitative studies on characterization of surface roughness of polyurethane materials are hard to find. It is believed that roughness of a material may affect its thrombogenicity.[50] Many biomaterials researchers evaluate roughness at a qualitative level by examination of Scanning Electron Micrographs. Shown in Figure 10 is a series of SEM pictures of a set of polyurethanes, including the base material after a number of chemical surface modifications. Free isocyanates were introduced onto the polyurethane through reaction with HMDI (PU-HMDI). This was reacted with dodecanediol to yield PU-DDO, or poly(ethyleneoxide) to yield PU-PEO200. PU-HMDI also was aminated (PU-NH2) followed by sulfonation with propane sulfone (PU-SO3). The PU-DDO and the PEO200 were reacted further with propane sulfone to produce PU-DDO-1 SO3 and PEO200-SO3 respectively. SEM methods are frequently employed to examine cell morphology after contact with biomaterials; many studies of platelet morphology to materials have been reported, and methods have been developed to quantify responses by examination of the length of pseudopodia of attached cells. Surface roughness also can be examined using optical interferometry.

Scanning Tunneling Microscopy (STM) and Atomic Force Microscopy are two scanning probe microscopic techniques that are contributing further to the examination of biomaterial surfaces. These techniques examine the morphology of surfaces at an atomic level. STM and AFM utilize a similar piezoelectric method for surface examination. STM can only be used on conducting surfaces whereas AFM can be used on insulating surfaces, and it is the latter technique that has greater relevance to studies of polyurethane surfaces. As the tip of the probe is moved across the surface, it responds to changes in the electron cloud density, and the force required to maintain a constant current is measured. One of the greatest advantages of AFM is that surface can be examined not only under vacuum conditions, but in air and under water. Difficulties arise in the examination of "soft" surfaces, due to frictional and viscoelastic effects. This has made examination of polyurethanes difficult, although AFM examination of Biomer has been performed.[51]

The texture of a surface is heavily influenced by the method of fabrication. The texture of a surface may be nonporous, woven, knitted, velour, fibrous etc. Surface texture also may be isotropic, as in the case of woven materials, or anisotropic, in the case of extruded materials. Surface texture can play an important role in biomedical applications, for example, vascular grafts made from polyethylene terephthalate PET, sold under the trade name Dacron®, are woven to provide the mechanical flexibility required for vascular applications; the woven texture has been shown to influence the biocompatibility of the device, in that woven fabrics contain pores that allow tissue ingrowth. Quantification of the texture of a surface is generally difficult. Biomer has been used in blood-contacting applications in both cast and extruded forms,[7] porous form,[52] woven form,[53] and as a suture material.[53] It was found to perform favorably in all applications, but no real comparison on the basis of texture alone can be made, due to the different experimental conditions that were employed.

The porosity of a surface also can be considered as a bulk property of the material. Pore cross sections will be present on the surface of a material. Pores can be created using a number of different techniques, such as sintering, salt leaching, foaming, stretching, casting and the use of solid-particulate material. Pores can vary according to their size, shape, number, and density. For biomedical applications, polymer pore sizes can range from one to 200 microns. SEM techniques lend themselves well to the examination of surface morphology and the examination of pore structures.

The porosity of materials for biomedical application can be extremely influential with respect to their biocompatibility; thus the ability to control porosity is important. In animal studies of small arterial prostheses, the porosity of the lumen allows the deposition of a thin layer of fibrin, which provides the basis for a pannus ingrowth of fibrous tissue, and the formation of a neointima

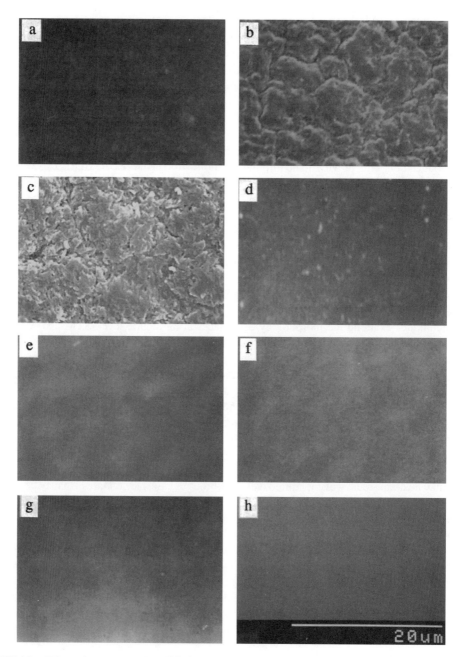

FIGURE 10 SEMs micrographs of modified polyurethane surfaces: (a) PU (b) PU-HMDI (c) PU-NH2 (d) PU-DDO (e) PU-PEO200 (f) PU-SO3 (g) PU-DDO-SO3 (h) PU-PEO200-SO3. From Han, D. K., Jeong, S.Y., Ahn, K., Kim, Y.H., and Min, B.G.: *J. Biomater. Sci., Polym. Ed.*, 4, 579, 1993. Reproduced with permission.

containing endothelial cells. The occurrence of fibrous ingrowth is often used to anchor implanted devices, such as percutaneous cardiovascular and orthopedic devices, transcutaneous pacemaker leads and artificial larynx devices. The porosity of the materials also can affect the blood compatibility. The formation of microbubbles in synthetic vascular grafts can contribute to thrombogenesis. Pores sizes in such applications should be large enough to allow cellular ingrowth, yet small enough to restrict blood flow through the wall and prevent periprosthetic hematoma. Optimal pore sizes for vascular grafts are considered to be within the range 20 to 50 microns, and for soft tissue ingrowth, 100 to 200 microns. Wilkes and Samuels have studied of the porosity of polyurethanes by examining a systematic series of well-defined polyetherurethanes and blends of the polyurethanes.[54] They found that the porosity of the polyurethanes was dependent on the casting conditions. More details on how the porosity of a polyurethane can be influenced by fabrication method are given in Chapter 3.

VI. SURFACE ELECTRICAL PROPERTIES

In the past the surface electrical properties of biomaterials were believed to be of importance in determining the biocompatibility of the material. This was based on the results of a number of investigations of biological systems. Early experiments showed that mammalian blood cells were cataphoretic, i.e., they migrated towards a positive electrode and were therefore negatively charged. Sawyer and Pate recorded that a thrombus would form at the anode when an electrical potential was applied across a blood vessel.[55] Studies by other researchers showed that the normal vascular surface is negatively charged, and that a decrease in this negative charge could lead to intravascular thrombosis. These studies have provided the basis of characterizing biomaterials on the basis of electrical charge. It was thus believed that negatively charged surfaces would possess superior blood contacting properties, as the negatively charged blood cells would be repelled by a similar charge; however, the intrinsic pathway of coagulation (also known as contact phase activation) may be promoted by negatively charged surfaces, and coagulation does appear to be enhanced on glass, celite, collagen kaolin and ellagic acid, all of which have negatively charged surfaces.

Measurable electrical parameters include surface charge, surface potential difference, resting potential and zeta (streaming) potential. Zeta potential measurements of polyurethanes for biomedical applications have been studied.[56-60] There is some uncertainty as to the importance of surface charge measurements as an indication of thrombogenicity. Baier has postulated that the surface electrical properties of a material do not significantly influence the initially adsorbed protein layers, due to the high ionic strength of the blood and plasma, and the rapid equilibrium that is established.[61] The presence of ionic groups in a polymer may alter the surface electrical properties. The presence of ionic groups bonded to the main polymer chain could also influence the properties through mediation of ionic interactions at the interface.

SUMMARY

Surface characterization has not only a role in improving our understanding of the surface structure at a molecular level, but also as a tool in biomaterials development and manufacture to quantitatively assess sample consistency and contamination. Evidence for large variations in biomaterial composition at the surface of similar polyurethane materials has been presented in this chapter. If such large variations in the surface compositions exist, then this may provide a partial explanation for the difficulties in comparing surface characterization and *in vitro* test results obtained by different research groups on closely related materials.

There is an ongoing drive to understand, at a molecular level, the nature of biomaterial surfaces, in order to probe one half of the elusive structure-property relationship. Each of the characterization techniques have their strengths and limitations, which must be considered when interpreting results from such studies. Complementary studies are therefore recommended in order to obtain as much information as possible about a surface, considering not only surface chemistry, but the density and orientation of functional groups. In addition, the mobility of the surface and the ability to rearrange in different environments must be considered. Surface characterization techniques and their application to biomaterials will advance the establishment of steadfast relationships between biomaterial structure and biological systems.

REFERENCES

1. Ratner B. D. "Surface characterization of biomaterials." *Cardiovasc. Pathol.,* 2:87S, 1993.
2. Vogler E. A. "Interfacial chemistry in biomaterials science." In *Wettability,* Ed. Berg J. C. Marcel Dekker, New York, 1993: 183.
3. Andrade J. D., Smith L. M., and Gregonis D. E. "The contact angle and interface energetics." In *Surface and Interfacial Aspects of Biomedical Polymers.,* Ed. Andrade J. D. Plenum Press, New York, 1985: 249.
4. Fox H. W. and Zisman W. A. "The spreading of liquids on low energy surfaces. III. Hydrocarbon surfaces." *J. Coll. Interf. Sci.,* 7:428, 1952.
5. Neumann A. W. and Good R. J. *Techniques of measuring contact angles.* Plenum Press, New York, 1979.
6. Hamilton W. C. "A technique for the characterization of hydrophilic solid surfaces." *J. Coll. Interf. Sci.,* 10:219, 1972.
7. Lelah M. D., Lambrecht L. K., Young B. R., and Cooper S. L. "Physicochemical characterization and *in vivo* blood tolerability of cast and extruded Biomer." *J. Biomed. Mater. Res.,* 17:1, 1983.
8. Giroux T. A. and Cooper S. L. "Surface characterization of plasma-derivatized polyurethanes." *J. Appl. Polym. Sci.,* 43:145, 1991.
9. Lelah M. D., Grasel T. G., Pierce J. A., and Cooper S. L. "*Ex vivo* interactions and surface property relationships of polyurethanes." *J. Biomed. Mater. Res.,* 20:433, 1986.
10. Boretos J. W., Pierce W. S., Baier R. E., Leroy A. F., and Donachy H. J. "Surface and bulk characteristics of a polyether urethane for artificial hearts." *J. Biomed. Mater. Res.,* 9:327, 1975.
11. Kaelble D. H. and Moacanin J. "A surface energy analysis of bioadhesion." *Polymer,* 18:475, 1977.
12. Marchant R. E., Anderson J. M., Hiltner A., Castillo E. J., Gleit J., and Ratner B. D. "The biocompatibility of solution cast and acetone-extracted Biomer." *J. Biomed. Mater. Res.,* 20:799, 1986.
13. Pitt W. G. and Cooper S. L. "FTIR–ATR studies of the effect of shear rate upon albumin adsorption onto polyurethaneurea." *Biomaterials,* 7:340, 1986.
14. Nyilas E. "Development of blood compatible elastomers. II. Performance of Avcothane blood contact surfaces in experimental animal implantation." *J. Biomed. Mater. Res.,* 3:97, 1972.
15. Lelah M. D., Pierce J. A., Lambrecht L. K., and Cooper S. L. "Polyether-urethane ionomers: surface property/*ex vivo* blood compatibility relationships." *J. Coll. Interf. Sci.,* 104:422, 1985.
16. Castner D. G., Ratner B. D., and Hoffman A. F. "Surface characterization of a series of polyurethanes by X-ray photoelectron spectroscopy and contact angle methods." *J. Biomater. Sci., Polym. Ed.,* 1:191, 1990.
17. Okkema A. Z., Yu X.-H., and Cooper S. L. "Physical and blood contacting properties of propyl sulphonate grafted Biomer." *Biomaterials,* 12:3, 1991.
18. Hergenrother R. W. and Cooper S. L. "Improved materials for blood-contacting applications: blends of sulphonated and non-sulphonated polyurethanes." *J. Mat. Sci., Mat. Med,* 3:313, 1992.
19. Grasel T. G. and Cooper S. L. "Surface properties and blood compatibility of polyurethaneureas." *Biomaterials,* 7:315, 1986.
20. Sung C. S. P. and Hu C. B. "Surface chemical analysis of segmented polyurethanes. Fourier Transform IR internal reflection studies." In *Multiphase Polymers,* Ed. Cooper S. L., Estes G. M. American Chemical Society, Washington, D.C., 1979: 63.
21. Gendreau R. M. and Jacobsen R. J. "Fourier transform infrared techniques for studying complex biological systems." *Appl. Spectr.,* 32:326, 1978.
22. Ihlenfeld J. V. and Cooper S. L. "Transient *in vivo* protein adsorption onto polymeric biomaterials." *J. Biomed. Mater. Res.,* 13:577, 1979.
23. Chittur K. K., Fink D. J., Leininger R. I., and Hutson T. B. "FT-IR/ATR studies of protein adsorption in flowing systems: approaches for bulk correction and compositional analysis of adsorbed and bulk proteins in mixtures." *J. Coll. Interf. Sci.,* 111:419, 1986.
24. Iwamoto R., Ohja K., Matsuda T., and Imachi K. :Quantitative surface analysis of Cardiothane 51 by FT–IR–ATR spectroscopy." *J. Biomed. Mater. Res.,* 20:507, 1986.
25. Srichatrapimuk V. W. and Cooper, S. L. "Infrared thermal analysis of polyurethane block copolymers." *J. Macromol. Sci.–Phys. B.,* 15:267, 1978.
26. Lyman D. J., Alb D., Jackson R., and Knutson K. "Development of small diameter vascular graft prostheses." *Trans. Am. Soc. Artif. Intern. Organs,* 23:253, 1977.

27. Knutson K. and Lyman D. J. "Morphology of block co-polyurethanes. II. FTIR and ESCA techniques for studying surface morphology." *Am. Chem. Soc. Div. Org. Coat. Plast. Chem. Prepr.,* 42:621, 1980.
28. Knutson K. and Lyman D. J. "The effect of polyether segment molecular weight on the bulk and surface morphologies of copolyether-urethane-ureas." In *Biomaterials: Interfacial Phenomena and Applications,* Ed. Cooper S. L., Peppas N. A. Advances in Chemistry Series, 1982: 109.
29. Grasel T. G. and Cooper S. L. "Properties and biological interactions of polyurethane anionomers: effect of sulfonate incorporation." *J. Biomed. Mater. Res.,* 23:311, 1989.
30. Grobe G. L., Gardella J. A., Chin R. L., and Salvati L. "Characterization of solution-cast extracts from Biomer by FT–IR and ESCA." *Appl. Spectr.,* 42:989, 1988.
31. Takahara A., Hergenrother R. W., Coury A. J., and Cooper S. L. "Effect of soft segment chemistry on the biostability of segmented polyurethanes. II. *In vitro* hydrolytic stability." *J. Biomed. Mater. Res.,* 26:801, 1992.
32. Takahara A., Coury A. J., Hergenrother R. W., and Cooper S. L. "Effect of soft segment chemistry on the biostability of segmented polyurethanes. I. *In vitro* oxidation." *J. Biomed. Mater. Res.,* 25:341, 1991.
33. Hearn M. J., Ratner B. D., and Briggs D. "SIMS and XPS studies of polyurethane surfaces 1. Preliminary Studies." *Macromolecules,* 21:2950, 1988.
34. Affrossman S., Barbenel J. C., Forbes C. D., MacAllister J. M. R., Meng J., Pethrick R. A., and Scott R. A. "Surface structure and biocompatibility of polyurethanes." *Clin. Mater.,* 8:25, 1991.
35. Okkema A. Z., Fabrizius D. J., Grasel T. G., Cooper S. L., and Zdrahala R. J. "Bulk, surface and blood-contacting properties of polyether polyurethanes modified with polydimethylsiloxane macroglycols." *Biomaterials,* 10:23, 1989.
36. Takahara A., Jo N. J., and Kajiyama T. "Surface molecular mobility and platelets reactivity of segmented poly(etherurethaneureas) with hydrophilic and hydrophobic soft segment components." *J. Biomater. Sci., Polym. Ed.,* 1:17, 1989.
37. Lin H.-B., Lewis K. B., Leach-Scampavia D., Ratner B. D., and Cooper S. L. "Surface properties of RGD-peptide grafted polyurethane block copolymers: variable take-off angle and cold-stage ESCA studies." *J. Biomater. Sci., Polym. Ed.,* 4:183, 1993.
38. Sung C. S. P. and Hu C. B. "ESCA studies of surface chemical composition of segmented polyurethanes." *J. Biomed. Mater. Res.,* 13:161, 1979.
39. Graham S. W. and Hercules D. M. "Surface spectroscopic studies of Biomer." *J. Biomed. Mater. Res.,* 15:465, 1981.
40. Feuerstein I. A. and Ratner B. D. "Adhesion and aggregation of thrombin prestimulated human platelets: evaluation of a series of biomaterials characterized by ESCA." *Biomaterials,* 11:127, 1990.
41. Coleman D. L., Meuzelaar H. L. C., Kessler T. R., McClennen W. H., Richards J. M., and Gregonis D. E. "Retrieval and analysis of a clinical total artificial heart." *J. Biomed. Mater. Res.,* 20:417, 1986.
42. Tyler B. J., Ratner B. D., Castner D. G., and Briggs D. "Variations between Biomer™ lots. 2. The effect of differences between lots on *in vitro* enzymatic and oxidative degradation of a commercial polyurethane. *J. Biomed. Mater. Res.,* 27:327, 1993.
43. Tyler B. J., Ratner B. D., Castner D. G., and Briggs D. "Variations between Biomer™ lots. 1. Significant differences in the surface chemistry of two lots of a commercial poly(ether urethane)." *J. Biomed. Mater. Res.,* 26:273, 1992.
44. Belisle J., Maier S. K., and Tucker J. A. "Compositional analysis of Biomer." *J. Biomed. Mater. Res.,* 24:1585, 1990.
45. Brunstedt M. R., Ziats N. P., Robertson S. P., Hiltner A., Anderson J. M., Lodoen G. A., and Payet C. R. "Protein adsorption to poly(ether urethane ureas) modified with acrylate and methacrylate polymer and copolymer additives." *J. Biomed. Mater. Res.,* 27:367, 1993.
46. Grobe G. L., Gardella J. A., Hopson W. L., McKenna W. P., and Eyring E. M. "Angular dependent ESCA and infrared studies of segmented polyurethanes." *J. Biomed. Mater. Res.,* 21:211, 1987.
47. Larsson N., Linder L.-E., Curelaru I., Buscemi P., Sherman R., and Eriksson E. "Initial platelet adhesion and platelet shape change on polymer surfaces with different carbon bonding characteristics (an *in vitro* study of Teflon, Pellethane and XLON intravenous cannulae)." *J. Mat. Sci., Mat. Med,* 1:157, 1990.
48. Graham S. W. and Hercules D. M. "Surface spectroscopic studies of Avcothane." *J. Biomed. Mater. Res.,* 15:349, 1981.
49. Gasieki E. *Surface Texture.* NIH, 1980.

50. Hecker J. F. "Thrombus formation of intravascular catheters and cannulas." In *Blood Compatibility.* CRC Press Inc, Boca Raton, FL, 1987: 79.
51. Nurdin N. and Descouts P. "Effect of toluene extraction on Biomer surface: An atomic force microscope study." *J. Biomater. Sci., Polym. Ed.,* 7:381, 1995.
52. Pollock E., Andrews E. J., Lentz D., and Sheikh K. "Tissue ingrowth and porosity of Biomer." *Trans. Am. Soc. Artif. Intern. Organs,* 27:405, 1981.
53. Wagner M., Reul G., Teresi J.. and Kayser K. L. "Experimental observations on a new and inherently elastic material for sutures and vascular prostheses." *Am.. J. Surg.,* 111:858, 1966.
54. Wilkes G. L. and Samuels S. L. "Porous segmented polyurethanes — possible candidates as biomaterials." *J. Biomed. Mater. Res.,* 7:541, 1973.
55. Sawyer P. N. and Pate J. W. "Bioelectric phenomena as an etiologic factor in intravascular thrombosis." *Am. J. Physiol.,* 175:118, 1953.
56. Murphy P., Lacroix A., and Merchant S. "Studies relative to materials suitable for use in artificial organs." *Artificial Heart Progress Conference,* 99, 1969.
57. Bruck S. D. "Biomaterials in medical devices." *Trans. Am. Soc. Artif. Intern. Organs,* 18:1, 1972.
58. Miller B. G., Dyer K. A., Taylor B. C., Wright J. I., and Sharp W. V. "Electrical conductivity; effect on intravascular performance of foams, velour, flock and fabric." *Trans. Am. Soc. Artif. Intern. Organs,* 20:91, 1974.
59. Voight A., Becher R., and Donath E. "Streaming potential and streaming current measurements to estimate surface conduction and electric double layer structure of biomaterials." *J. Biomed. Mater. Res.,* 18:317, 1984.
60. Taylor B. C., Sharp W. V., Wright J. I., Ewing K. L., and Wilson C. L. "The importance of zeta potential, ultrastructure, and electrical conductivity to the *in vivo* performance of polyurethane-carbon black vascular prostheses." *Trans. Am. Soc. Artif. Intern. Organs,* 18:317, 1971.
61. Baier R. E. "Key events in blood interactions at non-physiologic interfaces — a personal primer." *Artif. Organs,* 2:422, 1978.

6 Introduction to Host-Biomaterial Interactions

I. INTRODUCTION

Ultimately, biomaterials are employed in the clinic, to replace or augment the functions of host tissues. So far in this book, we have examined the fundamentals of polyurethane chemistry, synthesis, fabrication and properties. Medical devices fabricated from polyurethanes are employed in a diverse range of applications, and are thus in contact with blood and tissues at sites throughout the body. In the remainder of this book, we will consider this biological environment, and its interactions with polyurethanes in more detail, discussing the consequences of these interactions on both the host and the material. This includes sections on blood and soft tissue interactions, degradation and toxicity issues, and finally a review of the use of polyurethanes in biomedical applications. In this chapter we provide background information regarding plasma proteins and the fundamentals of protein adsorption, protein systems including coagulation and fibrinolysis, cells, inflammation, the foreign body response and the immune system.

II. PROTEIN ADSORPTION

A. The First Event

Blood consists of approximately 45% formed elements and 55% plasma. The formed elements include red and white blood cells, and platelets. Of the plasma, 93% is water. The remaining 7% is made up of ions, sugars, hormones, enzymes, amino acids and hundreds of proteins. Plasma protein adsorption to biomaterial surfaces is frequently considered to be the initial biological interaction with the host environment. Proteins are high molecular weight solutes that can be considered as copolymers of amino acids.[1] Proteins are heterogeneous molecules and contain regions of differing polarity, charge and hydrophilicity. Thus, proteins exhibit amphoteric and amphiphilic properties. The precise structure of a protein is not only determined by its specific sequence of amino acids, but by the secondary and tertiary structure that determines the conformation of the molecule and the distribution and orientation of the side groups. A protein may contain anywhere from fifty to over ten thousand residues with a specific chain sequence of amino acids. Proteins may assume a variety of conformations determined by the amino acid sequence (primary structure) which results in ordered secondary structures such as α-helices and β-sheets. The tertiary structure of a protein refers to the way in which unordered and ordered secondary structures combine to give the protein its characteristic three-dimensional shape, and it results largely from unfavorable interactions between the amino acids. In solution the three-dimensional shape attained by a protein will be one that minimizes the free energy of the system including the interactions between the protein and the surrounding medium.[1-2] The major driving force for the folding of a polypeptide in solution is dehydration of hydrophobic amino acid side chains.[1] Amino acids with hydrophobic side groups tend to be in the interior of the molecule, away from water. The amino acids with charged or polar side chains tend to be at the periphery of the molecule.[1] The net result is a spontaneously folding protein with a hydrophobic core and a complex irregular exterior surface formed by the polar or hydrophilic side chains.

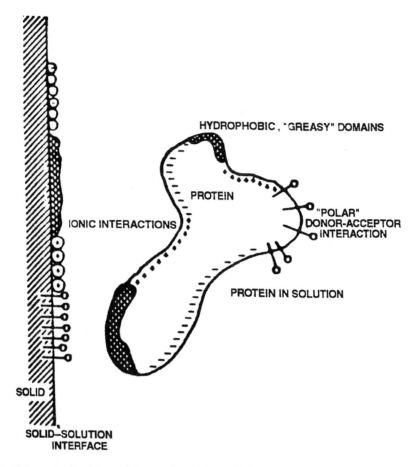

FIGURE 1 Schematic view of protein interacting with a well-characterized surface. The protein has a number of surface domains with hydrophobic, charged, and polar character. The solid surface has a similar domainlike character. From Andrade J. D. "Principles of protein adsorption." In *Surface and Interfacial Aspects of Biomedical Polymers,* Ed. Andrade, J. D., Plenum Press, New York, 1985. With permission.

Proteins generally prefer an aqueous environment. However, when a protein solution is contacted with another phase, there is a tendency for the protein molecules to accumulate at the interface. At a solid interface, the complex structure of proteins give rise to a number of interactions with the surface, involving hydrophobic, electrostatic and polar forces. The extent of these interactions is not only dependent on the nature of the surface and the nature of the protein, but also on the number and concentration of proteins in the contacting solution, the temperature of the system, the length of time of contact and rheological conditions. Thermodynamic driving forces may cause protein molecules to condense onto the surface. Adsorption to the surface may invoke conformational changes in the protein, or cause the protein to denature. Figure 1 illustrates the interactions generally considered to occur in protein adsorption.[3]

Adsorption is not a static event as adsorbed proteins can undergo conformational changes with time,[4-5] and exchange with other molecules in the contacting solution.[6-7] It is generally accepted that the adsorption of plasma proteins onto an artificial surface is the first event to occur when blood contacts a biomaterial, usually within a few seconds,[8] preceded only by the adsorption of water and inorganic ions. Blood platelets and other formed elements arrive at the surface shortly thereafter, and at that time, interact with a protein layer on the order of a few hundred Ångstroms.[6] It also is accepted that the adsorbed protein layer influences the nature of subsequent events, as other blood components such as blood cells must interact with this protein layer.[9-11] Adhesive proteins may act as bridging molecules for cellular adhesion. Thus, studies of protein adsorption onto biomaterial surfaces is not only relevant to gaining an understanding of blood-material interactions, but also is an important step in the design of improved materials for clinical applications. The concept of "controlled" protein adsorption to surfaces has been realized to an extent, enabling a reduction in protein adsorption, or favoring adsorption of specific types or conformations of proteins.[10]

1. Kinetics of protein adsorption

An important question in the study of interfacial phenomena is whether the rate is reaction or transport controlled. Protein adsorption is generally agreed to be transport limited when the fraction of the surface covered by the protein is low (less than 10% of monolayer coverage).[3,10] In this situation the flow conditions must be taken into account since convection as well as diffusion will be present.

The combined transport adsorption process may be modeled using the appropriate form of the convection-diffusion equation, Equation 1.1, with appropriate boundary conditions.[12]

$$\frac{\partial c}{\partial t} + v(y)\frac{\partial c}{\partial x} = D\frac{\partial^2 c}{\partial y^2} \tag{1.1}$$

where c   = concentration
       t   = time
       v(y) = velocity distribution across the flow path
       D   = protein diffusivity
       x   = axial co-ordinate (direction of flow)
       y   = radial co-ordinate perpendicular to the flow (e.g., in a tube).

An important boundary condition, Equation 1.2, applies at the surface:

$$D\frac{\partial c}{\partial y} = R(c) \tag{1.2}$$

Equation 1.2 states that the flux at the surface is equal to the intrinsic (kinetic) rate of adsorption, $R(c)$.

In general Equation 1.1 must be solved numerically. However, analytical solutions are possible for simple cases such as the transport limited case in a nonflowing system (diffusion limited). In this case the flux at the surface, i.e., the adsorption rate is given by Equation 1.3:

$$\frac{d\Gamma}{dt} = C_o \left(\frac{D}{\pi t}\right)^{1/2} \tag{1.3}$$

and the surface concentration is given by Equation 1.4:

$$\Gamma = 2C_o \left(\frac{Dt}{\pi}\right)^{1/2} \tag{1.4}$$

where Γ = surface concentration
       C_o = bulk concentration of the protein in solution
       D   = diffusivity
       t   = time

Equation 1.4 indicates the $t^{1/2}$ dependence expected from a diffusion controlled process.

When adsorption is kinetically limited, whether in a flowing or nonflowing system, the rate is given by the intrinsic kinetics, of the general form of Equation 1.5:

$$\frac{d\Gamma}{dt} = R(C_0) \tag{1.5}$$

As indicated, adsorption may initially be transport limited but as the surface sites become occupied, the intrinsic kinetics will determine the rate.[13]

2. Equilibria and isotherms

Theoretical and empirical models have been used to describe single protein adsorption.[14] Single protein adsorption isotherms can be reasonably well explained by the Langmuir model (theoretical) and the Freundlich model (empirical) which were developed for gas adsorption.

The Langmuir model assumes that only one molecule adsorbs per site (monolayer assumption), that there is only one type of site present (energetically uniform surface, constant heat of adsorption), that the adsorption of one molecule does not affect the adsorption of another, and that the adsorption is reversible (i.e., equilibrium between the adsorbate on the solid surface and in solution is assumed).[3,10,14] Several investigators have found that protein adsorption is essentially irreversible on a reasonable time scale.[13,15-16] Indeed the use of the terms "isotherm" and "equilibria" are questionable when applied to protein adsorption. However, despite these difficulties, the Langmuir model has been used extensively in the literature and provides a reasonably good fit to many adsorption data.[10,17] The success of the Langmuir model is surprising since the fundamental assumptions of this model are clearly not applicable to protein adsorption.

The Langmuir model can be derived using kinetic arguments.[18] Adsorption of protein P to surface site x may be described by:

$$P + x \underset{k_d}{\overset{k_a}{\rightleftharpoons}} Px \tag{1.6}$$

where k_a is the adsorption rate constant and k_d is desorption rate constant.

The rate of adsorption (R_{ads}) is given by:

$$R_{ads} = k_a C_p (1 - \theta) \tag{1.7}$$

where θ is the fraction of the surface area covered by adsorbed molecules at any time, and C_p is the protein concentration.

The rate of desorption is given by:

$$R_{des} = k_d \theta \tag{1.8}$$

At equilibrium:

$$k_d \theta = k_a C_p (1 - \theta) \tag{1.9}$$

Solving for θ:

$$\theta = \frac{KC_p}{1+KC_p} = \frac{\Gamma}{\Gamma_{max}} \quad (1.10)$$

where Γ = adsorption
Γ_{max} = adsorption at the plateau (monolayer adsorption)
K = k_a/k_d and is called the adsorption coefficient. The adsorption coefficient has the properties of an equilibrium constant.

A characteristic of this isotherm is that a plot of θ vs. concentration yields a curve that rises monotonically with increasing concentration to a plateau of constant surface concentration (θ = 1). This plateau level is assumed to represent complete coverage. Two limiting cases are generally considered when analyzing adsorption data which fits a Langmuir model. In the first case when the concentration is very low Equation 1.10 reduces to:

$$\theta \cong KC_p \quad (1.11)$$

The curve approximates a straight line and the slope of this line can be used to determine the adsorption coefficient. In the second case, at high concentration with θ approximately equal to one, the plateau adsorption can be used to calculate the monolayer concentration and the surface area occupied per molecule bound.

The other model frequently used to describe single protein adsorption is the Freundlich isotherm described by Equation 1.12. This empirical model was originally used to express the relationship between pressure and surface coverage in gas adsorption:[17,19]

$$\theta = kC_p^{\frac{1}{n}} \quad (1.12)$$

In Equation 1.12, θ is surface coverage, k and n are empirical constants characteristic of the system at a given temperature, and C_p is the bulk solution concentration of the protein. If it is assumed that the heat of adsorption falls exponentially as adsorption proceeds and that the decrease in heat of adsorption is due to surface heterogeneity, the Freundlich isotherm may be derived theoretically.[17,19]

Young, Pitt and Cooper investigated the adsorption isotherms of seven different proteins on four biomaterials. Figure 2 shows the surface concentrations of fibrinogen adsorbed to Biomer, vs. time. They found that the data fit a Langmuir isotherm in the regime of low protein solution concentrations.[17] However, at higher adsorption levels the authors found multilayer adsorption and that different models had to be applied to describe the adsorption isotherms. Moreno et al.[20] showed that protein adsorption could be fit to a Langmuir model but questioned the significance of the parameters obtained. These studies are but two examples of the extensive literature available on protein adsorption modelling and indicate the controversy surrounding this complex issue. The reader is referred to a series of excellent reviews by MacRitchie,[2] Andrade,[3] Brash,[10] and Norde,[1] for more detailed information.

3. Protein adsorption onto biomaterials

Thought to be the initiating event in the whole series of subsequent cellular interactions which occur when a polymer is implanted in the body, protein adsorption has been studied in some detail

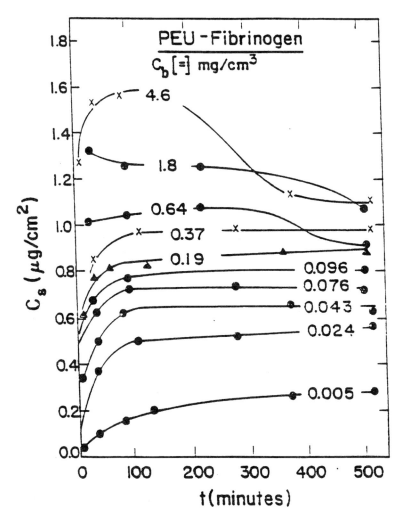

FIGURE 2 Fibrinogen adsorption to Biomer, surface concentration (Cs) vs. time. From: Young B. R., Ph.D. Thesis, University of Wisconsin – Madison, 1984.

over the last twenty years, particularly in the context of blood contacting applications. The proteins that are present in the blood in higher concentrations have been the most widely studied and are listed in Table 1. The molecular dimensions of proteins are 100–500Å. This is significant because many polyurethanes have the same order of magnitude of phase structure heterogeneity. Studies of protein adsorption have been focused on the identification of factors that determine the composition of a protein layer on a given surface. Adsorption from complex solutions such as blood plasma yield a protein layer of different composition than the fluid medium. Studies of the adsorption of the "big three" proteins, namely albumin, gamma-globulin (γ-globulin, IgG) and fibrinogen have dominated research into protein adsorption onto biomaterials. Albumin is the most abundant of the plasma proteins; it accounts for approximately half of the protein content of plasma. Its main functions are to maintain the colloidal stability of blood, act as a readily available protein reserve, and as a transport protein to carry bilirubin, lipids and hormones. It has been shown that the adsorption of albumin onto a polymer surface greatly improves its short term thromboresistance. Albumin is not a glycoprotein, and the lack of saccharide residues is thought to contribute to the lack of platelet adhesion to albuminated surfaces.[21] The preferential adsorption of albumin is

TABLE 1
Blood protein concentrations in plasma

Protein	Molecular weight	Concentration (g/l)
Albumin	66,300	35–55
Fibrinogen	340,000	2.0–4.5
IgG	150,000	8–18
IgA	150,000	0.9–4.5
IgM	900,000	0.6–2.5
IgE	190,000	2.5
α_2-Macroglobulin	760,000	1.6–3.7
C3	195,000	1.6
High Molecular Weight Kininogen	120,000	0.07–0.09
Fibronectin	450,000	0.3
Vitronectin	50,000	0.01
α_1-Lipoprotein (HDL)	200,000	3
β-Lipoprotein (LDL)	3200,000	1
Transferrin	79,500	2.0–4.0
More than 100 known minor proteins		<1

believed to reduce the extent of platelet interactions with the surface, improving the blood compatibility.[22–25] This observation has led to the development of materials that preferentially adsorb albumin, and materials that contain albumin molecules fixed to the surface.[25–27]

The adsorption of either gamma-globulin or fibrinogen onto a surface is considered to be unfavorable as the presence of these proteins has been correlated with increased platelet adhesion.[28–29] The globulins are a family of proteins with an antibody function, and play an important role in the host defence against infection. The adsorption of IgG promotes the platelet release reaction and thrombogenesis. IgG adsorbed onto a surface also may activate the classical pathway of complement.[30] Fibrinogen's most important function is the role it plays in thrombosis. During coagulation, two acidic residues are cleaved by thrombin from fibrinogen. Cleavage of these fibrinopeptides reveal polymerization sites on fibrinogen that will polymerize to form fibrin. Fibrinogen acts as a co-factor for the platelet release reaction and aggregation. Fibrinogen also is able to bind plasminogen, and "clump" *Staphylococcus aureus*, a strain of bacteria that is associated with infection of biomedical devices. The adsorption of fibrinogen greatly enhances thrombogenesis, and adsorbed fibrinogen has been shown to be adhesive for platelets. Large thromboembolytic events have been observed in a canine *ex vivo* shunt, on surfaces that were pre-adsorbed with fibrinogen.[31] The transient nature of fibrinogen adsorption, termed the Vroman Effect, has been widely studied, and this will be considered later in this chapter.

Other proteins that have been studied in the context of blood-material interactions include plasminogen, transferrin, lipoproteins, von-Willebrand factor and high molecular weight kininogen, although not all of these have been studied in detail in relation to adsorption onto polyurethane surfaces. Lipoproteins are macromolecular or micellar structures consisting of water insoluble lipids that are transported with specific proteins. Lipids include cholesterol, triglycerides and phospholipids. Each lipoprotein component has a characteristic density, and the presence of protein on the surface provides them with an electrical charge. Free fatty acids are transported by albumin. The proteins fibronectin and vitronectin are classified, like fibrinogen, as cell adhesive proteins, as they contain the RGD (Arg-Gly-Asp) peptide sequence that has been shown to be adhesive for platelets, and other cells including fibroblasts and endothelial cells. Albumin does not contain this tripeptide, but when grafted with a RGD residue, shows cellular adhesive activity comparable to fibronectin.[32]

Fibronectin is an adhesive glycoprotein that promotes the adhesion and spreading of platelets. Fibronectin can bind other substances present in blood, such as heparin, collagen and FXIIIa, and is incorporated into thrombi under physiological conditions. The many roles of this protein has stimulated interest with respect to hemocompatibility of biomaterials. It also has an affinity for, and associates with fibrinogen, although it has a greater affinity for fibrin. Vitronectin, also known as the complement S protein, is a multifunctional adhesive protein. It is able to bind heparin and participates in blood coagulation, in fibrinolysis and plays a role in the humoral system's response to invading organisms. Its role in the complement system of the blood is to protect the host cells from lysis by the membrane attack complex. Vitronectin also is adhesive to staphylococci and streptococci.[33]

B. COAGULATION SYSTEM

The coagulation system consists of a number of proteins that react in a cascade-like fashion,[9] and has been described as a biological amplifier with positive and negative feedback. The principal role of the coagulation system of the blood is to stabilize the platelet plug formed in the initial stages of hemostasis by the formation of a fibrin network from its precursor fibrinogen. Activation of the coagulation cascade can occur via one of two mechanisms; the intrinsic pathway, or the extrinsic pathway. The intrinsic pathway is activated on contact with surfaces such as glass or collagen. The extrinsic pathway is activated by tissue thromboplastin, or factor III (FIII), which is released into the blood on damage to blood vessels and surrounding tissues. Both activation mechanisms join a common pathway, terminating with the formation of the fibrin network. The system can be considered in three stages. The first is the generation of prothrombin activator (FXa), the second is the conversion of factor II (FII, prothrombin) to thrombin by the action of the prothrombin activator. The last step is the formation of fibrin from fibrinogen, (FGN, factor I, FI), catalyzed by thrombin. Fibrin formation is intimately related to platelet aggregation in the complex thrombus. Fibrin strands surround and link the platelet aggregates to stabilize the thrombus as it forms.

The intrinsic pathway also is referred to as contact phase activation. It is initiated by the actions of factor XII (FXII, Hageman factor), prekallikrein (PK) and high molecular weight kininogen (HMWK), when FXII contacts surfaces such as glass or collagen. FXII is activated to FXIIa, which acts as an enzyme, catalyzing the activation of factor XI (FXI) to FXIa. FXIa then acts in the presence of Ca^{2+} to activate factor IX (FIX). FIXa then activates FX, and at this stage the reaction proceeds along the common pathway. The common pathway commences with the activation of FX, which converts prothrombin (FII) to thrombin. Thrombin cleaves fibrinopeptides A and B from fibrinogen molecules, and the resulting fibrin monomers are then able to polymerize into a gel, forming the fibrin network required for the stabilization of the platelet plug. Thrombin and factor XIII (FXIII) stabilize the fibrin network by forming covalent bonds between fibrin molecules, essentially providing a crosslinked structure. An overview of coagulation is given in Figure 3.

C. FIBRINOLYTIC SYSTEM

The fibrinolytic system is responsible for the degradation of fibrin. The zymogen plasminogen is normally circulating in the blood and is activated to plasmin via the action of either FXIIa, tissue plasminogen activator (tPA), or urokinase. *In vivo*, plasminogen adheres to fibrin where it is activated and lyses the fibrin into smaller, more soluble polypeptides, termed fibrin degradation products. There are two primary pathways of plasminogen activation in blood, the extrinsic and the intrinsic. The extrinsic pathway is the more physiologically important; however, the intrinsic pathway is likely to be the pathway activated by blood contacting a biomaterial surface.[34-35] The fibrinolytic system is represented in Figure 4.

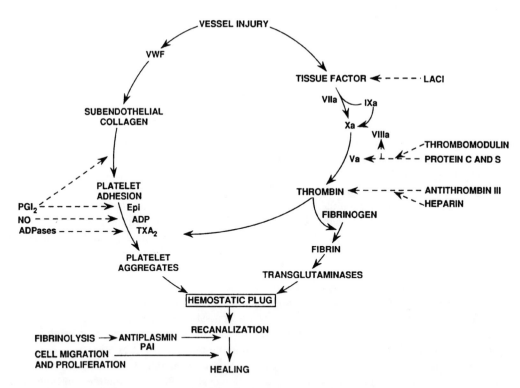

FIGURE 3 An overview of coagulation. The intrinsic and extrinsic pathways are shown. The extrinsic pathway is dominant under physiological conditions. Many of the enzymes of the extrinsic pathway require cell membranes for activation. From *Hemostasis and Thrombosis. Basic Principles and Clinical Practice.* R. W. Colman, V. J. Marder, E. W., Salzman, J. Hirsh. J. B. Lippincott Co., 1994. With permission.

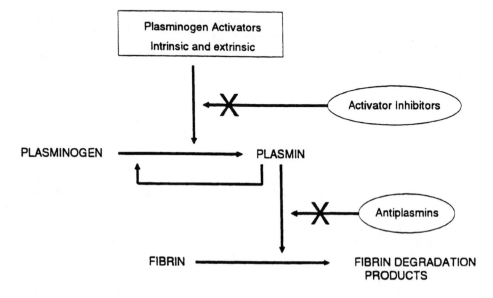

FIGURE 4 The fibrinolytic system. Adapted from Weitz, J. I. *Balliere's Clinical Haematology.* Woodhouse, K. A., Ph.D. Thesis, McMaster University, 1992.

III. CELLS, EXTRACELLULAR MATRIX AND CELLULAR INTERACTIONS

A. Platelets

Platelets are anuclear cells approximately 2-4μm in diameter. There are between 150,000 and 350,000 platelets per μl of blood, and they play an important role in thrombogenesis. Platelet reactions to vessel wall damage can be summarized as the induction of three responses, adhesion, release, and aggregation. Platelets are major participants in hemostasis and the induction of coagulation. Platelet adhesion and aggregation are thought to play an important role in thrombus formation on artificial surfaces *in vivo*. On contact with subendothelial collagen which is exposed on injury, the platelets undergo morphological changes, transforming from discoid cells to spherical structures with pseudopodia. Granules within the cell release a number of substances, including adenosine diphosphate (ADP), adenosine triphosphate (ATP), 5-hydroxytryptamine (5HT, serotonin), Ca^{2+}, platelet factor 4 (PF4), β-thromboglobulin (βTG) and fibrinogen. ADP induces other platelets near the site of injury to aggregate. A mass of platelets aggregate at the site of injury as a result, bridging the site of rupture.

Deposition of 70–100 platelets per 1000 μm^2 corresponds to a monolayer of platelets on artificial surfaces, depending on the degree of spreading. The platelets adhere via bridges of fibrinogen, for which there are receptors on the platelet surface. This crosslinking helps to strengthen the mass. In regions of low shear, low hydrostatic pressure or small discontinuities, the platelet plug alone may be sufficient to seal the rupture. However, in regions of higher hydrostatic pressure or high shear, reinforcement of the platelet plug is necessary to prevent the plug from being washed away. This reinforcement is one of the roles of the coagulation system. Platelet structure and function is represented schematically in Figure 5.

Platelet deposition onto artificial surfaces usually occurs after tens of seconds, when the protein layer is approximately 100–200Å deep.[36] The interaction of platelets with the artificial surface is influenced by the nature of the protein layer. Fibrinogen and γ-globulin have been shown to promote platelet adhesion,[22,28,37] whereas the presence of albumin on a surface can render it less thrombogenic by reducing the number of adherent platelets.[27,38] After deposition onto an artificial surface, platelets undergo morphological changes and release reactions as described above, flattening, degranulating, and extending pseudopodia. This is shown in Figure 6.

The rheological factors influencing platelet adhesion and interactions with foreign surfaces have been extensively studied *in vitro* by many investigators, including Turitto and coworkers.[39] These investigators found that at wall shear rates below 1000 s^{-1}, platelet adhesion is diffusion controlled, unless the surface adhesion reaction rate is very low or inhibited by a disease state.[40] At higher wall shear rates (>1000 s^{-1}) platelet attachment mechanisms dominate as the deposition rate is less than that predicted by diffusion.[41]

B. Erythrocytes

Erythrocytes, or red blood cells, are anuclear, biconcave disks approximately 8μm in diameter. The red blood cells constitute about 45% of the blood volume, averaging 5,000,000 cells per μl. The presence of red blood cells increases the frequency of collisions between platelets and the surface. In low shear regions, erythrocytes may become entrapped in the fibrin network, forming a red thrombus.[42] Red cells are believed to contribute only to its bulk, although Johnson has presented electron microscopic evidence that red blood cells participate actively in the formation of *in vitro* thrombi by undergoing hemolysis.[43] Their role in blood-materials interactions has not been intensively studied, but erythrocytes may interact with the surface, or influence the interaction of other

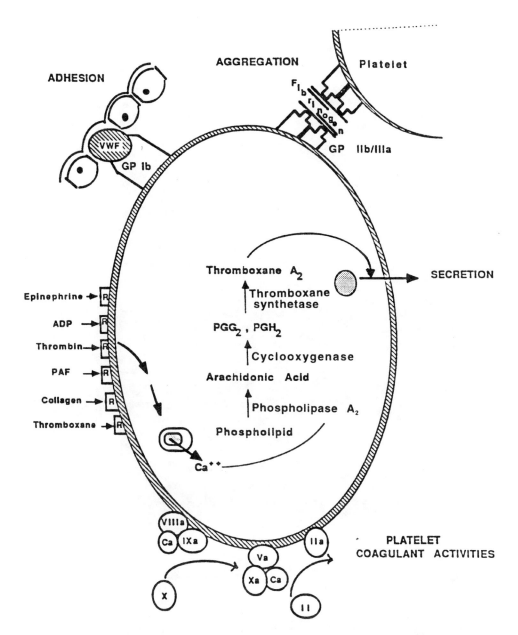

FIGURE 5 Platelet function. Adhesion to endothelial cells is mediated by Glycoprotein Ib (GPIb) which binds von Willebrand Factor (VWF) on the endothelial cells. Aggregation is mediated by glycoproteins IIb/IIIa (GPIIb/IIIa) bridged to GPIIb/IIIa on another platelet by fibrinogen. Various agonists, such as adenosine diphosphate (ADP) and platelet activation factor (PAF), are pictured as interacting with specific receptors. Mobilized intracellular Ca2+ leads to synthesis of thromboxane A2 (TXA2), which contributes to the stimulation and secretion of products of the granules. Platelet coagulant activity is generated by coagulation factors shown in Roman numerals: "tenase" (VIII, IXa, Ca2+) and "prothrombinase" (Va, Xa, Ca2+) form on the platelet external membrane phospholipid to convert prothrombin (II) to thrombin (IIa). Adapted from Rao, K., In Colman, R. W., Hirsh, J., Marder, V. J., Salzman E. W. For the sake of simplicity, only selected aspects of the platelet activation mechanisms are shown in this figure. Reproduced from *Hemostasis and Thrombosis. Basic Principles and Clinical Practice.* R. W. Colman, V. J. Marder, E. W, Salzman, J. Hirsh. J. B. Lippincott Co., 1994. With permission.

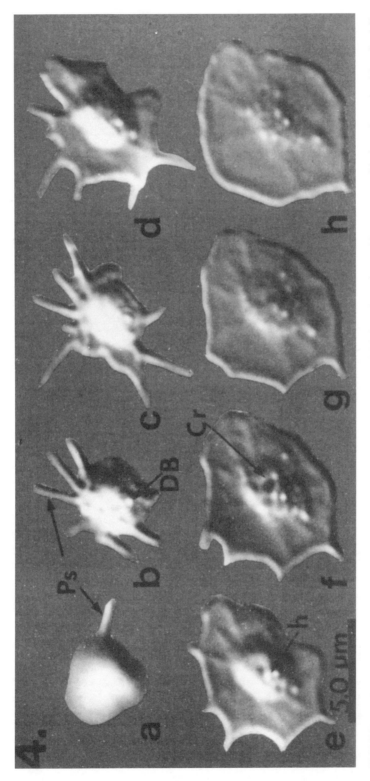

FIGURE 6 The same platelet at various stages in its transformation from a spheroidal form just after making contact with the substratum (a) to its fully spread form (h). The times at which micrographs were taken are 0,1,2,3,4,7,8, and 13 minutes for stages a-h. Structures visible include pseudopodia (Ps), dense bodies (DB) and craters (Cr). Note also some radial striations in the hyalomere of Figure 4h.

components with the surface. They interact with and adhere to the protein layer.[44] The presence of red blood cells in the contacting fluid has been shown to decrease the total amount of protein adsorbed onto artificial surfaces due to the deposition of red cell membrane components.[45] High shear flow may cause hemolysis; the released hemoglobin has a high affinity for surfaces,[46] and released ADP may activate platelets, promoting thrombus formation. Red blood cells also may influence the interaction of other components with the surface, such as platelets. Keller has studied flow-induced augmentation of platelet diffusion by red blood cells.[47] This enhanced diffusion effect is quite large and is a function of hematocrit (the fraction of the blood volume occupied by red blood cells).

C. Leukocytes

Leukocytes are the white blood cells. They provide the major defense against bacterial and fungal infection. Leukocytes can be divided into five classes; neutrophils, basophils, eosinophils, monocytes, and lymphocytes. They can be distinguished by morphological and staining characteristics. In a normal healthy adult, there are 4,000–10,000 white blood cells per μl of blood. Neutrophils, or polymorphonuclear leucocytes (PMNs) form the largest population — between 40 and 75%. The granulocytes (neutrophils, eosinophils and basophils) average 12–15 μm in diameter, and contain granular cytoplasm. They respond rapidly to chemotactic factors such as coagulation and complement factors, phagocytose invading organisms, and can migrate from the blood stream to the site of injury.

Basophils transition to mast cells when in the tissue. Mast cells reside in almost all vascularized peripheral tissue (especially the skin), and in the gastrointestinal and respiratory tracts. They have granules which contain inflammatory mediators including histamine, and have been implicated in hypersensitivity reactions, host response to parasites, nonspecific inflammatory responses, tissue remodeling and wound healing.[48] Mast cells produce and release a wide variety of multifunctional cytokines (cell messengers) including interleukins 1-6, granulocyte macrophage-colony stimulating factor (GM-CSF), and tumor necrosis factor (TNF-α). Their response to biomaterials has not been studied in detail. However, the rat peritoneal lavages used to isolate macrophages for *in vitro* investigation with biomaterials can contain a low level of mast cells.

Monocytes are slightly larger than granulocytes, 15–20 μm in diameter and are also phagocytes. They are produced in the bone marrow, remain in the circulation for approximately 12–32 days, and migrate into the tissue where they can remain for years as macrophages. Macrophages are multifunctional cells that can synthesize and release enzymes, and are able to replicate themselves *in situ*. In tissue, mature macrophages constitute what is now called the mononuclear phagocyte system and are present throughout connective tissue, around basement membrane, the lung, liver and lymph node sinuses. Macrophages are involved in inflammation, wound healing, and the immune response. They have been intimately associated with the foreign body response elicited by biomaterials.

Lymphocytes are the smallest of the leukocytes (6–20 μm in diameter). They are carried in the circulation to the tissue in response to an infection or foreign substance. There are two main types of lymphocytes, T-lymphocytes (T-cells) and B-lymphocytes (B-cells). These types in turn contain several different subclass of cells, each having different yet overlapping functions. B-cells are the antibody producing cells, where T-cells are involved in cell-mediated immunity. B-cells respond to the presence of antigen by differentiating into plasma cells and producing antibodies.[49-50] Each plasma cell produces a different antibody.

There are essentially four types of T-cells: (1) cytotoxic T-cells which are phagocytic and act directly to eliminate the foreign substance; (2) helper T-cells which enhance the immune response indirectly by secreting cytokines or interacting with other T-cells and B-cells through receptor binding to upregulate those cells. Helper T-cells signal the B-cells to divide.; (3) suppressor T-cells which downregulate the immune response; and (4) a cell that is involved in hypersensitivity reactions. In order for T-cells to be turned on and respond to a substance, the substance must be presented to them on the surface of another cell, usually a macrophage, in a very specific manner. Macrophages can digest very large pieces of the substance (antigen) and present them.

White cell responses to artificial surfaces are complex and include adhesion, aggregation, granule release, procoagulant and fibrinolytic activity and phagocytosis. The adhesion of leukocytes to artificial surfaces may occur through nonspecific phagocytosis, or through specific binding of cell receptors. Adhesion of leukocytes is often related to the inflammatory response. Leukocytes have been shown to adhere to polymer surfaces during clinical procedures such as hemodialysis,[51] hemofiltration,[52] cardiopulmonary bypass,[53] artificial heart implantation,[54] and leukopheresis.[55] Leukocyte alterations may result in the release of substances such as the superoxide radical, interleukin-1 (IL-1), interleukin-6 (IL-6), tumor necrosis factor (TNF) and platelet activating factor (PAF). Neutrophils and monocytes possess receptors for the anaphylatoxin C5a. White cell activation has been linked with complement activation during extracorporeal procedures.[51,56–57] Activated cells also adhere to the vascular surface and to each other, resulting in a drop in the white blood cell count. The interaction of leukocytes with an artificial surface also may induce changes in cell function. Damage to white cells can lead to impairment of phagocytic activities, and a reduced ability to combat infection.[58] White blood cells can adhere to fibrin in thrombus formation and contribute to platelet recruitment and fibrin formation. Granulocytes, and occasionally monocytes are also selectively incorporated into the thrombus.[59] White cells also participate in fibrinolysis through the release of enzymes.

Leukocyte adhesion to solid surfaces may be influenced by the surface free energy, hydrophilicity, chemistry, charge, protein adsorption, complement activation and adhesion of other cells, such as platelets. Morphological changes and release reactions can be observed when leukocytes interact with artificial surfaces, in a similar manner to alterations observed with platelets. Leukocyte function also appears to be sensitive to mechanical trauma. Exposure to shear stress can inhibit chemotactic responses and phagocytosis.[60]

D. THE EXTRACELLULAR MATRIX

In tissue, cells are contained in a support structure, the extracellular matrix. This matrix has a significant influence on the cellular response to injury, biomaterials, and general tissue health. It provides mechanical support for cells, modulates their growth, migration and differentiation, as well as influencing many aspects of wound repair. Its replacement after serious injury is extremely important. Although specific for the function of the tissue, generally the matrix is comprised of collagen and elastin fibers and a matrix of proteoglycans, solutes, water and other proteins.

Collagens are a family of related glycoproteins that have different forms, although all appear to share a triple helix within their structure. Different forms dominate in different tissues, for example, type I collagen is primarily found in the extracellular matrix of skin. Collagens are synthesized by fibroblasts and degraded by collagenases. Collagen fibers influence the mechanical properties of the tissue providing significant structural support.

Elastin is found in tissues requiring elastic recoil including the skin. Mechanically, elastin is extensible and can be stretched or deformed under an applied force. When the force is removed elastin will return to its undeformed state with very little hysteresis.[61] It is composed of two major components, a microfibrillar component and an elastin component. The microfibrillar component is made up of fibrillin, a microfibrillar associated glycoprotein (MAGP), a fibrillin-like glycoprotein, and other unknown molecules. It has been speculated that the microfibrillar component provides scaffolding for elastin deposition in the extracellular matrix, helping to align the elastin molecules and facilitate crosslinking *in vivo*.[62]

Glycosaminoglycans are another component of the extracellular matrix. They form an amorphous matrix supported by the collagen and elastin. They are usually found covalently linked to proteins, thus forming proteoglycans. The exception is the glycosaminoglycan hyaluronan. These proteoglycans along with the other nonfibrillar components such as fibronectin and laminin confer structural stability to the tissue, assist in water and solute balance, and influence cell adhesion, migration and differentiation via the interaction of cell membrane receptors with these matrix components.

E. CELL RECEPTORS AND MEDIATORS

There are many different structures and chemicals that influence the reactions of cells to injury, healing, each other and biomaterials. These include the cell receptors found on the cell membrane and the host of chemical and protein signals that result from cell-cell and cell-surface interactions.

1. Cell adhesion molecules

The interactions of cells with surfaces (including biomaterials) and with other cells are mediated by several different families of receptors.[63–66] Interest in adhesion receptors and their impact on biomaterial implants is growing in the research community because of the involvement of these receptors in wound healing, inflammation, and thrombogenesis. There are several different families of adhesion receptors. These families include: (1) Integrins which are involved in cell-cell and cell-surface interactions; (2) Members of the immunoglobulin superfamily which are involved in cell adhesion, particularly during wound healing and inflammation; (3) The LEC-cams that mediate white cell/endothelial cell adhesion; and (4) CD44, a leukocyte adhesion molecule responsible for lymphocyte binding to vascular endothelium.

The ligand/receptor binding that has been investigated most extensively, and in particular with polyurethanes (because of their frequent use in blood contacting applications), is the Arg-Gly-Asp (RGD) receptor binding sequence. The RGD peptide sequence is associated with the ligands fibrinogen, fibronectin and vitronectin and their binding to integrins such as the platelet glycoprotein gpIIb/IIIa receptor. Integrins appear to recognize certain amino acid sequences in their ligands (frequently extracellular matrix proteins). Not all integrins bind to the RGD containing parts of the matrix proteins such as fibrinogen and fibronectin and, in light of the potential of polymers to be used as substrates for tissue engineering and artificial organ development, significant research efforts are underway to explore interactions between surface-bound ligands and cell receptors.

2. Cytokines

Cells produce many polypeptide messengers called cytokines in response to stimulation or as a part of normal cell function. Nathan and Sporn define cytokines as "soluble (glyco)protein, non-immunologlobulin in nature, released by living cells of the host which act nonenzymatically in picomolar to nanomolar concentrations to regulate host cell function".[67] Cytokine functions frequently overlap and include stimulation of growth, cell differentiation and activation of functional responses of many of the protection systems within the body.[68–69] Certainly cytokine functions have implications for the interactions of biomaterials with tissues. Some cytokines and their known functions are listed in Table 2:

Many other families of molecules influence the interactions of cells. The reader is directed to the several fine books and articles on these topics for more details.[49–50, 63–67]

TABLE 2
Some cytokines: their sources and functions

Cytokine	Source	Function
IL-1 (13–17 kDa)	Macrophages Endothelium Keratinocytes Fibroblasts	Fibroblast collagen synthesis; T-and B-cell activation; acute phase response Induction of IL-6, IL-6, IFN-β1, GM-CSF; fever; induction of PEG_1, PEG_2 and cytokines by macrophage Induction neurophil and T-adhesion molecules on endothelial cells
IL-2 (15–5 kDa)	T-cells	Proliferation and differentiation of T, B, and LAK cells; activation of NK cells
IL-3 (28 kDa)	T-cells, NK cells, MC	Hemopoietic growth factor for myeloid, erythroid, and megakaryocytic lineage Mast growth
IL-4 (20 kDa)	T-cells, CD4 T, MC BM stroma	Proliferation and differentiation of B cells, isotype switching (IgE and IgG1), Proliferation of mast and T cell, antagonistic with IFN-γ Induction MHC class II and FcεR, IL-2R on T-cells Macrophage APC and cytotoxic function, macrophage fusion (migration inhibition)
IL-5 (45 kDa)	T-cells, CD4 T, MC	Proliferation and differentiation of B-cells and eosinophils; increased secretion of IgM, IgA and IgG from activated B-cells; expression IL-2R
IL-6 (23–30 kDa)	T-cells, MC, CD4 Macrophage, Monocytes Fibroblasts Endothelium	Acute phase protein; Proliferation and Ig secretion by activated B- and T-cell activating factor, and hemopoietic precursors
IL-7 (25 kDa)	Bone marrow stromal cells	Proliferation of large B, CD4 and CD8 cell progenitors, thymic maturation of T cells
IL-8 (14 kDa)	T cells, PMN Monocytes	T-cell chemotactic factor Neutrophils chemotactic and activated factor
IL-9	T-cells	Enhancing hemopoietic growth factor for Th, mast and erythroid cells (synergizes with IL-2, IL-3, and IL-4)
IL-10 (18 kDa)	T-cell, B-cells Monocytes/macrophages Keratinocytes	Immunosuppression: inhibits cytokine actions and expression, stimulates IL-1ra expression, stimulates proliferation of B-cells and mast cells
IL-11 (23 kDa)	Bone marrow stromal cells	Hemopoietic growth factor for megakaryocytes, myeloid progenitor cells, synergizes cytokines, stimulate acute cytotoxic activities of NK and LAK cells, growth factor for activated T-cells and NK cells
IL-12 (75 kDa)	B-lymphoblastoid cell line	Enhances cytotoxic activities of NK and LAK cells, growth factor for activated T-cells and NK cells
GM-CSF	T cells, MC, endothelium fibroblasts, macrophage	Proliferation and activation of granulocytes (PMN) and monocytes from bone marrow; macrophage colonies activates macrophage, neutrophils, eosinophils
G-CSF	Fibroblasts, endothelium	Growth mature granulocytes
M-CSF	Fibroblasts, endothelium epithelium	Growth macrophage colonies
TNF (17 kDa)	T-cells, NK Cells	Macrophage-activating factor (anti-microbial activity); giant cell formation; acts as a cofactor in the differentiation of cytolytic T-cells, B-cells and NK cells
TNF-α	Macrophage, T-cells	Tumour cytotoxicity
TBF-β	CD4 T-cells	Production of acute phase proteins Anti-viral and anti-parasitic activity Activation phagocytic cells Production several different cytokines

TABLE 2 (continued)
Some cytokines: their sources and functions

Cytokine	Source	Function
IFNα	Leucocytes	Anti-viral; expression MHC I
IFNβ	Fibroblasts	
IFNγ	T-cells (macrophage?)	Anti-viral; macrophage activation
		Expression MHC class I and II on macrophage and other cells
		Differentiation of cytotoxic T
		Synthesis IgG_2a by activated B
		Antagonism several IL/4 actions
TGF-β	T-cells, B-cells	Inhibition IL-2R upregulation and IL-2 dependent T- and B-cell proliferation;
		Inhibition (by TGF-β1) of IL-3 + CSF induced haematopoiesis
		Isotype switch to IgA
		Wound repair (fibroblasts chemotaxin) and angiogenesis
		Neoplastic transformation certain normal cells
CSIF	CD4 T-cell	Inhibits IFNγ secretion
LIF	T-cell	Proliferation embryonic stem cells without affecting differentiation
		Chemoattraction and activation of eosinophils

NK = natural killer cells; MHC = major histocompatibility complex; PG = prostaglandin; LAK = Lymphokine activated killer; APC =m Antigen helper cells; Th = T-helper cell; IFN = Interferon; G-CSF = granulocyte-colony stimulating factor; M-CSF = magrophage-colony stimulating factor

F. Hemostasis and Thrombosis

There are considered to be three phases of hemostasis; the constriction of blood vessels to reduce the blood flow, formation of a platelet plug, and the initiation of the coagulation cascade. Thrombosis is the formation of a thrombus or clot *in vivo*, and was first described by Virchow in 1846.[70] However, it was Welch who defined the thrombus as a "solid mass or plug formed in the living heart or vessels from constituents of blood."[71] *In vivo,* thrombi may form at sites where the endothelium of the blood vessel wall is damaged or in stagnation flow areas such as valve pockets or vein junctions.

In coagulation, erythrocytes and leukocytes may become entrapped within the thrombus. In regions of low shear, red cells adhere to fibrin to produce a red thrombus.[42,72] The entrapment of cells occurs to a lower extent in regions of high shear and a white, platelet rich thrombus results. The site of thrombus formation influences the composition of the thrombus. Arterial thrombi are formed in regions of high blood flow, and are composed predominantly of platelets, although a red tail of fibrin and red cells may be present. Thrombi formed under such conditions contain fewer entrapped red blood cells and are more compact than thrombi that form in slower venous currents.[73] Venous thrombi largely consist of fibrin, with red blood cells entrapped in the network. Thrombus formation and growth may lead to the total occlusion of the vessel with resulting stasis. Platelet aggregates or thrombi may be broken off by shear forces, or be removed from the surface through fibrinolytic mechanisms. These emboli can travel downstream, lodge in vital organs, and cause infarction of tissues.

Thrombosis also has been observed on artificial materials placed in contact with blood. During the 19th century, Hewson, Thackrah and Brücke postulated that the blood vessels exert a "vital or nervous principle" that prevents the blood from clotting in the human body. Further experiments and observations over time showed that blood components and the nature of the surface can influence the clotting process. A more recent view is that the nonthrombogenic nature of the endothelium is due to its ability to perform an active thromboresistant role.[9] This is in sharp contrast to, and beyond the capacity of artificial surfaces.

Virtually every physical and chemical characteristic of artificial materials has been suggested as being important in blood coagulation and thrombosis.[74] Surface properties that have been implicated in the blood compatibility of implant materials include surface charge, interfacial energy, albumin affinity, mobility, porosity, hydrophilicity, and surface texture.[75–78] Typically, these hypotheses have been developed based on empirical observations, where the relationship between blood compatibility and surface characterization of various polymers or families of polymers has been studied.

G. THE INFLAMMATORY RESPONSE

In response to injury, trauma, foreign material, or infection, the body initiates a series of interactions that result in the classic signs of inflammation: redness, swelling, heat, and pain.[69,79–84] Immediately after injury, the permeability of the blood vessels is altered, plasma is exuded into the wound, platelets aggregate, and several different biochemical pathways are initiated.[81,83] Wounds that do not create bleeding can still stimulate a local cellular inflammatory response.

Traditionally divided into acute and chronic stages, inflammation is a complex series of events involving different cells and biochemical pathways designed to contain or eliminate the cause of the injury and to begin tissue repair.[69,79–84] Acute inflammation precedes wound healing and is characterized by the presence of platelets, a fibrin matrix and white cell infiltrate. Chronic inflammation involves the presence of the macrophage and frequently results in pathological disruption of the tissue structure. The mediators of acute inflammation are shown in Table 3.

The early inflammatory phase is dominated by the influx of blood-borne cells and the subsequent release of their cytokines.[81] When tissue is injured, blood vessels are injured. The injury results in damage to the endothelial cells (cells lining the blood vessel) which exposes the underlying connective tissue components; proteins such as collagen, von Willebrand factor and fibronectin. Exposure of these elements triggers the adhesion and subsequent aggregation of platelets at the site of injury. Platelets in turn become activated and release a variety of products including cytokines and growth factors which lead to the infiltration of white cells into the site of injury.[85] The steps in white cell infiltration are illustrated in Figure 7.

In addition to platelet aggregation, activation of the platelets and exposure of the underlying subendothelium leads to coagulation, and subsequently the activation of fibrinolysis. The end product of coagulation, the fibrin clot, provides a matrix for the growing platelet clot, entrapment of the red cells, and the subsequent infiltration of macrophages and fibroblasts; cells involved in the events after acute inflammation.[86]

Leukocytes also play a dominant role in acute and chronic inflammation. PMNs appear very early in the process releasing products that modulate the inflammatory response. In addition, they are active phagocytes. During phagocytosis, the cells engulf the bacteria or foreign material (which may be a polymer fragment or wear debris) and "kill" or digest it through either an oxygen-dependent or oxygen-independent mechanism. These cells contain superoxide anions, hydrogen peroxide, hydroxyl radicals and a host of halogenating substances that are used for the oxygen dependent process. These substances also may contribute to the oxidative degradation of polyurethanes. The nonoxygen dependent mechanism appears to involve hydrolytic enzymes. Again, release of these enzymes also has been associated with polymer degradation *in vivo*. Neutrophils have been found in association with blood-contacting and soft-tissue applications implants.

Generally, neutrophils remain at the wound site for three–five days unless contamination occurs, which results in persistent neutrophil presence.[87] The granules of neutrophils contain enzymes, elastase and collagenase, that can degrade the extracellular matrix, removing dead tissue. These agents are released by the cell, not synthesized in the cell. This means that their production is

TABLE 3
Mediators of acute inflammation

Mediator	Origin	Actions
Histamine	Mast cells	Increased vascular permeability
	Basophils	Smooth muscle contraction
		Chemokinesis
5-hydroxy tryptamine (5HT)=serotonin	Platelets Mast Cells (rodents)	Increased vascular permeability Smooth muscle contraction
Platelet activating factor (PAF)	Basophils	Mediator release from platelets
	Neutrophils macrophages	Increased vascular permeability
		Smooth muscle contraction
		Neutrophil activation
Neutrophil chemotactic factor (NCF)	Mast cells	Neutrophil chemotaxis
IL-8	Lymphocytes	Monocyte localization
C3a	Complement C3	Mast cell degranulation
		Smooth muscle contraction
C5a	Complement C5	Mast cell degranulation
		Neutrophil and macrophage
		Chemotaxis, neutrophil activation
		Smooth muscle contraction
		Increased capillary permeability
Bradykinin	Kinin system (kininogen)	Vasodilation
		Smooth muscle contraction
		Increased vascular permeability
		Pain
Fibrinopeptides and fibrin breakdown products	Clotting system	Increased vascular permeability
		Neutrophil and macrophage
		Chemotaxis
Prostaglandin E2 (PGE2)	Cyclooxygenase pathway	Vasodilation
		Potentiate increased vascular permeability produced by histamine and bradykinin
Leukotriene B4 (LTB4)	Lipoxygenase pathway	Neutrophil chemotaxis
		Synergises with PGE2 in increasing vascular permeability
Leukotriene D4 (LTD4)	Lipoxygenase pathway	Smooth muscle contraction
		Increased vascular permeability

From Male, D., in *Immunology*, An Illustrated Outline, 2nd edition, Gower Medical Publishers, London, 1991, p. 79.

controlled; overproduction would result in tissue damage. Subsequent to these initial events, macrophages enter the injured area.

Like neutrophils, macrophages secrete a host of powerful inflammatory mediators including arachidonic acid metabolites, growth factors, cytokines and reactive oxygen intermediates (O_2^-, H_2O_2, OH^-). They scavenge foreign material and tissue debris and release factors which induce fibroblast and keratinocyte (skin cells) infiltration and proliferation.[81] Macrophages appear to play a pivotal role in "fine tuning" inflammation either up or down.

It is believed that the acute inflammatory phase is mediated by PMNs, and the chronic response by the macrophage. Generally, if the inflammatory stimulus is successfully removed during the acute response, tissue repair will begin. However, if not, as in the case of an implant, monocytes/macrophages continue to be recruited to the site. Here they also continue to secrete the

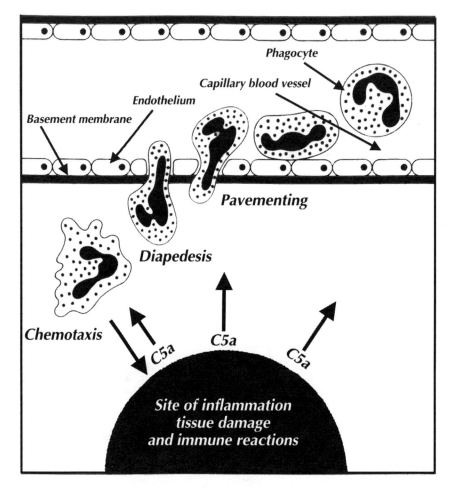

FIGURE 7 Stages of chemotaxis of white cells into the damaged tissue. From Male, D., Adapted from *Immunology: An Illustrated Guide*, 2nd edition, Gower Medical Publishers, London, 1991.

enzymes and other products that can ultimately cause significant tissue damage. Chronic inflammation is characterized by the presence of macrophages, some T-lymphocytes, increased vascular permeability, and the formation of granulation tissue. Granulation tissue is formed by fibroblasts and endothelial cells. Histologically it contains high levels of fibroblasts, macrophages and small blood vessels. It has a granular "look" and tends to be less ordered than normal tissue.

In the presence of a biomaterial, chronic inflammation differs from that found in wound healing or infection. Although granulation tissue is still formed, the cellular infiltration is different in both timing and type and the response is termed the foreign body response.

H. Foreign Body Response

It is possible that the concept of an acute inflammatory response followed by a chronic response may be too simplistic a model for biomaterial interactions with the body.[80,82] Anderson and others have shown that macrophages are present in the highest concentrations around an implant at the same time as the PMN concentration is highest.[79,82,88] This is different from the nonimplant case, where the macrophages follow the PMNs. Many investigators now use this phenomenon to differentiate between chronic inflammation and a foreign body response.

The typical foreign body response is characterized by the formation of granulation tissue and the presence of giant cells. The granulation tissue and granulatomous reactions associated with implants contain both epithelioid cells (flattened cells believed to be derived from macrophages), macrophages themselves, fibroblasts, and capillaries surrounded by a "cuff" of lymphocytes. Giant cells are believed to be formed from the fusion of many macrophages and/or epithelioid cells.[49,80] Macrophages and foreign body giant cells have been found attached to the surfaces of implanted materials.[82]

The foreign body response appears to depend on the surface of the implant. Smooth flat surfaces elicit a response which results in a few layers of macrophages; rough surfaces have both macrophages and foreign body giant cells present.[82] The response of the cells and the formation of granulation tissue generally results in the isolation of the material from the surrounding tissue through formation of a fibrous capsule.[79,82] The formation of a fibrous capsule is usually the end stage of healing in the presence of an implant, although again, this appears to be material and structure dependent. A schematic of the time variation in the acute inflammatory, chronic, granulation tissue development, and foreign body reaction to implanted biomaterials is illustrated in Figure 8.

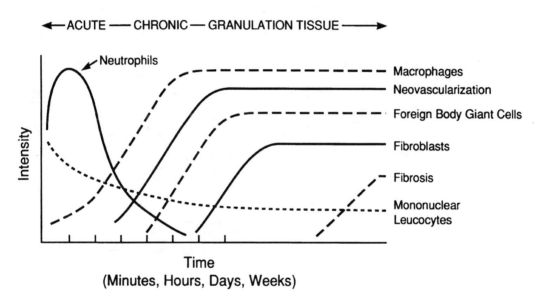

FIGURE 8 The temporal variation in the acute inflammatory response, granulation tissue development, and foreign body reaction to implanted biomaterials. Mechanisms of inflammation and infection with implanted devices. The intensity and time variables are dependent upon the extent of injury, the size, shape, structure and chemical and physical properties of the implant. Reprinted with permission from *Cardiovasc. Pathol* 2 Suppl. 3: J. M. Anderson, "Mechanisms of inflammation and infection with implanted devices 33S," 1993. Elsevier Science.

I. Wound Healing

In most situations where acute inflammation has been initiated, the body is trying to heal itself. Healing involves several different phases which involve inflammation, fibroblast proliferation, angiogenesis, wound contracture, scar contracture and epithelialization. The mechanisms vary slightly depending on the tissue. After the acute inflammatory response the following overlapping phases appear to occur.

1. Proliferation of fibroblasts

After injury, the normally quiet, sparsely distributed fibroblasts are activated to migrate into tissue. Here they proliferate and produce collage, elastin, and proteoglycans, constituents of the extracellular matrix (ECM).[89] They secrete cytokines which both upregulate and downregulate the healing response. The phase of healing associated with fibroblast secretion of collagen includes the influx of capillaries into the wound area. It is very similar to the granulation tissue formed in chronic inflammation; however, it differs in extent. It also is called the proliferative phase.

Angiogenesis (capillary growth and influx) also occurs in the proliferative phase to restore blood supply to the wound region. New vessel formation is stimulated by low oxygen tension, the presence of lactic acid (a cell metabolite), biogenic amines (produced by bacterial action), and growth factors released predominantly by macrophages.[87] The progression of wound healing in the dermal (inner) layer of the skin is shown in Figure 9. Gradually the wound becomes less cellular and the collagen is remodeled to increase the strength. Angiogenesis tends to be a very local phenomenon and stops once the wound has healed, although the exact mechanisms of its initiation and cessation are not known. Factors contributing to angiogenesis include growth factors, angiotensin and lack of oxygen.

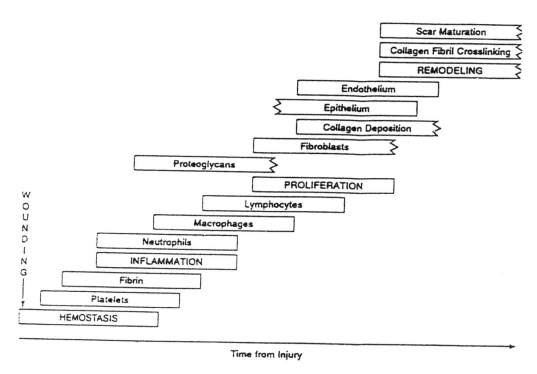

FIGURE 9 The progression of normal wound healing with time in the dermal region of skin. From Mast, B. A. *The skin. In Wound Healing: Biochemical and Clinical Aspects*. Eds. Cohen, I. K., Diegelmann, R. F., and Linbald, W .J., E. B. Saunders Co. Philadelphia, PA. Reproduced with permission.

2. Wound closure and scar contracture

Eventually the wound must close. The mechanisms by which this is accomplished are generated within the wound and collectively are termed wound contracture. Contracture results in the edges of wound being drawn toward the center. Some of the fibroblasts which have entered wound site alter their phenotype to become myofibroblasts which contain contractile proteins. The myofibroblasts then align along the lines of contraction and exhibit a unified contraction.[87] The amount of contraction varies with the depth of the wound and from species to species (less in humans).[81]

Wound contracture can be beneficial or produce large deformities impacting the function of the surrounding tissue. Usually smaller wounds that are not situated near joints close with relatively little deformation and damage. Contracture in larger wounds, whether internal or external is frequently problematic. The most familiar consequences of contracture are the disfiguring scars associated with extensive burns.

Polyurethane-based wound dressings and artificial skins are presently being designed to minimize the severe consequences of wound contracture in large wounds or wounds around joints. Materials that could mediate scar formation would be extremely beneficial to patient recovery and quality of life.

IV. IMMUNE RESPONSE

The immune system is designed to recognize foreign substances that may represent a threat to the body. The term immune response involves a variety of responses because of the complexity of the defense systems within the body. The immune response that is elicited by biomaterials, and specifically polyurethanes is the subject of ongoing research.

Generally, immune responses are defined as belonging to one of two types; innate or natural immunity and adaptive or acquired immunity. Classically the immune response has been divided into humoral and cell-mediated immunity. This division is becoming somewhat subjective because each "arm" of the immune response interacts with the other. For this discussion the nomenclature of Male,[49] and Roitt,[50] is used, which employs the terms innate and adaptive immunity. The components of each system are illustrated in Figure 10. As we learn more about the proection systems for our body, these divisions are becoming somewhat subjective, because each "arm" of the immune response interacts with the other.

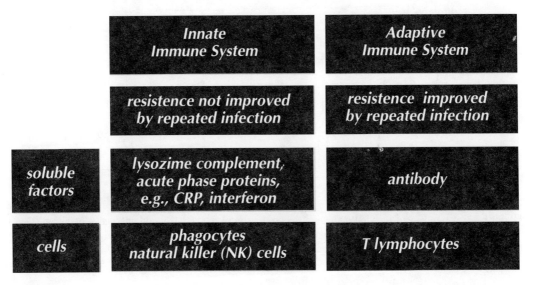

FIGURE 10 The innate and adaptive immune systems. Pg 47 Adapted from Male, D., in *Immunology: An Illustrated Guide*, 2nd edition, Gower Medical Publishers, London, 1991

A. INNATE IMMUNITY

Innate immunity is nonspecific, present in all individuals, provides the same response to any agent recognized as foreign, and does not improve with repeated exposures to the foreign substance (antigen). The innate system includes complement and its activation via the alternative pathway, phagocytes (white cells), and natural killer cells. It also includes the barrier systems of the body including the skin, and mucus membranes. These provide the first line of defense and do not distinguish between parasites, microbes or biomaterials.[49–50] Agents are recognized by the innate system by several different mechanisms including the opsonization (coating of the foreign substance in C3b or IgG) of abnormal surfaces, and through the chemoattractant mechanisms of C5a, another complement protein.

B. COMPLEMENT SYSTEM

The complement system is a collection of proteins that interact sequentially, usually after contact with antibody-antigen complexes, in order to lyse the membrane of the invading body and hence cause irreversible damage. The complement system regulates the immune response, facilitates opsonization and phagocytosis of invading species, and mediates the acute inflammatory response. Cleavage products of the complement pathway promote migration of leukocytes. Activation of the system occurs via one of two pathways, the classical pathway or the alternative pathway (Figure 11). The complement protein C3 plays a central role.

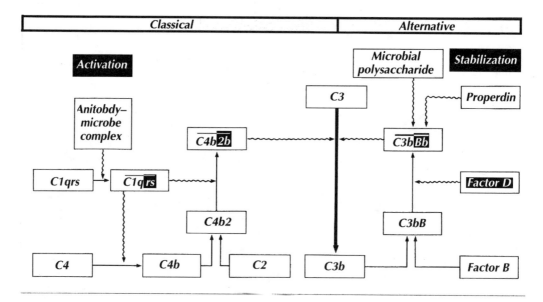

FIGURE 11 Complement reaction pathways. A comparison of the classical and alternative pathways. Generally the classical pathway requires antibodies and the alternative does not. The alternative may be activated by a biomaterial surface. Adapted from Roitt, I., *Essential Immunology*, 7th ed. Blackwell Scientific Publications, London, 1991.

The classical pathway is usually initiated by the presence of an antigen-antibody complex containing IgM or IgG. The alternative pathway involves the direct activation of C3.[90] Generally, complement activation by artificial surfaces is believed to occur through the alternative pathway, although this is not always the case. C3 is split into C3a and C3b, and in the presence of factor D, factor B is split into Ba and Bb. Bb binds onto the C3b fragment, which is stabilized by properdin (P). The C3bBbP complex is a C3 convertase, and fragments further C3 molecules. A further molecule of C3b can bind to the C3 convertase to produce the C5 convertase C3bBbP3b. However, if the C3b molecule associates with inhibitory factors H and I, formation of the C5a convertase is inhibited. Once C5 is cleaved; C5b binds to C6, C7, C8, and several C9 molecules to produce the terminal membrane attack complex (MAC). This can bind to cell walls resulting in cell destruction. Cleavage products C3a, C4a, and C5a are anaphylatoxins; C5a is the most potent. Anaphylatoxins are able to release histamine from mast cells and basophils, invoke contraction of smooth muscle and increase the permeability of capillaries. C5a also is involved in eliciting granulocyte responses, such as adhesion, aggregation, and the production of oxygen radicals, which can damage organ systems. It also can cause leukocytes to accumulate at sites of inflammation.[91]

Biomaterials, including polyurethanes have been shown to adsorb complement and activate it, producing C5a and C3b.[92] It is likely that biomaterials then trigger the innate immune system *in vivo*, and this is partially responsible for the foreign body reaction that is elicited. Complement also influences inflammation and cell-mediated immunity; however the mechanism is different from that of innate immunity and requires the antibodies, IgG or IgM, to initiate the classical complement cascade.[50,81,93-94] In the presence of the complement protein C5a, found at the injury site, neutrophil adhesion to endothelial cells is increased. Neutrophils recognize (among other stimulants for migration) complement proteins C3b and C3bi, as well as IgG. This may be important in the tissue response to polyurethanes. Monocytes are also attracted to the wound area by C5a.

C. Adaptive Immunity

Adaptive or acquired immunity is characterized by memory and specificity. It is specific for the antigen and improves on repeated exposure. Antigens are substances which are usually large (MW>4000–5000) and are foreign to the body, for example proteins. Specificity means that immunity acquired to one foreign substance (or organism) does not necessarily result in immunity to other substances. Memory results in the immune system being "primed" to recognize and mount a response to a substance which it has previously encountered, resulting in an accelerated and more effective elimination of that substance after the initial contact with the immune system.

The immune system accomplishes recognition, specificity and memory through a series of complex and interconnected interactions between cells that process and "present" antigen (usually macrophages), T-cells and B-cells which still are not fully understood. A very simplified overview of the two systems is shown in Figure 12.

Briefly, an antigen is processed by an antigen presenting cell (APC) which frequently is a macrophage. The processing provides the antigen in a form that can be recognized by B-cells and T-helper cells and the antigen is "presented" to them. The B-cell produces antibodies against that specific antigen under the influence of information from both the APC and the T-helper cell. The APC also can influence the T-helper cells to activate cytotoxic T-cells. As discussed previously, this subclass is phagocytic and can interact directly to eliminate the antigen. This overview is simplistic. How the cells react is dependent on the antigen itself, whether this is the first time the body has been exposed to the antigen, and the immune system of the individual. However, the hallmark of adaptive immunity is that the second time that a foreign substance evokes antibody and cellular responses these will be more rapid than the first time. Complement also influences cell-mediated immunity. However, the mechanism is different from that of innate immunity and requires the antibodies, IgG or IgM, to initiate the classical complement cascade.[50,81,93-94]

Traditionally, immunologists also have spoken about humoral and cell-mediated immunity. The inter-relationships between all four types is illustrated in Figure 13. The response of the immune system to biomaterials is controversial. Polyurethanes and other biomaterials do activate comple-

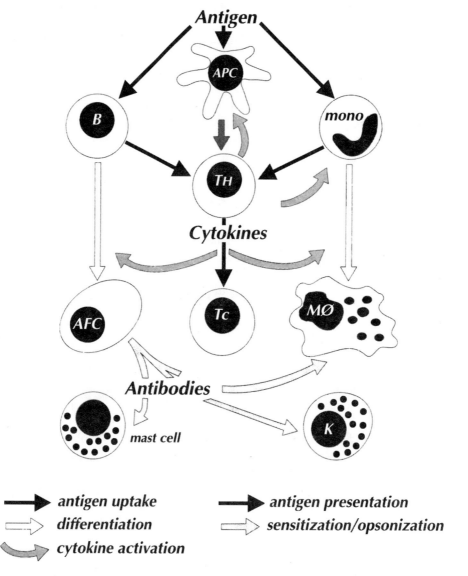

FIGURE 12 The cooperation between cells in the immune system including antigen presentation and cytokine production. AFC = antibody forming cells; APC = antigen presenting cells; TH = T helper cells; TC = cytotoxic T-cells; K = killer cells; MØ = macrophage. Adapted from: Male, D., *Immunology: An Illustrated Guide*. Gower Medical Publishers, London, 1991.

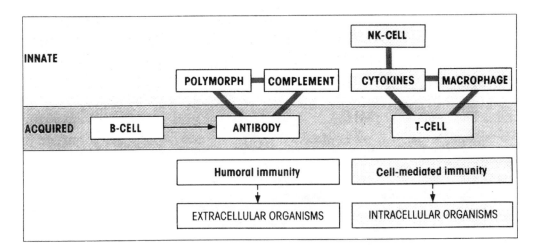

FIGURE 13 The two pathways linking innate and adaptive immunity. From: Roitt I. M. *Essential Immunology*. Blackwell Scientific Publications, Oxford, England, 1991. With permission.

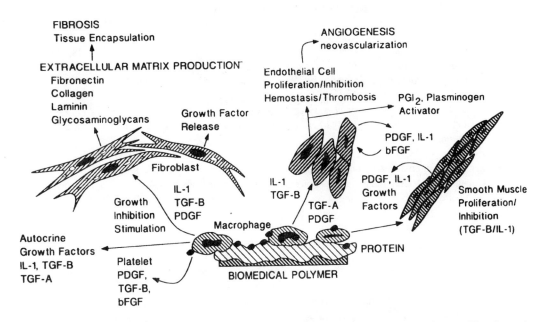

FIGURE 15 Polymer/protein/macrophage interfacial reactions leading to cellular activation, proliferation and synthesis. Cytokines and growth factors control cellular processes important in biocompatibility and the wound healing response. Reprinted with permission from *Cardiovasc. Pathol* 2 Suppl. 3: J. M. Anderson, "Mechanisms of inflammation and infection with implanted devices 33S," 1993. Elsevier Science.

ment. Therefore, an innate immune response can be evoked by implants. However, antigen processing and antibody production as a result of biomaterials in general and polyurethanes in particular has not been demonstrated and remains unproven *in vivo*.

Many of the possible interactions between the biomaterial/proteins/cells are illustrated in Figure 15. As our understanding of the interactions between materials and tissue increases, more details of the mechanisms involved will become known.

SUMMARY

The biological milieu is complex, aggressive and sophisticated in its response to damage and foreign substances. Implanting any biomaterial into this system and predicting the result is difficult. Significant amounts of research will need to be undertaken to design materials that can truly mimic and replace the various components of the body.

REFERENCES

1. Norde W. and Lyklema J. "Why proteins prefer interfaces." In *The Vroman Effect,* Ed. Bamford C. H., Cooper S. L., Tsuruta T. VSP, The Netherlands, 1992: 1.
2. MacCritchie F. "Proteins at interfaces." *Advances in Protein Chemistry,* 32:283, 1978.
3. Andrade J. D. "Principles of protein adsorption." In *Surface and Interfacial Aspects of Biomedical Polymers,* Ed. Andrade J. D. Plenum Press, New York, 1985: 1.
4. Gendreau R. M. and Jacobsen R. J. "Fourier transform infrared techniques for studying complex biological systems." *Appl. Spectr.,* 32:326, 1978.
5. Sato H., Kojima J., and Nakajima A. "Fibrinogen adsorption on artificial surfaces and its effect on platelets." *J. Disp. Sci. Tech.,* 14:117, 1993.
6. Baier R. E. "Key events in blood interactions at non-physiologic interfaces — a personal primer." *Artif. Organs,* 2:422, 1978.
7. Brash J. L. "Protein interactions with solid surfaces following contact with plasma and blood." In *Makromolecular Chemistry and Macromolecules Symposium.* 1988: 441.
8. Vroman L., Adams A. L., Klings M., Fischer G. C., Munoz P. C., and Solensky R. P. "Reactions of formed elements of blood with plasma proteins at interfaces." *Ann. N. Y. Acad. Sci.,* 283:65, 1977.
9. Szycher M. "Thrombosis, hemostasis and thrombolysis at prosthetic interfaces." In *Biocompatible Polymers, Metals and Composites,* Ed. Szycher M. Technomic, Lancaster, PA, 1983: 1.
10. Brash J. L. "Role of plasma protein adsorption in the response of blood to foreign surfaces." In *Blood Compatible Materials and Devices,* Ed. Sharma C. P., Szycher M. Technomic, Lancaster, PA, 1991: 3.
11. Mannhalter C. "Biocompatibility of artificial surfaces such as cellulose and related materials." *Sensors and Actuators B,* 11:273, 1993.
12. Lok B. K., Cheng Y. L., and Robertson C. R. "Protein adsorption on crosslinked polydimethylsiloxane using total internal reflection spectroscopy." *J. Coll. Interf. Sci.,* 91:104, 1983.
13. Cheng Y. L., Darst S. A., and Robertson C. R. "Bovine serum albumin adsorption and desorption rates on a solid surface with varying surface properties." *J. Coll. Interf. Sci.,* 82:217, 1987.
14. Silverberg A. "Modelling of protein adsorption." In *Surface and Interfacial Aspects of Biomedical Polymers,* Ed. Andrade J. D. Plenum Press, New York, 1985: 321.
15. Chan B. M. C. and Brash J. L. "Adsorption of fibrinogen on glass: reversibility aspects." *J. Coll. Interf. Sci.,* 82:217, 1981.
16. Norde W., MacCritchie F., Nowicka G., and Lyklema J. "Protein adsorption at solid-liquid interfaces: reversibility and conformational aspects." *J. Coll. Interf. Sci.,* 112:447, 1986.
17. Young B. R., Pitt W. G., and Cooper S. L. "Protein adsorption on polymeric biomaterials 1: Adsorption isotherms." *J. Coll. Interf. Sci.,* 124:28, 1988.
18. Moore W. J. *Physical Chemistry.* (4th Ed.): Prentice Hall, New Jersey, 1972.
19. Thomson S. J. and Webb G. *Heterogeneous Catalysis.* John Wiley & Sons, New York, 1968.
20. Moreno E. C., Kresak M., Kane J. J., and Hay D. I. "Adsorption of proteins peptides and organic acids from binary mixtures onto hydroxyapatite." *Langmuir,* 3:511, 1987.
21. Lee R. G. and Kim S. W. "The role of carbohydrate in platelet adhesion to foreign surfaces." *J. Biomed. Mater. Res.,* 8:393, 1974.
22. Mustard J. F., Glynn M. F., Nishizawa E. E., and Packham M. A. "Platelet-surface interactions: relationship to thrombosis and haemostasis." *Fed. Proc.,* 26:106, 1967.
23. Young B. R., Lambrecht L. K., Cooper S. L., and Mosher D. F. "Plasma proteins: their role in initiating platelet and fibrin desposition on biomaterials." In *Biomaterials: Interfacial Phenomena and Applications,* Ed. Cooper S. L., Peppas N. A. Adv. Chem. Ser. 199, 1982: 317.

24. Young B. R., Doyle M. J., Collins W. E., Lambrecht L. K., Jordan C. A., Albrecht R. M., Mosher D. F., and Cooper S. L. "Effect of thrombospondin and other platelet alpha-granule proteins on artificial-surface induced thrombosis." *Trans. Am. Soc. Artif. Intern. Organs,* 28:498, 1982.
25. Munro M. S., Eberhart R. C., Maki N. J., Brink B. E., and Fry W. J. "Thromboresistant alkyl derivatized polyurethanes." *ASAIO J.,* 6:65, 1983.
26. Joseph G. and Sharma C. P. "Prostacyclin immobilized albuminated surfaces." *J. Biomed. Mater. Res.,* 21:937, 1987.
27. Engbers G. H. M. "An *in vitro* study of the adhesion of blood platelets onto vascular catheters." *J. Biomed. Mater. Res.,* 21:613, 1987.
28. Packham M. A., Evans G., Glynn M. F., and Mustard J. F. "The effect of plasma proteins on the interaction of platelets with glass surfaces." *J. Lab. Clin. Med.,* 73:686, 1969.
29. Zucker M. B. and Vroman L. "Platelet adhesion induced by fibrinogen adsorbed onto glass." *Proc. Soc. Exp. Biol. Med.,* 131:318, 1969.
30. Uchida T., Hosaka S., and Murao Y. "Complement activation by polymer binding IgG." *Biomaterials,* 5:381, 1984.
31. Silver J. H., Lin H.-B., and Cooper S. L. "Effect of protein adsorption on the blood-contacting response of sulphonated polyurethanes." *Biomaterials,* 14:824, 1993.
32. Kishida A., Takatsuka M., and Matsuda T. "RGD-albumin conjugate: expression of tissue regeneration activity." *Biomaterials,* 13:924, 1992.
33. Preissner K. T. "The role of vitronectin as multifunctional regulator in the hemostatic and immune systems." *Blut,* 59:419, 1989.
34. Walker I. D. and Davidson J. F. "Fibrinolysis." In *Blood Coagulation and Haemostasis,* 1988: 208.
35. Weitz J. I. "Mechanism of action of the thrombolytic agents." In *Bailliere's Clinical Medicine,* Bailliere Tindall, 1990: 583.
36. Baier R. E. *Applied Chemistry at Protein Interfaces.* Vol. 145. American Chemical Society, Washington, DC, 1975.
37. Young B. R., Lambrecht L. K., Albrecht R. M., Mosher D. F., and Cooper S. L. "Platelet-protein interactions at blood-polymer interfaces in the canine test model." *Trans. Am. Soc. Artif. Intern. Organs,* 29:442, 1983.
38. Mosher D. F. "Influence of proteins on platelet-surface interactions." In *Interaction of the Blood with Natural and Artificial Surfaces,* Ed. Salzman EW. Marcel Dekker, New York, 1980: 85.
39. Turitto V. T., Weiss H. J., and Baumgartner H. R. "Rheological factors influencing platelet interaction with vessel surfaces." *J. Rheology,* 23:735, 1979.
40. Weiss H. J., Baumgartner H. R., Schopp T. B., and Turitto V. T. "Interaction of platelets with subendothelium." *Ann. N. Y. Acad. Sci.,* 283; 293, 1977.
41. Turitto V. T., Muggli R., and Baumgartner H. R. "Physical factors influencing platelet deposition on subendothelium: importance of blood shear rate." *Ann. N. Y. Acad. Sci.,* 283; 284, 1977.
42. Bruck S. D. *Properties of Biomaterials in the Physiological Environment.* CRC Press, Boca Raton, Florida, 1980.
43. Johnson S. A. "Role of blood vessels in thrombosis." In *11th Cong. International Dictionary of Haematology,* Ed. Blight VC. Sydney, 1966: 133.
44. Feijen J. "Thrombosis caused by blood-surface interaction." In *Artificial Organs,* Ed. Kenedi R. M., Courtney J, M., Gaylor J. D. S, Gilchrist T. MacMillan, London, 1977: 235.
45. Brash J. L. and Uniyal S. "Adsorption of albumin and fibrinogen to polyethylene in the presence of red cells." *Trans. Am. Soc. Artif. Intern. Organs,* 22:253, 1976.
46. Uniyal S. and Brash J. L. "Patterns of adsorption of proteins from human plasma onto foreign surfaces." *Thromb. Haemostas.,* 47:285, 1982.
47. Keller K. H. "The dynamics of the interaction of cells with surfaces." In *Interactions of the Blood with Natural and Artificial Surfaces,* Ed. Salzman EW. Marcel Dekker, New York, 1981: 119.
48. Gordon J. R., Burd P. R.. and Galli S. J. "Mast cells as a source of multifunctional cytokines." *Immunol. Today,* 1:458, 1990.
49. Male D. *Immunology: An Illustrated Guide.* Gower Medical Publishers, London, UK, 1991.
50. Roitt I. M. *Essential Immunology.* Blackwell Scientific Publications, Oxford, England, 1991.

51. Craddock P. R., Fehr J., Dalmaso A. P., Brigham K. L., and Jacob H. S. "Hemodialysis leukopenia: pulmonary vascular leukostasis resulting from complement activation by dialyzer cellophane membranes." *J. Clin. Inv.,* 59:879, 1977.
52. Bohler J., Dramer P., Gotze O., Schwartz O., and Scheler F. "Leukocyte counts and complement activation during pump-driven and arteriovenous haemofiltration." *Contr. Nephrol.,* 36:15, 1983.
53. Zimmerman G. A. and Armory D. W. "Transpulmonary polymorphonuclear leukocyte number after cardiopulmonary bypass." *Am. Rev. Respir. Dis.,* 126:1097, 1982.
54. Ryhanen P., Eleyva E., Hollman A., Naolinen R., Pihlajanieme R., and Saarela E. "Changes in peripheral blood leukocyte counts, lymphocyte subpopulations and *in vitro* transformation after heart valve replacement." *J. Thorac. Cardiovasc. Surg.,* 77:259, 1979.
55. Wright D. G. and Klock J. G. "Functional changes in neutrophils collected by filtration leukopheresis and their relationship to cellular events that occur during adherence of neutrophils to nylon fibers." *Exp. Hematol.,* 7:11, 1979.
56. Ringoir S. and Vanholder R. "An introduction to biocompatibility." *Artif. Organs,* 10:20, 1986.
57. Sundaram S., Courtney J. M., Taggart D. P., Tweddel A. C., Martin W., McQuiston A. M., Wheatley D. J., and Lowe G. D. O. "Biocompatibility of cardiopulmonary bypass: influence on blood compatibility of device type, mode of blood flow and duration of application." *Int. J. Artif. Organs,* 17:118, 1994.
58. Kusserow B., Larrow R., and Nichols J. "Perfusion and surface induced injury in leukocytes." *Fed. Proc.,* 30:1516, 1971.
59. Poole J. C. *Structural Aspects of Thrombosis.* Athlone Press, London, 1964.
60. Dewitz T. S., McIntire L. V., Martin R. R., and Sybers H. D. "Enzyme release and morphological changes in leukocytes induced by mechanical damage." *Blood Cells,* 5:499, 1979.
61. Viidik A. "Age-related changes in connective tissues." In *Lectures on Gerontology: On Biology and Aging,* Ed. Viidik A. Academic Press, New York, 1982: 173.
62. Mecham R. and Davis E. "Elastic fiber structure and assembly." In *Extracellular Matrix Assembly and Structure,* Ed. Yurchenco P. D., Birk D. E., Mecham R. P.. Academic Press, San Diego, CA., 1994: 281.
63. Hynes R. O. "Integrins: A family of cell surface receptors." *Cell,* 48:549, 1987.
64. Albelda S. M., Buck and A. C. "Cell Adhesion Molecules." *Fed. Am. Soc. Exp. Biol. J.,* 4; 2868, 1990.
65. Humphries M. J. "The molecular basis and specificity of integrin-ligand interactions." *J. Cell Sci.,* 97:55, 1990.
66. Patarroyo M. "Adhesion molecules mediating recruitment of monocytes to inflamed tissue." *Immunobiol.,* 191:474, 1994.
67. Nathan C. and Sporn M. "Cytokines in context." *J. Cell Biol.,* 113:981, 1991.
68. Shepard R., Rhind S., and Shek P. N. "Exercise and the Immune System." *Sports Med.,* 18:341, 1994.
69. Baruch A. B., Michiel D. F., and Oppenheim J. J. "Signals and receptors involved in recruitment of inflammatory cells," *J. Biol. Chem.,* 270:11703, 1995.
70. Virchow R. "Ueber die akute Entzudung der arterien." *Arch. Pathol. Anat.,* 1:272, 1846.
71. Welch W. H. "Diseases of blood vessels: Thrombosis." In *A System of Medicine,* Ed. Allbut T. D.. MacMillan, 1969, New York, 1899: 279.
72. Brash J. L. "Mechanism of adsorption of proteins to solid surfaces and its relationship to blood compatibility." In *Blood cOmpatible Polymers, Metals and Composites,* Ed. Szycher M. Technomic, Lancaster, 1983: 35.
73. French J. E. "Thrombosis." In *General Pathology,* Ed. Florey H. Saunders, Philadelphia, 1962: 234.
74. Andrade J. D., Nagaoka S., Cooper S. L., Okano T., and Kim S. W. "Surfaces and blood compatibility — current hypotheses." *Trans. Am. Soc. Artif. Intern. Organs,* 33:76, 1987.
75. Nagaoka S., Mori Y., Tanzawa H., Kikuchi Y., Inagaki F., Yokota Y., and Hoishiki Y. "Hydrated dynamic surfaces." *Trans. Am. Soc. Artif. Intern. Organs,* 33:76, 1987.
76. Cooper S. L. "Protein adsorption and preadsorption." *Trans. Am. Soc. Artif. Intern. Organs,* 33:78, 1987.
77. Okano T. "Surface morphology and microstructures." *Trans. Am. Soc. Artif. Intern. Organs,* 33:80, 1987.
78. Kim S. W. "Pharmaceutically active surfaces." *Trans. Am. Soc. Artif. Intern. Organs,* 33:82, 1987.

79. Ziats N. P., Miller K. M., and Anderson J. M. "*In vitro* and *in vivo* interactions of cells with biomaterials." *Biomaterials,* 9:5, 1988.
80. Anderson J. M. "Inflammatory response to implants." *Trans. Am. Soc. Artif. Intern. Organs,* 34:101, 1988.
81. Wahl L. M. and Wahl S. M. "I'nflammation, Wound healing:Biochemical and Clinical Aspects." In Eds. Cohen K., Dieglemann R. F., Lindblad W. J. W.B. Saunders Co., Philadelphia, 1992. (Authors check reference 81.)
82. Anderson J. M. "Mechanisms of inflammation and infection with implanted devices." *Cardiovasc. Pathol.,* 2:33S, 1993.
83. Baumann H. and Gauldie J. "The acute phase response." *Immunol. Today,* 15:74, 1994.
84. Zitelli J. "Wound Healing for the Clinician." *Adv. Dermatol.,* 2:243, 1987.
85. Gentry P. "The mammalian blood platelet: Its role in haemostasis, inflammation and tissue repair." *J. Comp. Path.,* 107:243, 1992.
86. Zitelli J. A. "Synthetic skin." *Adv. Dermatol.,* 4:323, 1989.
87. Kirsner R. S. and Eaglestein W. H. "The wound healing process." *Dermatol. Clinics,* 11:629, 1993.
88. Williams D. F. "Biocompatibility, an overview". In *The Concise Encyclopedia of Medical and Dental Materials,* Ed. Williams D. F. Pergamon Press, Oxford, UK, 1991.
89. Jordana M., Sarnstrand B., Sime P. J., and Ramis I. "Immune-inflammatory functions of fibroblasts." *Eur. Respir. J.,* 7:2212, 1994.
90. Law S. K. A. and Reid K. B. M. *Complement.* IRL Press, 1988.
91. Chenoweth D. E. "Complement activation produced by biomaterials." *Trans. Am. Soc. Artif. Intern. Organs,* 32:226, 1986.
92. Remes A. and Williams D. F. "Immune response in biocompatibility." *Biomaterials,* 13:731, 1992.
93. Colten H. R. "Tissue-specific regulation of inflammation." *J. Appl. Physiol.,* 72:1, 1992.
94. Quintans J. "Immunity and inflammation: The cosmic view." *Immun. Cell Biol.,* 72:262, 1994.

7 Protein, Cellular and Soft Tissue Interactions with Polyurethanes

I. INTRODUCTION

Protein interactions, thrombus formation, and platelet interactions are intimately involved in tissue interactions with materials. The human body's natural response to tissue injury is inflammation and wound healing. Implanting a biomaterial also results in inflammation; however this differs in several important features from that typically encountered in tissue damage. Although recent advances in biology, immunology, and biochemistry have increased our understanding of the tissue response to a biomaterial, the mechanisms still are not well understood. This chapter details the events that are involved in the biological response to a polyurethane including protein adsorption, blood and soft tissue interactions and immunologic complications. As the discussion of the biological interactions of polyurethane proceeds, reference will be made to the various types of tests used to evaluate these interactions. These are outlined below.

II. ASSESSMENT OF HOST-BIOMATERIAL INTERACTIONS

It is accepted that there is a need for new or improved biomaterials in clinical medicine. Information from clinical studies of devices is often limited in usefulness to the biomaterials scientist, partly due to the lack of adequate information about the materials used, but also due to the many factors in the clinic that can influence the final performance of the device. Researchers acknowledge the complexity of the biological responses, the integrated nature of the blood response, and the interrelationships between blood and tissue responses. Many test methods have been developed to investigate the biological responses to synthetic materials. As yet, there is no generally accepted test procedure for the investigation of biological responses to biomaterials, contrasting with the relatively well defined protocols that exist for the determination of mechanical properties. Many biological tests have been developed by investiagors involved in biomaterials research, and described in the literature. Some of these have been adapted directly from clinical hematological tests. Tests can be divided into four categories: *in vitro, ex vivo, in vivo* and clinical. Different tests are employed to study blood and tissue interactions. A brief discussion of the mthods is provided below.

A. IN VITRO TESTING

In vitro experiments involve the isolation of biological media from a suitable source, and its use in the laboratory. *In vitro* tests have an advantage as they are relatively inexpensive, rapid and versatile, when compared with other methods of evaluation. The laboratory environment also allows a greater control over experimental variables such as time and temperature than in other tests. The greatest limitation of *in vitro* tests is that the systemic response cannot be assessed. Furthermore, the relationship between data collected *in vitro* and clinical performance has not been established. However, *in vitro* tests are useful for screening during biomaterial development. *In vitro* methods also are playing an increasingly important role in performing controlled studies of the biological response to artificial surfaces, in the expectation that fundamental information on such interactions will facilitate the design of biomaterials with improved performance.

In vitro assessment of tissue compatibility employs cell, tissue and organ culture techniques. Cells or tissues are contacted with either the material, or extracts or eluates of the material under investigation. There are many variables that need to be considered when performing tests, such as the cell line or source of tissue, the medium used to incubate the cells and the physical form of the material, or nature of material extracts to be tested.[1,2] Furthermore, many cell responses may be inhibited *in vitro*, due, in part, to the lack of stimulating agents.

In the evaluation of blood compatibility, human blood is usually used, and options exist for the utilization of blood, plasma, serum or other less complex contact media, including suspensions of blood cells such as platelets. *In vitro* tests can be used as preliminary screening tests for the pre-selection of materials for further development in biomedical applications, or to conduct more detailed mechanistic studies into the blood response. Tests can be static or dynamic, depending on the absence or presence of blood flow respectively. Static tests involve the incubation of a finite amount of blood with the test surface. Analysis of the nature of the blood or the surface is then made, to determine any changes. Dynamic tests employ blood flow and are generally used to study cellular interactions,[3-5] although studies of protein activation under different shear rates also have been performed.[6] It has been shown that experimental conditions such as contact area, flow regime, method of anticoagulation and temperature can influence the blood response.[4,6-12] Such factors must be considered when conducting and assessing such studies. The main disadvantages of *in vitro* tests are the difficulties of obtaining fresh blood, the use of anticoagulants to prolong the "shelf life" of the blood, and contact with materials other than the test sample.

B. Ex Vivo Testing

Ex vivo studies are relevant to the study of blood-biomaterial interactions. *Ex vivo* procedures involve the extracorporeal contact of blood with the test material.[9,13-16] Blood usually flows directly onto or through the test piece. Blood contact may be single pass, where the blood is not returned to the donor, or recirculation, where the material is contained within a closed loop and the blood is returned to the donor. The presence of flow allows the study of thrombus formation and embolization, and the degree of occlusion of the test circuit. Although a single pass human *ex vivo* procedure has been reported,[9,16] animal models are predominantly used, which introduces differences between the hematological profiles of the respective model and human subjects.[17,18] Subhuman primate models are preferred for such studies, as this reduces the hematological and evolutionary differences. However, this is not always practical, on the grounds of the relative scarcity of such models and high cost. Canine and rabbit models have therefore been employed more widely, in such studies. Canine models are considered sensitive models for thrombus formation as the adhesion of canine platelets to biomaterials is significantly higher than human platelets. Therefore, studies in a canine model are considered to present a worst case scenario. Most *ex vivo* studies have examined protein adsorption, platelet deposition, or thrombus formation. Figure 1 shows a schematic of a canine *ex vivo* experiment.[15]

C. In Vivo Testing

The main purpose of *in vivo* tests is to evaluate the safety and biocompatibility of a device.[19] *In vivo* procedures generally involve the implantation of a section of test material into an animal followed by the subsequent explantation after a fixed period of time. Generally, the acquisition of short term data and continuous appraisal of a specific device is difficult. The site chosen for implantation depends on the intended use of the material. Materials also can be assessed in functional tests. This is more common in the testing of materials for cardiovascular and orthopedic applications. These can be more challenging technically, as miniature devices, appropriate for implantation into small animals, must be fabricated. The use of animal models makes correlation

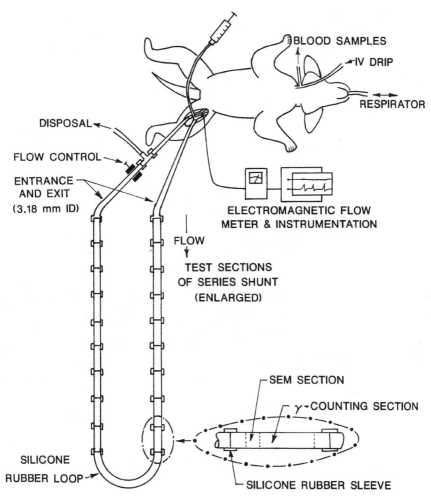

FIGURE 1 Schematic of canine *ex vivo* shunt experiment, showing catheter, instrumentation and shunt construction (enlarged).

of data to the human clinical application difficult, as different species have different hematological profiles.[17]

In vivo tissue responses to biomaterials involve the implantation of a sample of the material into an animal model. Many tissue tests involve the implantation of the material in a specific geometry into a nonfunctional site in an animal model. Apart from the inter-species differences impeding interpretation of the tissue response to a material, factors such as the size and location of the implant, and the surface chemistry and geometry also may influence the response.

In vivo tests for materials intended for cardiovascular use include the Vena Cava Ring Test,[20] and the Renal Embolus Test.[21] The degree of blood compatibility is generally based on the degree of thrombus formation. Thrombi can embolize and be transported to other sites by the circulating blood, and therefore, the apparent lack of thrombus formation on a surface does not necessarily infer that the material is blood compatible.[22] Patches of the test material also can be fabricated and implanted into the vascular system,[23] overcoming the technical difficulties in producing a small scale version of the final device.

D. CLINICAL EVALUATION

Clinical evaluation is the most relevant assessment of the biocompatibility of a material in a given application. Codes of conduct, ethical considerations and the perceived value of trials limit the extent and scope of clinical trials. In addition, the utilization of biomaterials in cardiovascular applications generally requires the presence of an anticoagulant, in order to maintain blood fluidity. Factors such as the device in which the material is used, the mode of application of the device, the disease state of the patient, and the use of pharmaceutical agents, including anticoagulant therapy may influence the performance of a material in the clinic.[24]

E. GUIDELINES FOR BIOLOGICAL TESTING OF MATERIALS

Development of medical devices requires that materials and devices are tested prior to clinical use, in order to evaluate the safety of the implant. The guidelines for evaluation have been produced by a number of organizations worldwide, and are constantly being modified and updated. In 1964, the National Institutes of Health (NIH) in the United States, initiated a biomaterials program, and in 1980, the NIH published two documents, outlining procedures for the physicochemical characterization and investigation of blood-materials interactions.[25,26] These guidelines were updated as the field expanded, with documents published in 1985,[27] and 1993.[28] In 1987, agencies in the United States, Canada and the United Kingdom compiled the Tripartite Biocompatibility Guidance for Medical Devices. The Tripartite document does not refer to specific tests, but recommends aspects of tests that should be considered. In 1990, the ASTM developed ASTM F748,[29] which presented a matrix of tests for the biological evaluation of materials and devices. Most recently, the International Standards Organization have produced a matrix of tests for the evaluation of materials.[30] This document gives guidance for testing, rather than defining specific tests, and is presented in 12 parts. Aspects of material testing are recommended on the basis of the intended application.

III. PROTEIN ADSORPTION ONTO POLYURETHANES

The investigation of protein adsorption to artificial surfaces has been significant in biocompatibility research. A large part of this research has been focused on glass, silicone rubber, and hydrogel surfaces. Protein adsorption studies on polyurethane surfaces have been relatively limited. Some studies have been carried out exclusively on polyurethanes in order to gain a better understanding of the effect of polyurethane surface chemistry or surface architecture on protein adsorption. Other studies have incorporated a polyurethane as one of many surfaces evaluated.

Radiolabeling, using ^{125}I, is generally the technique of choice for measuring protein adsorption, although immunochemical techniques also have been used. The use of FTIR–ATR to study protein adsorption in general, and adsorption to polyurethanes specifically, is becoming more widely used. For example, Bellissimo and Cooper studied albumin and fibrinogen adsorption using a flow cell where one surface was coupled to a thin film of Biomer coated on an ATR–IR crystal.[31] Albumin and fibrinogen absorption bands could be followed using this technique without flushing the system to take a measurement. Pitt et al. refined the technique and applied it to other polyurethanes.[32-34] Such studies have shown that the wall shear rate can influence the quantity of protein adsorbed, and the subsequent desorption of the protein.

Protein adsorption studies on polyurethanes have focused primarily on the adsorption of albumin, fibrinogen and the γ-globulins. Since albumin "passivates" while fibrinogen or γ-globulin "activates" surfaces, some investigators have studied competitive adsorption from mixed solutions, and have used albumin/fibrinogen or albumin/γ-globulin adsorption ratios as indicators of blood compatibility. The general consensus appears to be that these ratios are higher on polyurethanes than on other more thrombogenic surfaces such as glass, polyethylene, or polyvinylchloride, supporting the passivation/activation hypotheses. Kinetic adsorption data for fibrinogen, albumin, and γ-globulin from a mixed solution on an MDI/ED/PPO(1025) polyetherurethane urea showed that fibrinogen adsorption was greater than albumin adsorption and that albumin adsorption was more rapid and higher on the polyurethane than on the other polymer surfaces.[35] Brash et al. observed that albumin was adsorbed more rapidly on a hydrophilic PEO-based urethane than on a more hydrophobic PPO-based urethane.[36] More recently, it also has been reported that protein adsorption to polyurethanes containing polyethylene oxide soft segments is lower than on polyurethanes containing polytetramethylene oxide (PTMO) soft segments,[37] and other macroglycols.[38] Groth et al. have reported that plasma protein adsorption to polyurethane surfaces *in vitro* increases as the hard segment content increases.

The most complex protein solution used to study protein adsorption is blood. *In vivo* or *ex vivo* protein adsorption studies are clearly more difficult to design, perform and analyze than *in vitro* studies. Lyman et al. were among the early investigators to study blood contact in 9- to 10-mm ID recirculation polyurethane tubes anastomosed end-to-end to the descending aorta in dogs.[39] Adsorbed proteins were eluted from exposed surfaces using the detergent Triton-X 100 and proteins analyzed by polyacrylamide gel electrophoresis. Polyurethane surfaces studied include Biomer tubing and polyurethaneureas based on PPO which were coated on glass. Recirculation times were between 1 and 45 min. The urethane materials appeared free of thrombi. Electrophoretic analysis showed that Biomer and the 1025 m.w. PPO-based urethane, which were relatively nonthrombogenic, adsorb mostly albumin with small amounts of the globulins. The 710 m.w. PPO-based urethane was more thrombogenic and comparable to silicone rubber and Teflon surfaces, and adsorbed smaller amounts of albumin relative to the globulins. These results complement data from *in vitro* studies described earlier.

Experiments investigating protein adsorption have been performed in a canine *ex vivo* shunt, by Cooper and coworkers.[14,40-42] Sections of the test material are inserted into an aterio-venous (A-V) shunt as the animal is dosed with a quantity of radiolabeled protein and cells. The adsorption of blood components onto the test sections was then monitored over time. Generally, a peak in adsorption of fibrinogen and platelets was observed that was associated with the formation of thrombi, and subsequent embolization. Fibrinogen deposition was lowest on the more thromboresistant extruded Biomer surface,[40] in agreement with the results of Lyman et al.[39] In another set of experiments, the desorption of pre-adsorbed, radiolabeled fibrinogen, albumin, and γ-globulin was measured on Biomer, silicone rubber and PVC.[14] A time-dependent response over two hours of blood contact was observed. Biomer showed a high binding capacity of all three proteins; however, the initial fibrinogen levels were much lower than on the other more thrombogenic surfaces.

A. ALBUMIN

As discussed in previous sections, the adsorption of albumin onto glass surfaces has been shown to passivate the surface with respect to platelet adhesion and spreading. This property of the protein has been explored by modifying surfaces to either contain bound albumin, or to preferentially adsorb albumin from blood or plasma. Although protein molecules can be grafted onto a synthetic polymer, stability problems may arise in the long term. Albumin molecules directly grafted onto a surface are susceptible to denaturation and proteolysis by circulating enzymes, which may deactivate the protein and cause the surface to lose the desired passivating effect. Recently, Ryu et al. immobilized albumin onto a polyurethane substrate. *In vitro* studies showed a reduction in fibrinogen adsorption compared to the unmodified polyurethane. When tested *ex vivo* in a rabbit A-A shunt, the occlusion time was extended to 150 minutes, compared to 50 minutes for the untreated polyurethane, implying enhanced thromboresistance.[43]

Alkyl chains have been grafted onto polyurethane surfaces in order to promote albumin adsorption. Such a strategy is based on the hypothesis that since albumin transports fatty acids in the blood, alkyl chains grafted to a surface should provide a means of promoting albumin adsorption. Eberhart et al.[44] grafted aliphatic chains of 16-18 carbon atoms to adsorb and provide a regenerating layer of albumin. Adsorption of albumin onto the alkylated surfaces was enhanced and more rapid than on the unmodified polyurethane. Albumin adsorbed onto alkylated surfaces also was less susceptible to desorption by fluid shear and chemical means. Pitt et al. have used alkyl chain derivatized polyurethanes to show that the desorption rate of albumin decreased as the alkyl chain length increased from 2 to 18 methylene groups.[33] *Ex vivo* studies on alkylated materials have shown a short term improvement in blood contacting properties.[45] Polyurethane grafted with C_{18} chains reduced fibrinogen deposition and platelet deposition in an *ex vivo* canine shunt compared to the control polyurethane.[33,46] Adsorption to both the grafted and control polyurethanes was enhanced when delipidized albumin was used. Implantation studies of an alkylated polyurethane in a canine model showed improved thromboresistance.[47]

Keogh and Eaton have shown that Pellethane modified with a dextran-cibacron-blue adduct selectively and reversibly binds albumin.[48] Although the amounts of albumin adsorbed onto the modified and unmodified materials are similar, the grafted material shows greatly enhanced clotting times when compared with the unmodified material in an *in vitro* Chandler Loop test. No thrombi were observed after 16 hours of contact. Bacterial adhesion to the surface also was shown to be reduced. The reduction in adhesion of *S. epidermidis* was even greater after the surface was exposed to albumin. The researchers have proposed that this approach to bind albumin overcomes the problems associated with alkyl grafts, such as the hydrophobic nature of the alkylated surface, which may induce denaturation of the protein.

B. Fibrinogen

The adsorption of fibrinogen onto biomaterial surfaces is of interest, owing to the protein's role in mediating cellular responses, and as a coagulation protein. It has been postulated that it is not necessarily the amount of the protein that is adsorbed onto a given surface that is important, but also the conformation of the adsorbed protein. The precise conformation of a protein is partly determined by the length of time that the protein has resided on a surface. Fibrinogen has been shown to be less elutable by sodium dodecylsulfate from polyurethane surfaces as time increases.[49] The change in elutability may result from increased strength in the protein-surface bond. The increase in bond strength also may give rise to the reduced reactivity of the protein. Reduction in the α-helicity of fibrinogen desorbed from polyurethane surfaces, as well as from glass, has been reported.[50] Evidence of conformational changes has been provided by observing reductions in the levels of antibody binding with time.[51] Similar observations have been made on Biomer.[52] Large thromboembolytic events have been observed on surfaces pre-adsorbed with fibrinogen, and tested in a canine *ex vivo* shunt.[53,54]

Conflicting results exist concerning the effect of hard segment and soft segment domains on protein adsorption, which has extended to the study of fibrinogen adsorption. Several workers have reported that fibrinogen interacts with the hard segment,[55] and that the hard segment is a determinant of the thrombogenicity of polyurethane materials.[37,41] It also has been observed that as the hard segment concentration at the surface increases, the surface becomes less attractive to proteins.[51] The soft segment chemistry also has the capacity to influence adsorption. Fibrinogen adsorption was found to be increased on a polyurethane cast onto glass compared with the same material cast onto polyethyleneterephthalate. The authors explained this difference as arising from an increase in the soft segment polyether component at the surface of the polyurethane cast on glass.[56] An increase in polyether segments at the surface also has been reported to reduce the surface free energy and in turn reduce protein adsorption.[57] PTMO may adsorb more fibrinogen than a PEO soft-segment polyurethane, but these *in vitro* results do not correlate with *ex vivo* platelet interaction with the same materials, which demonstrated that the PEO polyurethane was more thrombogenic.[38,58] The molecular weight of the soft segment also has been shown to affect artificial surface induced thrombosis, which may be related to the degree of microphase separation in the bulk polymer. Fibrinogen, albumin and fibronectin have been observed to preferentially adsorb to the soft segment domains of a PEO polyurethane.[38]

Further *ex vivo* series shunt evaluations of polyetherurethaneureas,[42] solvent extracted polyetherurethanes,[59] polyetherurethanes modified with polydimethylsiloxane macroglycols,[60] and polyurethanes synthesized from nonether/nonester polyols,[61] have been published. For the polyurethaneureas, phase separation appeared to be a determinant for fibrinogen deposition (clearly observed with PPO and PTMO-based polyurethanes). Contrary to expectations, the surface properties and fibrinogen deposition on solvent extracted polyurethanes were minimally affected by the extractions. However, the data for the polyetherurethanes modified with PDMS showed that despite the variation in surface properties, fibrinogen deposition was not affected by the modifications. The PDMS based polyurethanes exhibited the lowest levels of fibrinogen deposition.

Lelah *et al.* examined *ex vivo* fibrinogen deposition on a series of polyurethanes of different hard-segment concentrations, chain extenders, soft segment polyethers, and soft segment molecular weights. This was followed by an evaluation of a series of polyurethane ionomers, including an anionomer, cationomer, and zwitterionomer.[62] Fibrinogen deposition was determined by ^{125}I-labeled fibrinogen. Extensive surface characterization was conducted on these polymers. In these studies, at early times (half minute of blood contact) a peak in fibrinogen deposition was observed, attributable to fibrinogen turnover at the polyurethane interface. A second fibrinogen peak, observed at 15 to 20 minutes of blood contact, occurred in parallel with a platelet deposition peak on all surfaces studied. Fibrinogen deposition was higher on a polyurethane cast from DMA than from THF. Fibrinogen deposition was observed to depend on both the hard and soft segment components and compositions. Fibrinogen deposition (and platelet deposition) was lowest on the high soft segment content urethane and on the anionomer and zwitterionomer.

Horbett, Ratner, and colleagues, have used a baboon model to study exposure of polymers to blood *in vivo*, and have focused on fibrinogen adsorption to various surfaces including Biomer, Pellethane, Renathane, Erythrothane, and Superthane.[63,64] They found that surface polarity correlates with a second stage of fibrinogen deposition that could be inhibited by heparin.[63] The pre-adsorption of plasma,[64] and albumin,[65] affected the adsorption of fibrinogen *in vivo*, the elutability of the adsorbed fibrinogen, the position of the platelet and fibrinogen deposition maxima, and altered antibody and platelet binding to the exposed surfaces. The authors have suggested that the adsorbed fibrinogen undergoes time dependent conformational changes which render it less reactive toward platelets and antibodies, and less elutable.

The presence of processing additives in commercially available polyurethanes may affect the protein adsorption profile of the polymer. The presence of Methacrol, an amphiphilic additive used in the manufacture of Biomer may reduce protein adsorption levels when compared with the additive-free polyurethane.[66] Reduced protein adsorption also was observed on a Biomer type polyurethane sample that contained an acrylic polymer additive when compared with the unmodified sample.[67] Reduced α-antisera deposition onto ethanol-extracted Pellethane compared to Pellethane also has been reported. Hari and Sharma have reported that external lubricants such as calcium stearate and silicone fluid may increase fibrinogen adsorption.[68]

Fibrinogen adsorption onto sulfonated polyurethanes has been the focus of recent investigation. Polyurethanes containing sulfonate ionic groups appear to adsorb high amounts of fibrinogen when tested *in vitro*,[69,70] and *ex vivo*.[71] This enhanced affinity is believed to be a direct effect of the sulfonate groups. Furthermore, the protein does not appear to be displaced by other blood proteins in a Vroman sequence of events.[72-74] Despite the high fibrinogen concentration at the surface in an *ex vivo* canine shunt, platelet deposition and thrombus formation onto these materials is reduced. Sulfonation has been reported to confer a degree of thromboresistance to a surface. This provides further support for the hypothesis that the conformation of an adsorbed protein is more important in determining subsequent events than the type of protein.[75,76]

C. Fibronectin

Fibronectin is believed to be a highly mutable protein, a property which may allow maximal interaction between the protein and the surface. Fibronectin also has the ability to multimerize which facilitates multi-layer adsorption; it is possible that under such circumstances, protein-protein interactions will dominate subsequent events, rather than the protein-surface interactions. Zilla *et al.* precoated polyurethane surfaces with fibronectin to affect the proliferation of endothelial cells.[77] Other researchers have reported that adsorption of fibronectin was greater on a PTMO containing polyurethane than a polyurethane containing PEO, although the fibronectin was eventually displaced from the surface by other proteins present in the plasma. Pitt *et al.*, using an FTIR–ATR technique, observed that adsorption of fibronectin occurred more rapidly onto a polyurethane with PDMS in the soft segment than on a PEO-polyurethane.[78] The total amount of protein adsorbed after 120 minutes correlated with the adsorption kinetics. Greater conformational changes were observed on the PDMS polyurethane sample than on the other two materials studied. Adsorption of fibronectin also has been shown to favor thrombogenesis.[53,54,76] The presence of either intact or fragmented fibronectin has been implicated in promoting adhesion of *S. aureus* to polyurethane catheters.[79]

D. Vitronectin

Adsorption of vitronectin onto a polyurethane surface has been shown to increase the number of adherent platelets, and to increase the degree of shape change in attached cells.[80] The incubation time of vitronectin with the surface was shown to affect the thrombogenicity of the protein.[80] Exposure of polymeric materials to a quaternary mixture of albumin, fibrinogen, fibronectin and vitronectin, revealed that vitronectin adsorption was enhanced on the polyurethane surfaces, at a higher ratio than present in the contacting solution. Vitronectin adsorption did not appear to be strongly influenced by surface wettability since it adsorbed equally well to hydrophilic and hydrophobic surfaces.

E. Lipoproteins

The adsorption of lipids to polyurethane surfaces, and absorption of lipids into the material have been associated with biodegradation phenomena and environmental stress cracking of polyurethane implants.[81] Possible interactions between lipoproteins and the microdomains of a polyurethane surface may facilitate their adsorption. Absorption into the bulk may then follow, affecting the mechanical properties. Studies by Takahara *et al.* of the adsorption of phosphatidylcholine and cholesterol on polyurethanes of differing soft segment chemistry also demonstrated that lipids are adsorbed onto the surface and into the bulk.[82] The more hydrophilic PEO segment was associated with higher adsorption of phosphatidylcholine. Competitive adsorption studies between phosphatidylcholine and cholesterol revealed that the more hydrophobic cholesterol was selectively adsorbed to the more hydrophobic polyurethanes.

F. Coagulation System

Evaluation of coagulation by measuring clotting times is based on the premise that a less thrombogenic material produces an extension of the clotting time. Polyurethanes have performed well in comparison to other biomaterials, and studies show that the clotting times are comparable to, or better than, those of silicone rubber. There appears to be little difference between the clotting times of the blood exposed to different polyurethanes.[83] The adsorption of coagulation proteins, particularly those involved in the contact phase of coagulation, is an aspect of protein adsorption relevant to thrombus formation on artificial surfaces. The main interest in the system has focused upon the interactions of FXII, high molecular weight kininogen (HMWK), FXI and prekallikrein (PK). Van der Kamp and van Oeveren have shown that the amounts of kallikrein and activated FXII generated by polyurethanes are much lower than on glass, although once again, only small differences between different polyurethanes were observed.[84]

Attempts to circumvent the thrombogenicity of artificial surfaces have involved the grafting of heparin, a naturally occurring anticoagulant, on to polymer surfaces. Heparin catalyses the neutralization of thrombin and FXa by antithrombin III (AT III). Polyurethanes have been heparinized,[85,86] and other molecules such as PEO and albumin have been incorporated as spacer arms, to enhance the effect of the heparin.[87-89] In vitro studies of these materials have shown reduced protein deposition and platelet adhesion, and increased occlusion times ex vivo. Thrombomodulin, a protein sythesized by the vascular endothelium that inhibits coagulation, also has been used to moderate the action of thrombin.[90] Sulfonated polyurethanes have been shown to possess anticoagulant properties.[69] The presence of alkyl chains on the surface can alter the protein adsorption profile, favoring the adsorption of albumin, and thus reduce the thrombogenicity of polyurethane surfaces.[45]

G. Fibrinolytic System

Although little attention has been paid to alterations in fibrinolytic activity imposed by contact with artificial surfaces, polyurethanes have been shown to adsorb plasminogen from plasma. The amount of plasminogen adsorbed is increased when the polyurethane is sulfonated, or derivatized with lysine.[91] Fibrinolytic agents such as urokinase,[92] and lumbrokinase,[93] also have been used to promote fibrinolytic activity on polyurethane surfaces. Studies have shown reduced platelet adhesion to these modified surfaces in vitro. It is possible that the reduction in platelet adhesion results from the degradation of fibrinogen by the fibrinolytic agent, which effectively reduces the number of binding sites for platelets. Lumbrokinase grafted materials also have been shown to increase the occlusion time in A-A shunts ex vivo, when compared with the unmodified polyurethane.[94]

H. Complement System

Complement activation induced by polyurethanes has not been as widely studied as it has been for other biomaterials considered for blood contacting applications. Generally, polyurethanes have been shown to be low activators of complement when compared to other materials, such as regenerated cellulose.[95-97] Coating the lumen of PVC blood tubing with polyurethane has been shown to reduce C3a generation.[98] Variations in polyurethane structure also can influence the degree of complement activation. Increasing amounts of oxyethylene units in the polymer has been shown to increase the complement hemolytic activity.[99] The grafting of sulfonate groups onto the polyurethane has been shown to reduce C3a generation in vitro,[100] although it was proposed that the observed reduction in C3a measurements in the fluid phase is due to the adsorption of the cationic C3a fragment onto the polyurethane surface. Complement activation in vitro also has been shown to be reduced on alkylated surfaces.[97,101]

I. The Vroman Effect

The composition of the adsorbed protein layer deposited from plasma or a multi-component protein solutions is time-dependent with respect to composition.[102] The most widely studied compositional change of the protein layer adsorbed from plasma has been termed the "Vroman Effect". This phenomenon first was reported by Vroman & Adams,[102] who found that although fibrinogen was adsorbed from plasma onto glass in the initial course of events, it was later "converted" and could no longer be detected. This "conversion" was actually the displacement of adsorbed fibrinogen by high molecular weight kininogen (HMWK), a low abundance protein with a higher affinity than fibrinogen for the glass surface (Figure 2).[103] The majority of studies of the Vroman Effect have been conducted on glass. It is now believed that the Vroman Effect is only part of a sequence of protein deposition and displacement; the proteins adsorb to the surface according to an order that is determined by their relative concentration and transport rates in the blood, and displaced by

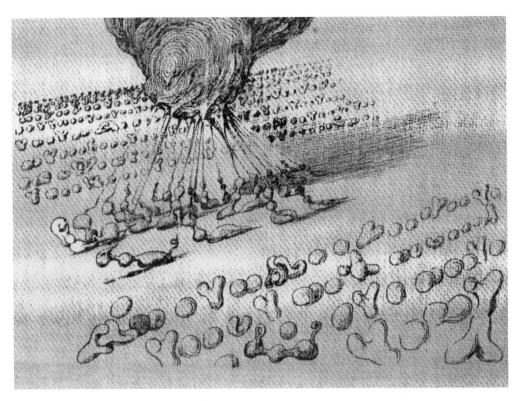

FIGURE 2 Concentrations and activities of plasma proteins related to platelet adhesion. An audience of 500 albumin molecules and 250 globulin molecules watches passively as 25 molecules of adsorbed fibrinogen (shown as rather flexible players, each consisting of 3 spheres on a rod) attract a platelet (the balloon floating above them), while a single high molecular weight kininogen molecule (white, carrying a molecule of Factor XI) disengages one fibrinogen molecule from the glass-like field. The proportions of albumin:globulins:fibrinogen:HMWK are approximately 500:250:25:1. From Vroman L. Protein/surface interaction. In *Biocompatible Polymers, Metals and Composites,* Ed. Szycher M. Technomic, Lancaster, PA, 1983.

lower concentration proteins with higher affinity for the particular surface. Albumin, the most abundant protein, adsorbs first and unless the surface has a high affinity for this protein over the other proteins present, albumin will be replaced with IgG, then fibrinogen, and HMWK.[104] It is expected that other trace proteins in the blood are also adsorbed and replaced, and the sequence of adsorption and replacement will terminate when a minimum in surface free energy is achieved.[105] Investigations into the Vroman Effect on polymer surfaces have involved studies of the maximum in fibrinogen adsorption that is observed on a surface upon plasma dilution, and the surface concentration of fibrinogen against time. Some results are shown in Figures 3 and 4. The observed maximum is material dependent and it should be noted that differences in the concentration at which maximum protein adsorption occurs to a given material have been reported.[64] Maximum fibrinogen adsorption onto polyurethane surfaces occurs at a 0.5-1.0% plasma solution;[52,74,106] for glass it is 1%, for polyethylene, 0.1%, and for Teflon, 10%.[63] Both the observed displacement of fibrinogen from glass by HMWK and the unusual concentration dependence of fibrinogen adsorption from plasma can be explained in terms of mass action effects. The competition between proteins for binding sites on a surface increases as the number of vacant binding sites decreases.[107]

The Vroman Effect also has been observed from blood, and limited studies suggest that adsorption and displacement phenomena are similar in blood and plasma. *In vitro* studies have shown that the presence of cells does not influence fibrinogen adsorption from plasma, so it is likely that the Vroman Effect occurs *in vivo*. The desirability of the Vroman Effect in relation to

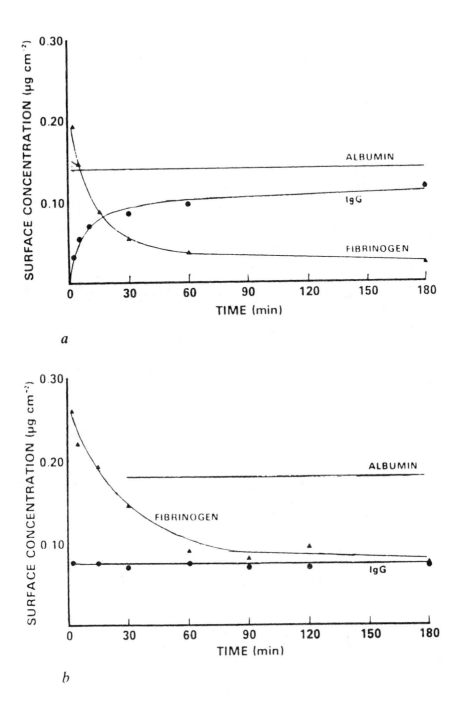

FIGURE 3 Adsorption of albumin, fibrinogen and IgG from diluted ACD plasma to (a) polyethylene and (b) siliconized glass, showing transient adsorption of fibrinogen. From Uniyal S. and Brash J. L. *Thromb. Haemost.*, 47(3):285, 1982. With permission.

thromboresistance is still being considered. A minimal Vroman Effect would minimize the replacement of fibrinogen by other proteins, but may promote platelet adhesion to adsorbed fibrinogen. On the other hand, promotion of the Vroman Effect may lead to the exchange of fibrinogen for other coagulation proteins, such as HMWK, which also favors thrombus formation.

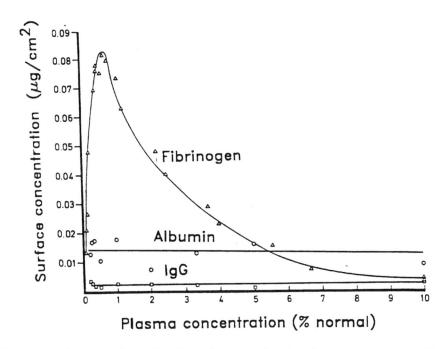

FIGURE 4 Adsorption of proteins to glass from plasma as a function of plasma concentration. Plasma was diluted with isotonic TRIS, pH 7.35 and adsorptions were for five minutes. From Brash J. L. and Hove P. T., *Thromb. Haemost.*, 51:326, 1984. With permission.

IV. CELLULAR RESPONSES TO POLYURETHANES

A. Platelets

Comparisons between different types of soft segments have shown that the polyethylene oxide (PEO) soft segment polyurethanes retain fewer platelets in an *in vitro* bead column test than the corresponding polypropylene oxide (PPO) or polytetramethylene oxide (PTMO) based polyurethanes. Merrill et al.[108] have hypothesized that the hydrophilic ether carbon groups are relatively unreactive in their interaction with blood elements. Thus the higher the ratio of ether carbons to aliphatic carbons, the more favorable the interaction with platelets. These researchers have extended this concept by showing that the PEO segment alone is very thromboresistant. Takahara et al.[109] have shown that an increase in molecular weight of the PEO soft segment can reduce the extent of platelet adhesion *in vitro*. The same researchers also investigated platelet adhesion to a series of polymers with increasing numbers of methylene units in the diamine chain extender. Platelet adhesion *in vitro* was lower on materials containing even numbers of methylene units than those with odd numbers of methylene units.[110] It is believed that this difference in platelet adhesion is a result of the differences in crystallinity of the hard segments. The materials with an even number of carbon atoms crystallize more readily than those with an odd number. Figures 5 and 6 show platelet attachment and spreading on polyurethane surfaces.

Merrill et al. also have found that polyurethanes with crystalline segments tend to be less blood compatible, as measured by an *in vitro* platelet retention test. A comparison of MDI/TDI/ED/PTMO 2000 and MDI/ED/PTMO 2000 polyurethanes showed the latter polyurethane to be both less crystallizable and more blood compatible. In addition, Merrill et al. have found that soft segments containing mixtures of PEO, PPO, and diblocks of PEO-PPO show low platelet retention, suggesting that molecular disorder is a useful soft-segment characteristic. Such molecular disorder can be induced through the use of low-molecular-weight soft segments, modifications in the hard segment,

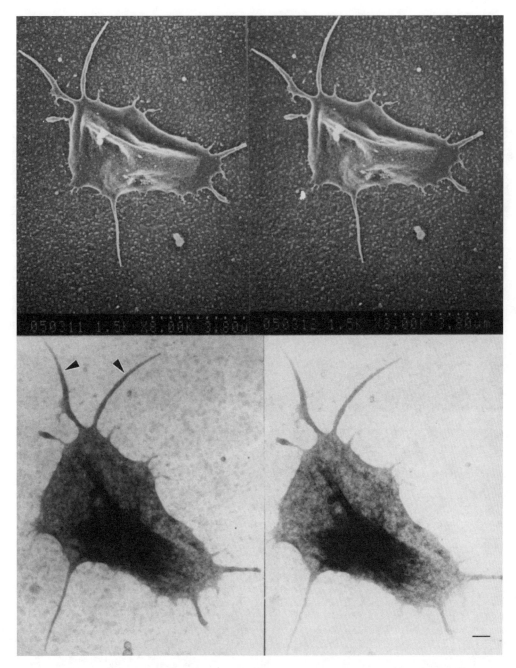

FIGURE 5 Correlative low voltage scanning electron micrograph of a platelet on 20% sulfonated polyurethane. The platelet membrane has collapsed and the pseudopodia (indicated by arrows) have become thin and drawn. (Bar = 1 µm). From Lai, Q.J., Ph.D. Thesis. University of Wisonsin–Madison. 1992.

and through the use of soft-segment blends or block copolymers. On the other hand, Harker et al.[111] have observed the opposite trends, and Takahara et al.[112] have found minimal *in vitro* platelet shape change at an intermediate soft-segment molecular weight range. Conflicting results for the effect of surface soft-segment concentration on blood compatibility could be accounted for by differences in the methods of assessing platelet alterations. The experiments of Hanson *et al.* involve platelet consumption as opposed to platelet deposition measurements. This in itself brings up an

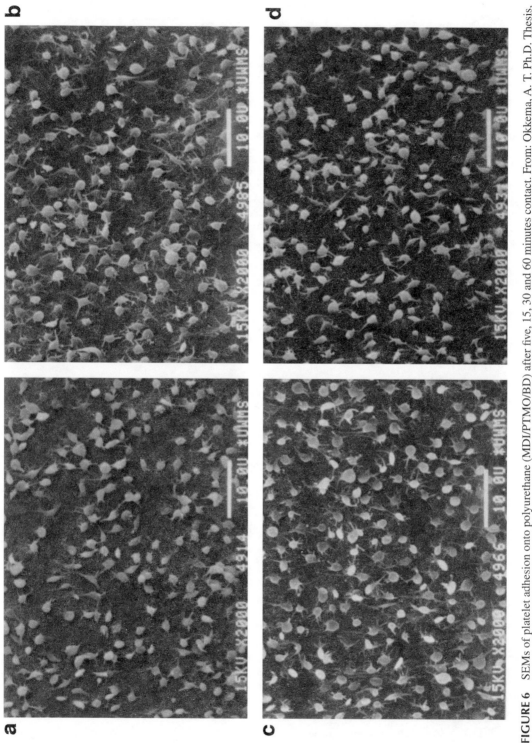

FIGURE 6 SEMs of platelet adhesion onto polyurethane (MDI/PTMO/BD) after five, 15, 30 and 60 minutes contact. From: Okkema, A. T. Ph.D. Thesis, Univerity of Wisconsin – Madison, 1990.

interesting question concerning the definition of blood compatibility. Most researchers assume that lower platelet deposition, minimal platelet activation, and lower thrombus formation are indicative of good blood compatibility. However, the platelet-consumption experiments may address a different aspect of blood compatibility than does the measurement of platelet deposition. It remains apparent that the relationship between polyurethane surface soft-segment concentration and blood compatibility is incompletely understood.

Surface modification of polyurethanes to reduce platelet adhesion has been performed by grafting antiplatelet agents onto the surface. Prostaglandin analogues that significantly inhibit platelet aggregation have been grafted onto polyurethane structures, with favorable results *in vitro*.[113,114] Alkylated polyurethanes also have demonstrated reduced platelet adhesion during blood contact.[45]

B. Leukocytes

Adhesion of leukocytes to polyurethane surfaces can be increased with the incorporation of ethyleneimine groups, acrylic acid groups,[115] or sulfonate groups.[116] Adhesion to sulfonate groups also leads to an observable increase in the degree of spreading of polymorphonuclear cells. Once adhered, degradation of the polymer can occur, possibly through the release of elastase.[117] Superoxide production *in vitro* has been shown to be enhanced within 30 minutes of contact with polyurethane; the level of activity diminished with prolonged contact, a feature that may contribute to compromised white cell function *in vivo*.[118]

Recently, materials grafted with phosphorylcholine moieties have been synthesized, based on the observation that the red blood cell membrane, which is largely composed of phosphorylcholine, presents a nonthrombogenic surface. These materials are characterized by low protein adsorption, low complement activation and enhanced thromboresistance.[119-122] This approach has recently been extended to polyurethanes, which show reduced levels of platelet adhesion and activation of platelets and neutrophils,[123,124] and bacterial adhesion.[125]

C. Thrombus Formation on Polyurethanes

The overall thrombogenicity of biomaterials in general and polyurethanes in particular has been the most widely studied aspect of blood-material interactions. Generally, these investigations suggest that polyurethanes tend to be more blood compatible than most other polymer materials. This has sustained the interest and development of polyurethane elastomers for blood-contacting devices. Some studies have shown the polyurethanes as a class to be as compatible or better than silicone rubber. The more hydrophilic polyurethanes also tend to be more inert to blood components than the hydrophobic polyurethanes. Surface analysis by ESCA shows *in vitro* blood compatibility to be related to surface soft-segment concentration. Fabrication technique is important, as discussed in Chapter 3, as differences in processing can result in different surface properties, potentially producing alteration in the blood compatibility. Nyilas and Ward,[126] and Picha et al.[127] found that *in vitro* blood compatibility was affected by fabrication method. In spite of this variability, a large number of polyurethanes were found to be relatively blood compatible *in vitro* by many different research groups.

The relationship between polyurethane surface chemistry and thrombogenicity also is of interest. It would be expected that the degree of microphase separation of the soft and hard segments, and the relative surface concentration of the soft-segment phase would be an important surface property affecting interactions with blood. It has been shown that the higher the degree of microphase separation, the better the blood compatibility.[128] The soft segment chemistry also can influence the blood response.[42,129] The number of methylene units in the diamine chain extender can affect the mechanical properties of the material, as well as the blood compatibility of the surface.[110] In a number of *in vitro, ex vivo* and *in vivo* investigations, the surface soft segment

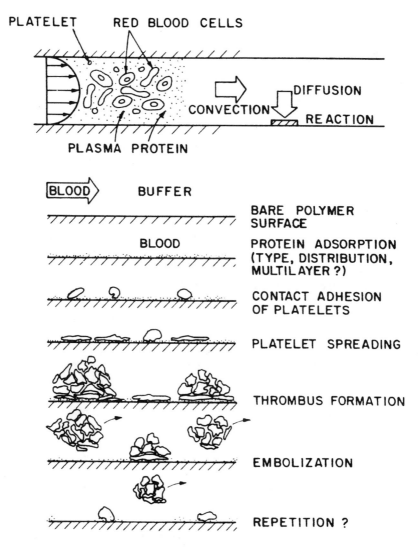

FIGURE 7 Schematic of protein adsorption, platelet deposition, thrombus formation and embolization on an artificial surface placed in the blood stream. From Lelah M.D. and Cooper, S.L., *Polyurethanes in Medicine.* CRC Press, Boca Raton, FL. 1986. With permission.

concentration correlated well with some measure of blood compatibility. In addition, in other studies using polyurethanes with different soft-segment molecular weights where no surface characterization was performed, the materials with high bulk soft-segment concentrations were most thromboresistant.

Ex vivo investigations into the thrombogenicity of polyurethane surfaces have been performed by Cooper and coworkers, providing information regarding the process of thrombus formation on synthetic materials. By observing levels of fibrinogen and platelet deposition onto surfaces in a canine *ex vivo* series shunt, the processes of protein adsorption, platelet deposition, thrombus generation and embolization have been studied. Thrombus formation and growth on a synthetic biomaterial may lead to occlusion of the vessel, leading to stasis of blood flow. Alternatively, platelet aggregates or emboli may be detached from a surface by mechanical forces or fibrinolytic activity; thrombi may travel downstream, and if large enough, may lodge in vital organs and cause transient ischemia, infarction or stroke. Figure 7 illustrates the sequence of events occurring when flowing blood contacts a foreign surface. Initially proteins are adsorbed onto the polymer surface, and studies performed using the canine *ex vivo* series shunt model have shown that platelet deposition, activation and aggregation usually parallels fibrinogen deposition. Fibrinogen is then converted to fibrin, forming a network with the platelets, and other cellular elements, such as leukocytes. Clot retraction is believed to precede embolization;[130] embolization in experiments of this nature is associated with a peak in the levels of fibrinogen and platelets attached to the surface. This generally occurs after 15-30 minutes of blood contact. Growth of new thrombi may be initiated, but it has been noted that these form on new sites, not sites where there were previously thrombi. This implies that the surface has somehow been passivated, although this is temporary, as the failure of shunts in chronic blood contact due to occlusion is a major problem in clinical medicine. Precisely how the surface becomes transiently unreactive to further thrombus formation, and the length of time of passivation is not known. Platelet adhesion alone is insufficient for thrombus generation; platelet spreading must occur to provide a stable base for platelet accretion, and thrombus formation.[3,75,131] It also has been postulated that the size of embolus detaching from a surface is influenced by the strength of adhesion between the adsorbed protein and the polymer surface.[75]

Thrombus formation on a number of polyurethanes of different chemistries has been studied, using the canine *ex vivo* series shunt. Cooper and coworkers have studied the effect of the hard segment, soft segment, chain extender, presence of ionic groups and method of fabrication. The hard segment content is believed to influence the overall thrombogenicity of these materials. Although a hard segment analog tested in the shunt proved to be thrombogenic, the presence of the hard segment at the surface of a block copolymer has been shown to improve the blood compatibility. The soft segment surface concentration and chemistry are also influential factors of blood compatibility.[132] A polyethylene oxide soft segment of molecular weight of 600 was found to produce a more thrombogenic polymer than similar materials containing PEO chains of 1450 and 8000 molecular weight. Little difference between these last two materials was reported.[37] A PEO soft segment also has been shown to be more thrombogenic than a PPO or a PTMO soft segment in a similar test.[60,129] Differences in thrombogenicity also have been observed while comparing chain extenders; an ethylene diamine extended polyurethane demonstrated more thromboresistance than a 1,4 butanediol extended polymer. Thus, it is postulated that the degree of phase separation of the material is an important feature of polyurethanes which influences the blood-contacting properties of these materials. Once a certain amount of phase separation is achieved, alterations in the blood compatibility profile become less apparent, possibly due to inadequacies in measurement techniques. The microphase separation of hard and soft segments that is characteristic of polyurethanes is an important contributor to the superior performance of polyurethanes in biomedical applications.

The incorporation of ionic groups into a polyurethane has been shown to influence the degree of phase separation of these materials as discussed in Chapter 4. Incorporation of such structures also affects the blood-contacting surface of the polymers. The presence of cationic amine in the hard segment increased the thrombogenicity of the polyurethane, when compared with the unmodified material. The grafting of sulfonate groups improved the thromboresistance of the base material, as did incorporation of both anionic and cationic groups to create zwitterionic functionality. The enhanced thromboresistance of the anionic and zwitterionic materials was attributed to the presence of sulfonate groups at the surface as determined by ESCA measurements.[132] Further studies of the sulfonated polyurethanes, including sulfonated Biomer, have shown that although these materials induce deposition of high quantities of fibrinogen, this is not paralleled by high levels of platelet deposition or activation. Consequently, these sulfonated materials show enhanced thromboresistance, with thrombus formation reduced by an order of magnitude compared to the unsulfonated counterparts.[54,71]

Investigations also have been conducted to evaluate the effect of fabrication on the blood-contacting properties of polyurethanes.[41,133] The presence of a polysiloxane polyurethane copolymer additive to a polyurethane at a level of 0.5% enhanced the thrombogenicity of the material. Surface analysis showed that the additive had migrated to the surface. The same investigation revealed that solvent polishing did not affect the blood-compatibility of the material. Lelah et al.[129] have demonstrated that solvent cast extruded grade Biomer is more thrombogenic than the same material formed by extrusion. Comparison between the materials implied a correlation between the increase in soft segment concentration at the surface and thromboresistance.[41]

D. SOFT TISSUE INTERACTIONS WITH POLYURETHANES

The biocompatibility of implanted materials is affected by interactions at the tissue-implant surface. Less is known about the ways in which soft tissue responds to polyurethanes than about polyurethane interactions with blood. However, in the past few years more investigators have studied polyurethanes and soft tissue primarily as a consequence of new techniques that have made studying tissue-polymer interactions easier.

The first event in soft tissue interactions is the adsorption of protein onto the surface followed by an acute inflammatory response characterized by the presence of PMNs.[134-136] The interesting consequence of the adsorbed protein layer on the biomaterial is that cells never actually come in contact with the material itself. Subsequent to protein adsorption an acute response is followed by chronic inflammation which includes wound healing mechanisms and foreign body reactions and involves both macrophages and fibroblasts. Polyurethanes like many other biomaterials, elicit a foreign body response as determined by the presence of multinucleated giant cells found in contact with their surfaces.[134] It has been hypothesized by both Anderson and co-workers.[134] that these giant cells form via the activation of macrophages and their coalescence into large cells. There is in vitro evidence that this does indeed happen in the presence of many polymers including polyurethanes.[137] In addition, investigators have found that polyurethanes, like many other materials, become encapsulated in a fibrous capsule.[134,138-139] Epigard, an older skin substitute made of polyurethane is rapidly infiltrated with tissue, macrophages and giant cells,[140] and studies on explanted breast implants coated in polyurethane foam indicate a foreign body reaction, fibrous capsule formation, and subsequent degradation.[141-145]

During the inflammatory response to an implanted material, monocytes are recruited to the implant site and macrophages become actively involved in maintaining a chronic inflammatory response.[146,147] Many investigators have shown that macrophages adhere to polymeric materials.[134,148-150] Marchant et al.[151] found that macrophages appear after PMN's in the presence of the polyurethane Biomer, and that the macrophages appear to preferentially adhere to the polyurethane. Other investigators also have found that polyurethanes cause an intense inflammatory response with sustained PMN concentrations for abnormally long periods.[135,152,153] Marois et al.[154] found that the extent and type of inflammatory response can be material dependent. They compared the cellular response of a microporous polyurethane vascular graft and Mitrathane® (Matrix Medical) vascular graft with an e-PTFE graft and found differences in both the pattern of inflammatory response and the T-cell populations at the sites. The polyurethane graft and Mitrathane showed an acute inflammation that lasted for two weeks, some formation of foreign body giant cells and encapsulation. The PTFE material showed chronic inflammation and foreign body giant cells still present after 6 weeks. The grafts were encapsulated by a thin collagen layer. The authors hypothesized that the polyurethanes modified the T-cell populations and induced a prolonged acute response.[154]

Investigators tested several polymers including a polyurethane and found that they activated macrophages to different extents and stimulated prostanoid release.[150] Several clinical abnormalities have been associated with the loading of macrophages with polymeric particles including polyurethanes.[155] Interestingly, Bonfield et al.[156-158] found that Biomer did not enhance macrophage activation as much as other polymers tested. They also found that protein adsorbed to the surface influenced the production of growth factors by the macrophages. Other effects on the function of macrophages by polyurethanes include expression and release of enzymes,[159] the selective activation of fibroblasts,[157] and encapsulation of catheter tips in tissue.[160]

One of the most important mediators of inflammation and wound healing is the cytokine interleukin-1 (IL-1) and as a consequence it has been studied in more detail than other cytokines. It has been implicated in the regulation of fibroblast growth and function, as well as the breakdown of the ECM. IL-1 performs many roles, including the regulation of fibroblast proliferation, growth, and collagen production. Miller et al.[149,150] found that that blood monocytes cultured in the presence of different polymers released factors that stimulated fibroblast proliferation and collagen synthesis. Interestingly, in this work, the polyurethane tested, Biomer, did not stimulate fibroblast proliferation but was able to stimulate greater production of collagen, most likely via the release of IL-1 from the monocytes.[150] Proliferation of fibroblasts was found to be suppressed on cationic polyurethanes but unaffected on other types,[161] and occurred at the highest rate on materials with contact angles of 70°.[162] Polyurethanes also have been shown to suppress IL-1 activity in monocytes in the presence of preadsorbed proteins but to stimulate IL-1 in the absence of the proteins.[156]

Biomaterials interact with tissue in what appears to be a material dependent manner.[147] Many factors including the implant chemistry, size, shape, the tissue surrounding the implant and the length of time it has been in place, have been implicated.[135,136,161] As previously discussed, surface chemistry and the relative hydrophobicity and hydrophilicity of polyurethanes has been found to influence the proteins adsorbed to the surface and this ultimately influences the subsequent cell migration and function.[161,163-165] Various authors have found that the surface hydrophobicity and chemistry affects the spreading, adhesion and function of endothelial cells either by altering the fibronectin conformation (ligand/integrin binding) or some other mechanism.

Mohanty et al.[166] and others[160] have found a relationship between pore size and the infiltration of macrophages into a polyurethane implant. Mohanty found that different microstructures within polyurethanes affected the cellular response.[166] Biomer was used to prepare materials of different microstructures, these were implanted *in vivo* and subsequently the cellular response was quantified. The different microstructures and cellular infiltrate are illustrated in Figure 8. In this study, the investigators found that a pore size of 5-10 µm inhibits cellular infiltration of the material while larger pore sizes (200-300 µm) encouraged cell infiltration.

The surface texture of the implant also can affect the response to the material. Indeed it is this concept of surface texture and characteristics that lead to the use of polyurethane coated breast implants. All breast implants, coated with polyurethane or not, are subject to potential problems.[167] These problems include fibrous capsules surrounding the implant thick enough to require surgical removal (4–20%), breast asymmetry (1–10%), and capsular contracture (30–40% for smooth implants, 2–10% for polyurethane covered).[167]

Previously, smooth walled breast implants (nonpolyurethane) were shown to have side effects including formation of a capsule around the implant followed by contracture and calcification.[168-171] There is clinical evidence that the polyurethane covered implants were successful at *delaying* the incidence of capsule formation,[169,172-173] and contracture.[168,174-179] Interestingly, laboratory evidence from at least one group suggested that capsular contracture did occur in polyurethanes but would not likely be clinically significant because it was of a mild degree.[180] Why polyurethanes reduced the amount of contracture associated with the implants is still not clearly understood. However, it is speculated that the covering may have disrupted the formation of the capsule by integrating into the surrounding tissue and being degraded. In addition, the foam was porous. Mohanty's work indicates that the porosity of the material may have influenced capsule formation. Bucky et al.[181] found that textured silicone implants had firmer capsules around them after one year of implantation in rabbits compared to smooth surface silicone implants or polyurethane materials. The capsules around the polyurethanes were found to be the most compliant. The textured materials also showed a significant inflammatory response with the capsules around the polyurethanes having the least fibrous tissue deposition.[181]

The positive impact on contracture in comparison to the smooth breast implants appears to have been limited to short term clinical findings (less than 6 years). In a 19 year study, the authors found that after the initial low incidence of contracture associated with polyurethane foam-coated

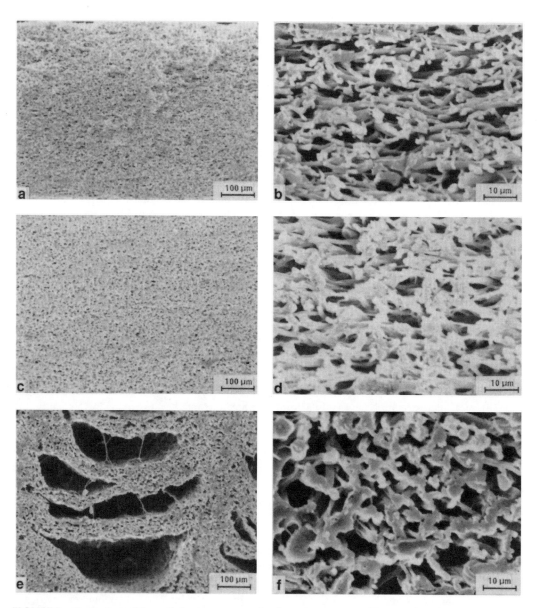

FIGURE 8 Evaluation of the soft tissue response of polyurethane ureas using scanning electromicrographs. Samples of different microstructures are shown in cross-section. A Sample A (original magnification ×100); b. Sample B (original magnification ×100); c. Sample G (original maginification ×100); d. Sample B (original magnification ×1000), e. Sample original magnification ×36) f. Sample C (original magnification ×1000); From Mohanty M., Hunt J. A., Doherty P. J., Annis D. and Williams D. F. Biomaterials, 13:651, 1992. Reproduced with permission from Elsevier Inc.

implants in the first five–six years, the rate approached that for smooth implants over five–10 years, and decreased after year 15.[182] Other clinicians found complications including prolonged foreign body reactions with granulomas,[183–184] late pain,[172,184] breast deformities,[183] and skin lesions.[185] It would appear that whatever initially reduced the fibrous capsule formation and contracture around polyurethane coated implants compared to smooth implants, be it texture, porosity or some other parameter, is lost after a long period of time. Other reactions of polyurethane-covered implants, including the degradation of the foam, are discussed in Chapter 8.

E. NEOINTIMA FORMATION

When a biomaterial is implanted into tissue, granulation tissue is laid down onto porous implant surfaces, followed by encapsulation into a fibrous capsule. A comparable phenomenon occurs at the blood-biomaterial interface. The biological layer that is formed at the blood-contacting interface is referred to as a neointima or pseudointima. Neointima formation results from the ingrowth of cellular material over a bed of fibrin. Fibrin forms on the surface as a result of coagulation, and traps formed elements. Within 24 hours, the entire graft surface is coated with platelets, thrombi and fibrin. Smooth muscle cells may migrate from the native artery. Some of these cells can then differentiate into endothelial cells and fibroblasts. This comprises the neointima. The nutrient supply from flowing blood can sustain a neointima approximately 500 μm thick.[186]

Differences have been observed in the degree of neointima formation in different animals. *In vivo* studies have shown that complete coverage of vascular grafts occurs in rats and partial coverage by a neointima occurs in dogs and pigs. This partial coverage is more representative of the degree of neointima formation in humans; complete endothelialization has not been observed in humans. In humans, the rate of cellular ingrowth is approximately one millmete per week, and the degree of growth into the vessel is limited to one to two centimeters from the anastomosis. There are many inter-species hematological and physiological differences and these make extrapolation of *in vivo* animal studies to the human situation very difficult.

The formation of a stable, thin neointima is a desirable characteristic for blood-contacting implants, where the long term implantation of the device may lead to thrombus formation. The vascular endothelium forms the most thromboresistant surface known, and it is believed that this property results from the synthesis of a number of agents by these cells. If a neointima can develop on the implant surface, with a confluent layer of endothelial cells that can perform all the metabolic and synthetic functions of the endothelium, it is reasonable to assume that the long term thrombogenicity of the implant and the risks of thrombus formation and embolism associated with this can be significantly reduced. The formation of a neointima also is perceived to be the only way to inhibit colonization by bacteria and hence reduce the risk of a device-centered biomaterial infection. Most of the clinical interest in neointima formation has been associated with development of vascular grafts and the total artificial heart. It is believed that the surface of a vascular prosthesis will remain patent if a stable, viable neointima can develop. The thickness of the neointima also becomes important, as if the neointima is allowed to thicken, or if the graft is of very small diameter, blockage of the vessel may result. The formation of a stable neointima may advance the application of the total artificial heart as a long term organ replacement option, rather than as a bridge to transplantation, by reducing the risk of thromboembolic events.

In order to promote the ingrowth and re-endothelialization of devices, biomaterials are fabricated with pores to promote tissue ingrowth. The texture of the surface, which can be imparted through flock-linings or pores can provide anchorage for fibrin and the formed elements and promote neointima formation. There have been numerous studies where the texture of the graft has been shown to be more important to tissue ingrowth than polymer surface chemistry.[187-190] Porous surfaces may provide better anchoring of fibrin and other material and thus promote neointima formation. There also is a contention that a neointima may not be able to perform all of the physiological functions of the normal endothelium,[77] which account for the thromboresistant properties of the vascular wall. Attempts to improve the endothelialization of polyurethanes in blood-contacting applications also have been tried by seeding device surfaces with endothelial cells prior to implantation,[191] pretreating surfaces with growth factors and proteins,[77,192] or through coating with extracellular matrix components prior to seeding.[193-195] A specific peptide sequence, Arg-Gly-Asp (RGD), found in adhesive proteins, also has been grafted onto polyurethane and evaluated by endothelial cell growth *in vitro*.[196] Most of these methods have had success *in vitro*, and increased surface coverage by endothelial cells has been observed. SEMs of endothelial cells on these surfaces are shown in Figure 9. The presence of polymeric additives also has been shown to influence endothelial

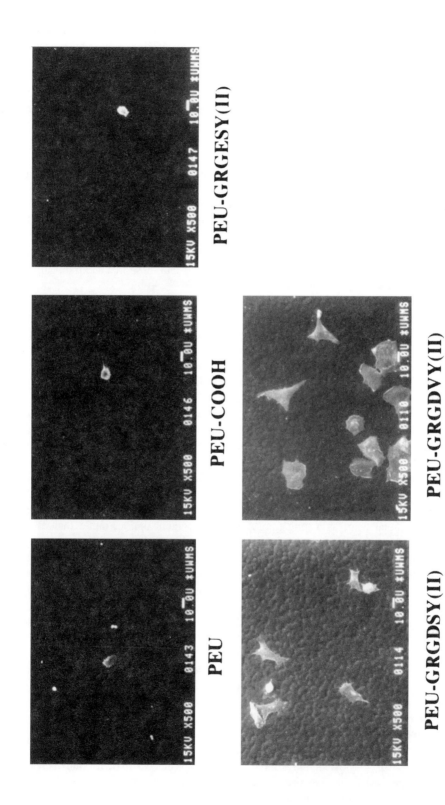

FIGURE 9 SEMs of HUVECs attached to polyurethanes. Base polyurethane (PEU), carboxylated polyurethane (PEU-COOH), RGE-grafted polyurethane (PEU-GRGESY), RGD grafted polyurethane (PEU-GRGDSY and PEU-GRGDVY). From Lin H.-B., Garcia-Echeverria C., Asakura S. Sun, W., Mosher, D.F., and Cooper, S.L., *Biomaterials*, 13:905, 1992. With permission of Elsevier, Inc.

cell proliferation *in vitro*.[197] *In vivo* studies of endothelialization on polyurethanes are discussed in more detail in Chapter 9, under consideration of vascular grafts.

F. Immunological Response to Polyurethanes

Whether or not polyurethanes invoke an "immune" response is controversial. As discussed, biomaterials activate complement in blood-contacting applications; sensitivity (immune reaction) to metals may result in loosening of some metallic implants; and IL-1 release is stimulated in the presence of polymers.[198] Complement is part of the innate immune response and inflammation and IL-1 is a pluripotent mediator which acts on macrophages, a cell at the center of both chronic inflammation and cell-mediated immunity.

As discussed in Chapter 6, agents are recognized by the innate system through several different mechanisms including the opsonization (coating of the foreign substance in C3b or IgG), abnormal surfaces, and through the chemoattractant mechanisms of C5a. Biomaterials, including polyurethanes have been shown to adsorb complement and activate it, producing C5a and C3b.[198] Therefore, it is likely that polyurethanes can trigger the innate immune system *in vivo*, and this is partially responsible for the foreign body reaction that is elicited by these materials. Complement also influences inflammation and cell-mediated immunity. However, the mechanism is different from that of innate immunity and requires the antibodies, IgG or IgM, to initiate the classical complement cascade.[199–202]

Polyurethanes have been implicated in downregulating the immune systems of test animals.[152–153] The investigators found that a polyetherurethane had a significant effect on the proliferation of lymphocytes in the presence of tumor cells and as previously mentioned, polyurethanes appear to influence the T-cell population around the implant.[154] However, there has been no direct link made between polyurethanes and a specific cell or antibody mediated immune response *in vivo* in humans whether through complement activation, T-cell interactions or the effect of the material on macrophages.

G. Infection

Biomaterials, particularly in long-term implants are associated with bacterial infection. The implant appears to offer an attractive site for bacterial colonization. Indeed, after thrombosis, infection is the most common cause of implant failure in blood-contacting applications.[203] In cardiovascular prostheses, thrombosis and infection are associated with protein adsorption and cellular adhesion to the surfaces, most likely involving similar mechanisms.[138] Infection also is a serious problem for devices which are implanted in the abdomen including vascular grafts, ventriculoperitoneal shunts, and peritoneal dialysis catheters and feeding tubes.[204,205] Mora et al.[204] have shown that even when the biomaterial is sterile at the time of implantation into the peritoneal cavity (i.e., contamination did not occur during implantation), the material itself will cause bacteria to move from an intact normal bowel wall onto the prosthesis. Any contamination by bacteria in the peritoneal area is very hard to remove from the catheter material by any cleaning method.[205] Certain types of bacteria, particularly gram negative bacteria, are associated with biomaterials infections.

Coagulase-negative staphylococcal bacteria are the most common pathogens found in association with biomaterials including polyurethanes.[203,206] These bacteria have certain characteristics that include slime production and the secretion of proteins that protect against phagocytosis.[207] These properties in association with a biomaterial, contribute to their pathogenicity. Although all the factors which result in the pathogenicity are not clearly understood, there is general agreement that coagulase negative staphylococci can cause severe infections. The clinical manifestations associated with biomaterials are endocarditis, septicemia, infection of the biomaterial, and urinary tract infection. Predisposition towards a coagulase-negative staphylococcus infection includes the presence of an implant or indwelling catheter. Infections due to coagulase-negative staphylococci have been associated with shunts for hydrocephalus, heart valves, pacemakers, continuous ambulatory peritoneal dialysis (CAPD) catheters and intravascular catheters.[208]

1. Staphylococcus epidermidis

Staphylococcus epidermidis is a normal constituent of the flora of human skin. It rarely causes infections in normal hosts but in susceptible people, such as those who are immunocompromised or have implants or catheters, it is the most common cause of infection. It adheres to polymer surfaces, including polyurethanes and produces a slime which is believed to protect the bacteria from antibiotics.[209,210] Prolonged infection ultimately leads to septicemia and/or an inflammatory tissue reaction resulting in implant failure. The infections caused by *S. epidermidis* are persistent and resistant to treatment and because of this, diagnosis of an infection in a cardiovascular implant where *S. epidermidis* is involved, generally requires surgical removal of the implant.[138]

S. epidermidis is felt to be associated with both acute and chronic infections and syndromes related to the presence of biomaterials, including aseptic loosening in hip implants.[207,208,211] Investigators now believe that *S. epidermidis* first adheres to the polymer surface and then secretes its slime.[207,208] Neither the mechanism of adhesion nor slime production on biomaterial surfaces is clearly understood; however adhesion seems to be both bacteria and material dependent. There is evidence that protein adsorption may play an important role in bacterial adhesion.[212-225, 217] Mohammad *et al.*[212] found enhanced bacterial adhesion to polyurethanes, polyvinylchloride and glass coated with fibrinogen and fibronectin, and reduced adhesion when serum was used. Others have obtained similar results associated with catheters.[214,218]

In a normal response to infection, the bacteria are eliminated from the body by white cells which phagocytose them. However, at a biomaterial surface this mechanism is not effective, probably due to the slime which surrounds the bacteria. This slime also protects the bacteria from antibiotics. Martinez-Martinez *et al.*[219] found that nonmucoid and mucoid (slime producing) strains of *Pseudomonas aeruginosa* adhered to polyvinyl chloride, polyurethane and siliconized latex. They found that initially the nonmucoid forms adhered but were replaced with the mucoid strains over time.

2. Gram positive bacteria

Gram positive bacteria also are associated with infection including osteomyelitis and burn infections. *S. aureus* is one of the most common bacterial infections associated with burns and the most common in osteomyelitis.[208,220]

Bakker *et al.*[221] found that Estane, a polyether urethane, was a better porous middle ear implant material to use in the presence of an infection compared to a polyester polyether copolymer. In order to decrease the rate of infection associated with implanted polyurethanes various strategies have been applied. Antibiotics and antimicrobials have been incorporated into the material,[222,223] applied as varnishes on teeth and covered with polyurethane sealants.[224]

SUMMARY

Adsorption of proteins at the interface between a solution and an artificial surface occurs within seconds. There is only a limited understanding of the factors that influence protein adsorption, and there is not yet the ability to predict the precise sequence of proteins that will adsorb to a given biomaterial surface, or the conformation that they will adopt. One interesting consequence of the rapidity of protein adsorption from blood to a polyurethane surface is that subsequent interactions with cells are mediated by this protein layer. The complexity of blood, cellular and tissue responses to biomaterials means that it is difficult to predict the result of contact between the two. The chemistry, physical characteristics and mechanical properties of polyurethanes can ultimately influence the biocompatibility of the material. Therefore, focusing on the "right" area to investigate is almost impossible. Generally, polyurethane elastomers possess good blood compatibility. The blood compatibility is comparable to or better than silicone rubber, which is considered to be one of the most blood compatible synthetic materials. The relative tissue compatibility of polyurethanes also is higher than most other synthetic polymer materials.

Despite the large number of groups investigating the biological interactions between polyurethanes and indeed many other biomaterials, and the biological environment from all different aspects, we are still at the very beginning of our understanding. With the rapid changes taking place in the fields of molecular biology, microbiology, biochemistry, immunology and genetics, tools and information are added each day. It is likely that it will require interdisciplinary research to reach a more complete understanding of biomaterial interactions with that most complex of environments, the human body.

REFERENCES

1. Black J. *Biological Performance of Materials. Fundamentals of Biocompatibility.* (2nd Ed.): Marcel Dekker Inc., New York, 1992.
2. Rae T. "Tissue culture techniques in biocompatibility testing." In *Techniques of Biocompatibility Testing*, Ed. Williams D. F. CRC Press, Boca Raton, FL, 1986: 81.
3. Baumgartner H. R. and Muggli R. "Adhesion and aggregation: Morphological demonstration and quantitation *in vivo* and *in vitro*." In *Platelets in Biology and Pathology*, Ed. Gordon J. L. Elsevier, Amsterdam, 1976: 23.
4. Richardson P. D., Mohammad S. F., and Mason R. G. "Flow chamber studies of platelet adhesion at controlled, spatially varied shear rate." *Proc. Eur. Soc. Artif. Organs*, 4:175, 1977.
5. Cozens-Roberts C., Quinn J. A., and Lauffenburger D. A. "Receptor-mediated adhesion phenomena. Model studies with the Radial-Flow Detachment Assay." *Biophys. J.*, 58:107, 1990.
6. Lamba N. M. K. *Blood-biomaterial interactions: application of a parallel plate flow cell to investigate blood responses* in vitro [Ph.D.]. University of Strathclyde, 1994.
7. Friedman L. I. and Leonard E. F. "Platelet adhesion to artificial surfaces: consequences of flow, exposure time, blood condition and surface nature." *Fed. Proc.*, 30:1641, 1971.
8. Vienken J. and Baurmeister U. "Improved biocompatibility of dialyzers by reduced membrane surface area." *Artif. Organs*, 11:272, 1987.
9. Mahiout A., Meinhold H., Kessel M., Schulze H., and Baurmeister U. "Dialyzer membranes: effect of surface area and chemical modification of cellulose on complement and platelet activation." *Artif. Organs*, 11:149, 1987.
10. Chenoweth D. E. and Henderson L. W. "Complement activation during hemodialysis: laboratory evaluation of hemodialysers." *Artif. Organs*, 11:155, 1987.
11. Chang G., Absolom D. R., Strong A. B., Stubley G. D., and Zingg W. "Physical and hydrodynamic factors affecting erythrocyte adhesion to polymer surfaces." *J. Biomed. Mater. Res.*, 22:13, 1988.
12. Siemssen P. A., Garred P., Olsen J., Aasen A. O., and Mollnes T. E. "Activation of complement, kallikrein-kinin, fibrinolysis and coagulation systems by urinary catheters. Effect of time and temperature in biocompatibility studies." *Brit. J. Urol.*, 67:83, 1991.
13. Schultz J. S., Goddard J. D., Ciakowski A., Penner J. A., and Lindenauer S. M. "An *ex vivo* method for the evaluation of biomaterials in contact with blood." *Ann. N. Y. Acad. Sci.*, 283:494, 1977.
14. Ihlenfeld J. V. and Cooper S. L. "Transient *in vivo* protein adsorption onto polymeric biomaterials." *J. Biomed. Mater. Res.*, 13:577, 1979.
15. Lelah M. D., Lambrecht L. K., and Cooper S. L. "A canine ex vivo series shunt for evaluating thrombus deposition on polymer surfaces." *J. Biomed. Mater. Res.*, 18:475, 1984.
16. Spencer P. C., Schmidt B., Samtleben W., Bosch T., and Gurland H. J. "*Ex vivo* model of hemodialysis membrane biocompatibility." *Trans. Am. Soc. Artif. Intern. Organs*, 31:495, 1985.
17. Grabowski E. F., Didisheim P., Lewis C. J., Franta J. T., and Stropp J. Q. "Platelet adhesion to foreign surfaces under controlled conditions of whole blood flow: human vs. rabbit, dog, calf, sheep, macaque and baboon." *Trans. Am. Soc. Artif. Intern. Organs*, 23:141, 1977.

18. Dodds W. J. "Platelet function in animals:species specificities." In *Platelets: a mutlidisciplinary approach*, Ed. Gaetano G. D., Garattini S. Raven Press, 1978: 45.
19. Anderson J. M. "Perspectives on in vivo testing of biomaterials, prostheses, and artificial organs." *J. Am. College Toxicol.*, 7:369, 1988.
20. Gott V. L., Koepke D. E., Gaggett R. L., Zamstorff W., and Young W. P. "The coating of intravascular plastic prostheses with colloidal graphite." *Surgery*, 50:382, 1961.
21. Kusserow B., Larrow R., and Nichols J. "Perfusion and surface induced injury in leukocytes." *Fed. Proc.*, 30:1516, 1971.
22. Bruck S. D. "On the evaluation of medical plastics in contact with blood." *Biomaterials*, 3:121, 1982.
23. Recum A. F. V., Imamura H., Freed P. S., Kantrowitz A., Chen S. T., Ekstrom M. E., Baechler C. A., and Barnhart M. I. "Biocompatibility tests of components of an implantable cardiac assist device." *J. Biomed. Mater. Res.*, 12:743, 1978.
24. Courtney J. M., Sundaram S., Lamba N. M. K., and Forbes C. D. "Monitoring of the blood response in blood purification." *Artif. Organs*, 17:260, 1993.
25. NHLBI. *Guidelines for Physicochemical Characterization of Biomaterials.* National Institutes of Health, 1980.
26. NHLBI. *Guidelines for Blood Materials Interactions.* National Institutes of Health, Bethesda, MD, 1980.
27. NHLBI. *Guidelines for Blood-Material Interactions.* National Institutes of Health, 1985.
28. NHLBI. "Cardiovascular Biomaterials and Biocompatibility: A Guide to the study of Blood-tissue-material interactions." *Cardiovasc. Pathol.*, 2, 1993.
29. ASTM. "Standard Practice for Selecting Generic Biological Test Methods for Materials and Devices." In *1990 Annual Book of ASTM Standards*, Ed. ASTM, Philadelphia, PA, 1990: 227.
30. ISO-10993. *Biological Testing of Medical Devices.* International Standards Organisation, 1993.
31. Bellissimo J. A. and Cooper S. L. "Fourier Transform infrared spectroscopic studies of plasma protein adsorption under well-defined flow conditions." *Trans. Am. Soc. Artif. Intern. Organs*, 30:359, 1984.
32. Pitt W. G. and Cooper S. L. "FTIR–ATR studies of the effect of shear rate upon albumin adsorption onto polyurethaneurea." *Biomaterials*, 7:340, 1986.
33. Pitt W. G. and Cooper S. L. "Albumin adsorption on alkyl chain derivatized polyurethanes: I. The effect of C-18 alkylation." *J. Biomed. Mater. Res.*, 22:359, 1988.
34. Pitt W. G., Grasel T. G., and Cooper S. L. "Albumin adsorption on alkyl chain derivatized polyurethanes: II. The effect of alkyl chain length." *Biomaterials*, 9:36, 1988.
35. Kim S. W., Lee R. G., Oster H., Coleman D., Andrade J. D., Lentz D. J., and Olsen D. "Platelet adhesion to polymer surfaces." *Trans. Am. Soc. Artif. Intern. Organs*, 20:449, 1974.
36. Brash J. L., Uniyal S., and Samak Q. "Exchange of albumin adsorbed on polymer surfaces." *Trans. Am. Soc. Artif. Intern. Organs*, 20:69, 1974.
37. Silver J. H., Myers C. W., Lim F., and Cooper S. L. "Effect of polyol molecular weight on the physical properties and haemocompatibility of polyurethanes containing polyethylene oxide macroglycols." *Biomaterials*, 15:695, 1994.
38. Goodman S. L., Simmons S. R., Cooper S. L., and Albrecht R. M. "Surface morphology and protein adsorption properties of polyurethanes." *Trans. Soc. Biomaterials*, 15:201, 1989.
39. Lyman D. J., Metcalf L. C., Albo D., Richards V. K., and Lamb J. "The effect of chemical structure and surface properties of synthetic polymers on the coagulation of blood. III. *In vivo* adsorption of proteins on polymer surfaces." *Trans. Am. Soc. Artif. Intern. Organs*, 20:474, 1974.
40. Ihlenfeld J. V., Mathis T. R., Barber T. A., Mosher D. F., Riddle L. M., Hart A. P., Updike S. J., and Cooper S. L. "Transient *in vivo* thrombus deposition onto polymeric biomaterials: role of plasma fibrinogen." *Trans. Am. Soc. Artif. Intern. Organs*, 24:727, 1978.
41. Lelah M. D., Lambrecht L. K., Young B. R., and Cooper S. L. "Physicochemical characterization and *in vivo* blood tolerability of cast and extruded Biomer." *J. Biomed. Mater. Res.*, 17:1, 1983.
42. Grasel T. G. and Cooper S. L. "Surface properties and blood compatibility of polyurethaneureas." *Biomaterials*, 7:315, 1986.
43. Ryu G. H., Han D. K., Kim Y. H., and Min B. "Albumin immobilized polyurethane and its blood compatibility." *ASAIO J.*, 38:M644, 1992.

44. Eberhart R. C., Lynch M. E., Bilge F. H., Wissinger J. F., Munro M. S., Ellsworth S. R., and Quattrone A. J. "Protein adsorption on polymers; visualization, study of fluid shear and roughness effects, and methods to enhance albumin binding." In *Biomaterials: Interfacial Phenomena and Applications*, Ed. Cooper S. L., Peppas N.A. Adv Chem Ser, 199; 293. 1982.
45. Munro M. S., Eberhart R. C., Maki N. J., Brink B. E., and Fry W. J. "Thromboresistant alkyl derivatized polyurethanes." *ASAIO J.*, 6:65, 1983.
46. Grasel T. G., Pierce J. A., and Cooper S. L. "Effects of alkyl grafting on surface properties and blood compatibility of polyurethane block copolymers." *J. Biomed. Mater. Res.*, 21:815, 1987.
47. Eberhart R. C., Munro M. S., Williams G. B., Kulkarni P. V., Shannon W. A., Brink B. E., and Fry W. J. "Albumin adsorption and retention on C18-alkyl-derivatized polyurethane vascular grafts."*Artif. Organs*, 11:375, 1987.
48. Keogh J. R. and Eaton J. W. "Albumin binding surfaces for biomaterials."*J. Lab. Clin. Med.*, 124:537, 1994.
49. Rapoza R. J. and Horbett T. A. "Changes in the SDS elutability of fibrinogen adsorbed from plasma to polymers." *J. Biomater. Sci., Polym. Ed.*, 1:99, 1989.
50. Chan B. M. C. and Brash J. L. "Conformational changes in fibrinogen desorbed from glass surface." *J. Coll. Interf. Sci.*, 84:263, 1981.
51. Slack S. M., Rapoza R. J., and Horbett T. A. *Changes in the state of fibrinogen adsorbed to biomaterials*. The Third World Biomaterials Congress. Kyoto, Japan. 1988: 95.
52. Chinn J. A., Posso S. E., Horbett T. A., and Ratner B. D. "Residence time effects in surface bound fibrinogen as indicated by changes in SDS elutability, antibody binding and platelet adhesion."*Trans. Soc. Biomaterials*, 16:242, 1990.
53. Pitt W. G., Park K., and Cooper S. L. "Sequential protein adsorption and thrombus deposition on polymeric biomaterials." *J. Coll. Interf. Sci.*, 111:343, 1986.
54. Silver J. H., Lin H.-B., and Cooper S. L. "Effect of protein adsorption on the blood-contacting response of sulphonated polyurethanes." *Biomaterials*, 14:824, 1993.
55. Lenk T. J., Chittur K. K., and Ratner B. D. "Infrared detection of time-dependent changes in fibrinogen adsorbed to polyurethanes." *Trans. Soc. Biomaterials*, 15:134, 1989.
56. Stupp S. I., Kauffman J. W., and Carr S. H. "Interactions between segmented polyurethane surfaces and the plasma protein fibrinogen." *J. Biomed. Mater. Res.*, 11:237, 1977.
57. Price T. M. and Rudee M. L. "Early stages of plasma protein adsorption" In *Proteins at Interfaces. Physicochemical and Biochemical Studies*, Ed. Brash J. L., Horbett T. A. Vol. 343. American Chemical Society, Washington, DC, 1987.
58. Collins W. E., Fabrizius D. J., and Cooper S. L. "Plasma protein adsorbed to polyurethane block copolymers." *Trans. Soc. Biomaterials*, 15:112, 1989.
59. Grasel T. G., Lee D. C., Okkema A. Z., Slowinski T. J., and Cooper S. L. "Extraction of polyurethane block copolymers: effects on bulk and surface properties and biocompatibility."*Biomaterials*, 9:383, 1988.
60. Okkema A. Z., Fabrizius D. J., Grasel T. G., Cooper S. L., and Zdrahala R. J. "Bulk, surface and blood-contacting properties of polyether polyurethanes modified with polydimethylsiloxane macroglycols." *Biomaterials*, 10:23, 1989.
61. Takahara A., Okkema A. Z., Cooper S. L., and Coury A. J. "Effect of surface hydrophilicity on ex vivo blood compatibility of segmented polyurethanes." *Biomaterials*, 12:324, 1991.
62. Lelah M. D., Pierce J. A., Lambrecht L. K., and Cooper S. L. "Polyetherurethane ionomers: surface property/*ex vivo* blood compatibility relationships." *J. Coll. Interf. Sci.*, 104:422, 1986.
63. Horbett T. A., Cheng C. M., Ratner B. D., Hoffman A. S., and Hanson S. R. "The kinetics of baboon fibrinogen adsorption to polymers: *In vitro* and *in vivo* studies." *J. Biomed. Mater. Res.*, 20:739, 1986.
64. Chinn J. A., Horbett T. A., and Ratner B. D. "Baboon fibrinogen adsorption and platelet adhesion to polymeric materials." *Thromb. Haemost.*, 65:608, 1991.
65. Chinn J. A., Posso S. E., Horbett T. A., and Ratner B. D. "Postadsorptive transitions in fibrinogen adsorbed to Biomer: changes in baboon platelet adhesion, antibody binding and sodiumdodecylsulfate elutability." *J. Biomed. Mater. Res.*, 25:535, 1991.
66. Brunstedt M. R., Ziats N. P., Robertson S. P., Hiltner A., Anderson J. M., Lodoen G. A., and Payet C. R. "Protein adsorption to poly(ether urethane ureas) modified with acrylate and methacrylate polymer and copolymer additives." *J. Biomed. Mater. Res.*, 27:367, 1993.

67. Tengvall P., Lundstrom I., Freij C., Kober M., and Wesslen B. "Ellipsometric studies of antisera binding onto medical polyurethanes immersed in human plasma *in vitro*." *J. Mater. Sci., Mater. Med*, 4:305, 1993.
68. Hari P. R. and Sharma C. P. "Protein adsorption — effect of external lubricants at the interface." *J. Biomaterial Appl.*, 7:375, 1993.
69. Silver J. H., Hart A. P., Williams E. C., Cooper S. L., Charef S., Labarre D., and Jozefowicz M. "Anticoagulant effects of sulphonated polyurethanes." *Biomaterials*, 13:339, 1992.
70. Santerre J. P., Hove P. T., vanderKamp N. H., and Brash J. L. "Effect of sulfonation of segmented polyurethanes on the transient adsorption of fibrinogen from plasma: possible correlation with anticoagulant behavior." *J. Biomed. Mater. Res.*, 26:39, 1992.
71. Okkema A. Z., Yu X.-H., and Cooper S. L. "Physical and blood contacting properties of propyl sulphonate grafted Biomer." *Biomaterials*, 12:3, 1991.
72. Santerre J. P., VanderKamp N. H., and Brash J. L. "Effect of sulfonation of segmented polyurethanes on the transient adsorption of fibrinogen from plasma: possible correlation with anticoagulant behavior." *Trans. Soc. Biomaterials*, 15:113, 1989.
73. Fabrizius-Homan D. J. and Cooper S. L. "Competitive adsorption of vitronectin with albumin, fibrinogen, and fibronectin on polymeric biomaterials." *J. Biomed. Mater. Res.*, 25:953, 1991.
74. Han D. K., Ryu G. H., Park K. D., Jeong S. Y., Kim Y. H., and Min B. G. "Adsorption behavior of fibrinogen to sulfonated polyethyleneoxide-grafted polyurethane surfaces." *J. Biomater. Sci., Polym. Ed.*, 4:401, 1993.
75. Park K. D., Mosher D. F., and Cooper S. L. "Acute surface-induced thrombosis in the canine ex vivo model: importance of protein concentration of the initial monolayer and platelet activation."*J. Biomed. Mater. Res.*, 20:589, 1986.
76. Collins W. E., Mosher D. F., Diwan A. R., Murthy K. D., Simmons S. R., Albrecht R. M., and Cooper S. L. "*Ex vivo* platelet deposition on fibronectin-preadsorbed surfaces." *Scanning Electron Microscopy*, 1:1669, 1987.
77. Zilla P., Fasol R., Grimm M., Fischlein T., Eberl T., Preiss P., Krupicka O., Oppell U. V., and Deutsch M. "Growth properties of cultured human endothelial cells on differently coated artificial heart materials." *J. Thorac. Cardiovasc. Surg.*, 101:671, 1991.
78. Pitt W. G., Weaver D. R., and Cooper S. L. "Fibronectin adsorption kinetics on phase segregated polyurethaneureas." *J. Biomater. Sci., Polym. Ed.*, 4:337, 1993.
79. Vaudaux P., Pittet D., Haeberli A., Lerch P. G., Morgenhaler J. J., Proctor R. A., Waldvogel F. A., and Lew D. P. "Fibronectin is more active than fibrin or fibrinogen in promoting Staphylococcus aureus adherence to inserted intravascular catheters." *J. Infectious Dis.*, 167:633, 1993.
80. Fabrizius-Homan D. J., Wabers H. D., and Cooper S. L. "The biological activity of adsorbed vitronectin." *Trans. Soc. Biomaterials*, 16:138, 1990.
81. Dong D. E., Andrade J. D., and Coleman D. L. "Low density lipoprotein (LDL) adsorption to cardiovascular biomaterials." *Polymer Prepr.*, 24:40, 1983.
82. Takahara A., Takahashi K., and Kajiyama T. "Effect of polyurethane surface chemistry on its lipid sorption behavior." American Chemical Society Division of Polymer Chemistry. *J. Biomater. Sci., Polym. Ed.*, 5:183, 1993.
83. Boretos J. W. and Pierce W. S. "Segmented polyurethane: a polyether polymer. An initial evaluation for biomedical applications." *J. Biomed. Mater. Res.*, 2:121, 1968.
84. Kamp K. W. "Factor XII fragment and kallikrein generation in plasma during incubation with biomaterials." *J. Biomed. Mater. Res.*, 28:349, 1994.
85. Heyman P. W., Cho C. S., McRea J. C., Olsen D. B., and Kim S. W. "Heparinized polyurethanes: *in vitro* and *in vivo* studies." *J. Biomed. Mater. Res.*, 19:419, 1985.
86. Ito Y. "Antithrombogenic heparin-bound polyurethanes." *J. Biomater. Appl.*, 2, 1987.
87. Engbers G. H. M. "An *in vitro* study of the adhesion of blood platelets onto vascular catheters." *J. Biomed. Mater. Res.*, 21:613, 1987.
88. Park K. D., Okano T., Nojiri C., and Kim S. W. "Heparin immobilization onto segmented polyurethaneurea surfaces — effect of hydrophilic spacers." *J. Biomed. Mater. Res.*, 22:977, 1988.
89. Nojiri C., Okano T., Park K. D., and Kim S. W. "Suppression mechanisms for thrombus formation on heparin-immobilized segmented polyurethane-ureas." *Trans. Am. Soc. Artif. Intern. Organs*, 34:386, 1988.

90. Kishida A., Ueno Y., Fukudome N., Yashima E., Maruyama I., and Akashi M. "Immobilization of human thrombomodulin onto poly(ether urethaneurea) for developing antithrombogenic blood-contacting biomaterials." *Biomaterials*, 15:848, 1994.
91. Woodhouse K. A. and Brash J. L. "Adsorption of plasminogen to lysine-derivatized polyurethane surfaces." *Biomaterials*, 13:1103, 1992.
92. Kitamoto Y., Tomita M., Kiyama S., Inoue T., Yabushita Y., Sato T., Ryoda H., and Sato T. "Antithrombotic mechanisms of urokinase immobilised polyurethane." *Thromb. Haemost.*, 65:73, 1991.
93. Ryu G. H., Park S., Kim M., Han D. K., Kim Y. H., and Min B. "Antithrombogenicity of lumbrokinase-immobilized polyurethane." *J. Biomed. Mater. Res.*, 28:1069, 1994.
94. Ryu G. H., Han D. K., Park S., Kim M., Kim Y. H., and Min B. "Surface characteristics and properties of lumbrokinase-immobilized polyurethane." *J. Biomed. Mater. Res.*, 29:403, 1995.
95. Sevestianov V. I. and Tsetjlina E. A. "The activation of the complement system by polymer materials and their blood compatibility." *J. Biomed. Mater. Res.*, 18:969, 1984.
96. Yu J., Sundaram S., Weng D., Courtney J. M., Moran C. R., and Graham N. B. "Blood interactions with novel polyurethaneurea hydrogels." *Biomaterials*, 12:119, 1991.
97. Lim F., Yu X.-H., and Cooper S. L. "Effects of oligoethylene oxide monoalkyl(aryl) alcohol ether grafting on the surface properties and blood compatibility of a polyurethane." *Biomaterials*, 14:537, 1993.
98. Branger B. "Biocompatibility of blood tubings." *Int. J. Artif. Organs*, 13:697, 1990.
99. Ikeda Y., Kohjiya S., Yamashita S., and Fukumura H. "Activation of complement in human serum by polyurethane having PEO-PTMO-PEO as soft segment." *J. Mater. Sci. — Mater. Med.*, 2:110, 1991.
100. Wabers H. D., McCoy T. J., Okkema A. T., Hergenrother R. W., Wolf M. F., and Cooper S. L. "Biostability and blood-contacting properties of sulfonate grafted polyurethane and Biomer." *J. Biomater. Sci., Polym. Ed.*, 4:107, 1992.
101. Eberhart R. C., Munro M. S., Frautschi J. R., Lubin M., Clubb J. F., Miller C. W., and Sevestianov V. I. "Influence of endogenous albumin binding on blood-material interactions." *Ann. N. Y. Acad. Sci.*, 516:78, 1987.
102. Vroman L. and Adams A. L. "Identification of rapid changes at plasma-solid interfaces." *J. Biomed. Mater. Res.*, 3:43, 1969.
103. Vroman L., Adams A. L., Fischer G. C., and Munoz P. C. "Interaction of high molecular weight kininogen, factor XII and fibrinogen at plasma interfaces." *Blood*, 55:156, 1980.
104. Leonard E. F. and Vroman L. "Is the Vroman Effect of importance in the interaction of blood with artificial materials?" *J. Biomater. Sci., Polym. Ed.*, 3:95, 1991.
105. Brash J. L. "Protein interactions with solid surfaces following contact with plasma and blood." In *Makromolecular Chemistry and Macromolecules Symposium*, Ed. 1988: 441.
106. Fabrizius-Homan D. J. and Cooper S. L. "A comparison of the adsorption of three adhesive proteins to biomaterial surfaces." *J. Biomater. Sci., Polym. Ed.*, 3:27, 1991.
107. Horbett T. A. "Mass action effects in competitive adsorption of fibrinogen from hemoglobin solutions and from plasma." *Thromb. Haemost.*, 51:174, 1984.
108. Merrill E. W., Costa V. C. S. D., Salzman E. W., Brier-Russell D., Kuchner L., Waugh D. F., Trudel G., Stopper S., and Vitale V. "A critical study of segmented polyurethanes." In *Biomaterials: Interfacial Phenomena and Applications*, Ed. Cooper S. L., Peppas N. A. Adv. Chem. Ser. 199, 1982:
109. Takahara A., Tashita J., Kajiyama T., and Takayanagi M. "Interaction between blood components and surface of segmented poly(urethaneurea) with various soft segment length." *Rep. Progr. Polym. Phys. Japan*, XXIV:737, 1981.
110. Takahara A., Tashita J., Kajiyama T., Takayanagi M., and MacKnight W. J. "Microphase separated structure and blood compatibility of segmented poly(urethaneureas) with different diamines in the hard segment." *Polymer*, 26:978, 1985.
111. Harker L. A., Hanson S. R., and Hoffman A. S. "Platelet kinetic evaluation of prosthetic material *in vivo*." *Ann. N. Y. Acad. Sci.*, 283:317, 1977.
112. Takahara A., Kajiyama T., and Takayanagi M. "Effect of hydrophilic property of polyether components of segmented poly(urethane ureas) on their surface structure and blood compatibility." *Rep. Prog. Polym. Phys. Japan.*, 26:665, 1983.
113. Bamford C. H., Middleton I. P., and Satake Y. "Grafting and attachment of anti-platelet agents to poly(ether-urethanes)." *Polymer Prepr.*, 25:27, 1984.

114. Joseph G. and Sharma C. P. "Prostacyclin immobilized albuminated surfaces." *J. Biomed. Mater. Res.*, 21:937, 1987.
115. Bruil A., Terlingen J. G. A., Beugeling T., Aken W. G. V., and Feijen J. "*In vitro* leukocyte adhesion to modified polyurethane surfaces." *Biomaterials*, 13:915, 1992.
116. Lim F. and Cooper S. L. "Effect of sulphonate incorporation on in vitro leucocyte adhesion to polyurethanes." *Biomaterials*, 16:457, 1995.
117. Labow R. S., Erfle D. J., and Santerre J. P. "Neutrophil-mediated degradation of segmented polyurethanes." *Biomaterials*, 16:51, 1995.
118. Kaplan S. S., Basford R. E., Mora E., Jeong M. H., and Simmons R. L. "Biomaterial-induced alterations of neutrophil superoxide production." *J. Biomed. Mater. Res.*, 26:1039, 1992.
119. Ishihara K., Aragaki R., Ueda T., Watanabe A., and Nakabayashi` N. "Reduced thrombogenicity of polymers having phospholipid polar groups." *J. Biomed. Mater. Res.*, 24:1069, 1990.
120. Ishihara K., Ziats N. P., Tierney B. P., Nakabayashi N., and Anderson J. M. "Protein adsorption from human plasma is reduced on phospholipid polymers." *J. Biomed. Mater. Res.*, 25:1397, 1991.
121. Chapman D. "Biocompatible surfaces based upon the phospholipid asymmetry of biomembranes." *Biochem. Soc. Trans.*, 21:258, 1993.
122. Yu J., Lamba N. M. K., Courtney J. M., Whateley T. L., Gaylor J. D. S., Ishihara K., Nakabayashi N., and Lowe. G. D. O. "Polymeric biomaterials: influence of phosphorylcholine polar groups on protein adsorption and complement activation." *Int. J. Artif. Organs*, 17:499, 1994.
123. Ishihara K., Hanyuda H., and Nakabayashi N. "Phospholipid polymers having a urethane bond in the side chain as coating material on segmented polyurethane." *Trans. Soc. Biomaterials*, 18:83, 1995.
124. Lamba N. M. K., Yung L. L., and Cooper S. L. "Leukocyte adhesion to polyurethane surfaces under well-defined flow conditions." *Polymers in Medicine and Surgery.* Glasgow, Scotland. 1996: 81.
125. Nagel J. A., Dickinson R. B., and Cooper S. L. "Bacterial adhesion to polyurethane surfaces in the presence of pre-adsorbed high molecular weight kininogen." *J. Biomater. Sci., Polym. Ed.*, 7:769, 1996.
126. Nyilas E. and Ward R. S. "Development of blood compatible polymers. V. Surface structure and blood compatibility of Avcothane elastomers." *Polymer Prepr.*, 16:681, 1975.
127. Picha G. J., Gibbons D. F., and Auerbach R. A. "Effect of polyurethane morphology on blood coagulation." *J. Bioeng.*, 2:301, 1978.
128. Takahara A., Tashita J., Kajiyama T., Takayanagi M., and MacKnight W. J. "Microphase separated structure, surface composition and blood compatibility of segmented poly(urethaneureas) with various soft segment components." *Polymer*, 26:987, 1985.
129. Lelah M. D., Grasel T. G., Pierce J. A., and Cooper S. L. "*Ex vivo* interactions and surface property relationships of polyurethanes." *J. Biomed. Mater. Res.*, 20:433, 1986.
130. Lelah M. D., Jordan C. A., Pariso M. E., Lambrecht L. K., Cooper S. L., and Albrecht R. M. "Morphological changes occurring during thrombogenesis and embolization on biomaterials in a canine *ex-vivo* series shunt." *Scanning Electron Microscopy*, 4; 1983.
131. Salzman E. W. and Merrill E. W. "Interaction of blood with artificial surfaces." *In Hemostasis and Thrombosis: Basic Principles and Clinical Practice*, Ed. Colman R. W., Hirsch J., Marder V. J., Salzman E. W. J. B. Lippincott Co., Philadelphia, 1983: 931.
132. Lelah M. D., Pierce J. A., Lambrecht L. K., and Cooper S. L. "Polyether-urethane ionomers: surface property/*ex vivo* blood compatibility relationships." *J. Coll. Interf. Sci.*, 104:422, 1985.
133. Hergenrother R. W. and Cooper S. L. "Improved materials for blood-contacting applications: Blends of sulphonated and non-sulphonated polyurethanes." *J. Mat. Sci., Mat. Med.*, 3:313, 1992.
134. Ziats N. P., Miller K. M., and Anderson J. M. "*In vitro* and *in vivo* interactions of cells with biomaterials." *Biomaterials*, 9:5, 1988.
135. Anderson J. M. "Mechanisms of inflammation and infection with implanted devices." *Cardiovasc. Pathol.*, 2:33S, 1993.
136. Tang L. and Eaton J. W. "Inflammatory responses to biomaterials."*Am. J. Clin. Pathol.*, 103:466, 1995.
137. Spargo B. J., Rudolph A. S., and Rollwagen F. M. "Recruitment of tissue resident cells to hydrogel composites: in vivo response to implant materials." *Biomaterials*, 15:853, 1994.
138. Anderson J. M. "Inflammatory response to implants."*Trans. Am. Soc. Artif. Intern. Organs*, 34:101, 1988.
139. Bakker D., van Blitterswijk C. A., Hesseling S. C., Daems W. T., and Grote J. J. "Tissue/biomaterial interface characteristics of four elastomers. A transmission electron microscopical study." *J Biomed. Mater. Res.*, 24:277, 1990.

140. Lexander J. W. "Clinical evaluation of Epigard, a new synthetic substitute for homograft and heterograft skin." *J. Trauma*, 13:374, 1973.
141. Imber G., Schwager R. G., Guthrie R. H., and Gray G. F. "Fibrous capsule formation after subcutaneous implantation of synthetic materials in experimental animals." *Plastic Reconstr. Surg.*, 54:183, 1974.
142. Cocke W. M., Leathers H. K., and Lynch J. B. "Foreign body reactions to polyurethane covers of some breast prostheses." *Plastic Reconstr. Surg.*, 56:527, 1975.
143. Smahel J. "Tissue reactions to breast implants coated with polyurethane." *Plastic Reconstr. Surg.*, 61:82, 1978.
144. Brand K. G. "Foam-covered mammary implants." *Plastic Reconstr. Surg.*, 15:533, 1988.
145. Brohim R. M., Foresman P. A., Hildebrandt P. K., and Rodeheaver G. T. "Early tissue reaction to textured breast implant surfaces." *Ann. Plast. Surg.*, 28:354, 1992.
146. Vince D. G., Hunt J. A., and Williams D. F. "Quantitative assessment of the tissue response to implanted biomaterials." *Biomaterials*, 12:731, 1991.
147. Hunt J. A., Abrams K. R., and Williams D. F. "Modelling the pattern of cell distribution around implanted materials." *Anal. Cell. Pathol.*, 7:43, 1994.
148. Marchant R. E., Zhao Q., Anderson J. M., Hiltner A., and Ward R. S. "Surface degradation of polyurethanes." In *Surface Characterization of Biomaterials*, Ed. Ratner B. D. Elsevier Science Publishers, Amsterdam, 1988: 297.
149. Miller K. M. and Anderson J. M. "*In vitro* stimulation of fibroblast activity by factors generated from human monocytes activated by biomedical polymers." *J. Biomed. Mater. Res.*, 23:911, 1989.
150. Miller K. M., Huskey R. A., Bigby L. F., and Anderson J. M. "Characterization of biomedical polymer-adherent macrophages: Interleukin-1 generation and scanning electron microscopy studies." *Biomaterials*, 10:187, 1989.
151. Marchant R. E., Miller K. M.. and Anderson J. M. "*In vivo* biocompatibility studies. V. *In vivo* leukocyte interactions with Biomer." *J. Biomed. Mater. Res.*, 18:1169, 1984.
152. Habal M. B. and Powell R. D. "Biophysical evaluation of the tumorigenic response to implanted polymers." *J. Biomed. Mater. Res.*, 14:447, 1980.
153. Habal M. B., Powell M. L., and Schimpff R. D. "Immunological evaluation of the tumorigenic response to implanted polymers." *J. Biomed. Mater. Res.*, 14:455, 1980.
154. Marois Y., Roy R., Marois M., Guidoin R. G., von Maltzahn W. W., Kowligi R., and Eberhart R. C. "T-lymphocyte modification with the UTA microporous polyurethane vascular prosthesis: in vivo studies in rats." *Clin. & Inv. Med*, 15:141, 1992.
155. Bommer J., Gemsa D., Waldherr R., Kessler J., and Ritz E. "Plastic filling from dialysis tubing induces prostanoid release from macrophages." *Kidney Int.*, 26:331, 1984.
156. Bonfield T. L., Colton E., and Anderson J. M. "Cellular induction of interleukin-1 in the presence of protein adsorbed biomedical polymers." *Trans. Soc. Biomaterials*, 15:91, 1989.
157. Bonfield T. L., Colton E., and Anderson J. M. "Fibroblast stimulation by monocytes cultured on protein adsorbed biomedical polymers. I. Biomer and polydimethylsiloxane." *J. Biomed. Mater. Res.*, 25:165, 1991.
158. Bonfield T. L., Colton E., Marchant R. E., and Anderson J. M. "Cytokine and growth factor production by monocytes/macrophages on protein preadsorbed polymers." *J. Biomed. Mater. Res.*, 26:837, 1992.
159. Chignier E., Guidollet J., Freyria A. M., Ardail D., McGregor J. L., and Louisot P. "Dacron vascular biomaterial triggers macrophage ectoenzyme activity without change in cell membrane fluidity." *J. Biomed. Mater. Res.*, 27:1087, 1993.
160. Wilkins E. S. "Tissue reaction to intraperitoneally implanted catheter materials." *J. Biomed. Eng.*, 13:173, 1991.
161. Ito Y., Imanishi Y., and Sisido M. "Attachment and proliferation of fibroblast cells on polyetherurethane urea derivatives." *Biomaterials*, 8:464, 1987.
162. Tamada Y. and Ikada Y. "Effect of preadsorbed proteins on cell adhesion to polymer surfaces." *J. Coll. Interf. Sci.*, 155:334, 1993.
163. Schakenraad J. M., Kuit J. H., Arends J., Busscher H. J., Feijen J., and Wildevuur C. R. H. "*In vivo* quantification of cell-polymer interactions." *Biomaterials*, 8:207, 1987.
164. Lim F. and Cooper S. L. "The effect of surface hydrophilicity on biomaterial-leukocyte interactions." *Trans. Am. Soc. Artifi. Int. Org.*, 37:M146, 1991.

165. Brunstedt M. R., Ziats N. P., Schubert M., Stack S., Rose-Caprara V., Hiltner A., and Anderson J. M. "Protein adsorption and endothelial cell attachment and proliferation on PAPI-based additive modified poly(ether urethane ureas)." *J. Biomed. Mater. Res.*, 27:499, 1993.
166. Mohanty M., Hunt J. A., Doherty P. J., Annis D., and Williams D. F. "Evaluation of soft tissue response to a poly(urethane urea)." *Biomaterials*, 13:651, 1992.
167. Boyes D. C., Adey C. K., Bailar J. et al. "Safety of polyurethane-covered breast implants." *Can. Med. Assoc. J.*, 145:1125, 1991.
168. Hester T. R., Nahai F., Bostwick J., and Cukic J. "A 5-year experience with polyurethane-covered mammary prostheses for treatment of capsular contracture, primary augmentation mammoplasty and breast reconstruction." *Clin. Plast. Surg.*, 15:569, 1988.
169. Melmed E. P. "Polyurethane implants: A 6-year review of 416 patients." *Plastic Reconstr. Surg.*, 82:285, 1988.
170. Gayou R. and Rudolph R. "Capsular contraction around silicone mammary protheses." *Ann. Plast. Surg.*, 2:62, 1979.
171. McGrath M. H. and Burkhardt B. R. "The safety and efficacy of breast implants for augmentation mammaplasty." *Plastic Reconstr. Surg.*, 74:550, 1984.
172. Capozzi A. "Long-term complications of polyurethane-covered breast implants." *Plastic Reconstr. Surg.*, 88:458, 1991.
173. Pennisi V. R. "Polyurethane-covered silicone gel mammary prosthesis for successful breast reconstruction." *Aesthet. Plast. Surg.*, 9:73, 1985.
174. Eyssen J. E., von Werssowetz A. J., and Middleton G. D. "Reconstruction of the breast using polyurethane-coated prostheses." *Plastic Reconstr. Surg.*, 73:415, 1984.
175. Schatten W. E. "Reconstruction of breasts following mastectomy with polyurethane-covered gel-filled prostheses." *Ann. Plast. Surg.*, 12:147, 1984.
176. Shapiro M. A. "Smooth vs. rough: an 8-year survey of mammary prosthesis." *Plastic Reconstr. Surg.*, 84:449, 1989.
177. Melmed E. P. "Treatment of breast contractures with open capsulotomy and replacement of gel prostheses with polyurethane-covered implants." *Plastic Reconstr. Surg.*, 86:270, 1990.
178. Handel N., Silverstein M. J., Jensen J. A., and Collins A. "Comparative experience with smooth and polyurethane breast implants using the Kaplan-Meier method of survival analysis." *Plastic Reconstr. Surg.*, 88:475, 1991.
179. Gasperoni C., Salgarello M., and Gargani G. "Polyurethane-covered mammary implants: A 12-year experience." *Ann. Plast. Surg.*, 29:303, 1992.
180. Caffee H. H. and Hathaway C. "Polyurethane foam-covered implants and capsular contracture: A laboratory investigation." *Plastic Reconstr. Surg.*, 86:708, 1990.
181. Bucky L. P., Ehrlich H. P., Sohoni S., and May J. W. J. "The capsule quality of saline-filled smooth silicone, textured silicone, and polyurethane implants in rabbits: A long-term study." *Plastic Reconstr. Surg.*, 93:1123, 1994.
182. Cohney B. C., Cohney T. B., and Hearne V. A. "Nineteen years' experience with polyurethane foam-covered mammary prosthesis: A preliminary report." *Ann. Plast. Surg.*, 27:27, 1991.
183. Berrino P., Galli M., Rainero M. L., and Santi P. L. "Long-lasting complications with the use of polyurethane-covered breast implants." *Brit. J. Plast. Surg.*, 39:549, 1986.
184. Jabaley M. E. and Das S. K. "Late breast pain following reconstruction with polyurethane-covered implants." *Plastic Reconstr. Surg.*, 78:390, 1986.
185. Dunn K. W., Hall P. N., and Khoo C. T. K. "Breast implant materials: sense and safety." *Brit. J. Plast. Surg.*, 45:315, 1992.
186. Sharp W. V., Gardner D. L., and Anderson G. T. "Electrolour: a new vascular interface." *Trans. Am. Soc. Artif. Intern. Organs*, 14:73, 1968.
187. Bernhard W. F., Colo N. A., Wesolowski J. S., Szycher M., Fishbein M. C., Parkman R., Franzblau C. C., and Haudenschild C. C. "Development of collagenous linings on impermeable prosthetic surfaces." *J. Thorac. Cardiovasc. Surg.*, 79:552, 1980.
188. Hess F., Jerusalem C., and Braun B. "A fibrous polyurethane microvascular prothesis. Morphological evaluation of the neo-intima." *J. Cardiovasc. Surg.*, 24:509, 1983.
189. Whalen R. "Improved textured surfaces for implantable prostheses." *Trans. Am. Soc. Artif. Intern. Organs*, 34:887, 1988.

190. Kogel H., Vollmar J. F., and Proschek P. "New prostheses for venous substitution." *J. Cardiovasc. Surg.*, 32:330, 1991.
191. Wachem P. B. v., Stronck J. W. S., Koers-Zuideveld R., Dijk F., and Wildevuur C. R. H. "Vacuum cell seeding: a new method for the fast application of an evenly distributed cell layer on porous vascular grafts." *Biomaterials*, 11:602, 1990.
192. Soldani G., Steiner M., Galletti P. M., Lelli L., Palla M., and Giusti P. "Development of small-diameter vascular prostheses which release bioactive agents." *Clin. Mater.*, 8:81, 1991.
193. Bordenave L., Baquey C., Bareille R. et al. "Endothelial cell compatibility testing of three different Pellethanes." *J. Biomed. Mater. Res.*, 27:1367, 1993.
194. Lee Y., Park D. K., Kim Y. B., Seo J. W., Lee K. B., and Min B. "Endothelial cell seeding onto the extracellular matrix of fibroblasts for the development of a small diameter polyurethane vessel."*ASAIO J.*, 39:M740, 1993.
195. Miwa H., Matsuda T., Tani N., Kondo K., and Iida F. "An *in vitro* endothelialized compliant vascular graft minimizes anastomotic hyperplasia." *ASAIO J.*, 39:M501, 1993.
196. Lin H.-B., Garcia-Echeverria C., Asakura S., Sun W., Mosher D. F., and Cooper S. L. "Endothelial cell adhesion on polyurethanes containing covalently attached RGD peptides." *Biomaterials*, 13:905, 1992.
197. Brunstedt M. R., Ziats N. P., Rose-Caprara V., Hiltner A., Anderson J. M., Lodoen G. A., and Payet C. R. "Attachment and proliferation of bovine aortic endothelial cells onto additive modified poly(ether urethane ureas)." *J. Biomed. Mater. Res.*, 7:483, 1993.
198. Remes A. and Williams D. F. "Immune response in biocompatibility." *Biomaterials*, 13:731, 1992.
199. Roitt I. M. *Essential Immunology.* Blackwell Scientific Publications, Oxford, England, 1991.
200. Wahl L. M. and Wahl S. M."Inflammation Wound healing:Biochemical and Clinical Aspects." In Eds. Cohen K., Dieglemann R. F., Lindblad W. J. W. B. Saunders Co., Philadelphia, 1992:
201. Colten H. R. "Tissue-specific regulation of inflammation." *J. Appl. Physiol.*, 72:1, 1992.
202. Quintans J. "Immunity and inflammation: The cosmic view." *Immun. Cell Biol.*, 72:262, 1994.
203. Wadstrom T., Eliason I., Holder I., and Ljungh A. *Pathogenesis of Wound and Biomaterial-Associated Infections.* Springer–Verlag, London, 1990.
204. Mora E. M., Cardona M. A., and Simmons R. L. "Enteric bacteria and ingested inert particles translocate to intraperitoneal prosthetic materials." *Arch. Surg.*, 126:157, 1991.
205. Anderton A. and Nwoguh C. E. "Re-use of enteral feeding tubes — a potential hazard to the patient? A study of the efficiency of a representative range of cleaning and disinfection procedures."*J. Hospital Infec.*, 18:131, 1991.
206. Reid G., Khoury A. E., Preston C. A. K., and Costerton J. W. "Influence of dextrose dialysis solutions on adhesion of staphylococcus aureus and pseudomonas aeruginosa to three catheter surfaces."*Am. J. Nephrol.*, 14:37, 1994.
207. Gristina A. G., Hobgood C. D., and Barth E. "Biomaterial specificity, molecular mechanisms and clinical relevance of S. epidermidis and S. aureus infections in surgery." In *Pathogenesis and Clinical Significance of Coagulase-Negative Staphylococci*, Ed. Pulverer G., Quie P. G., Peters G. Gustav Fischer Verlag, Stuttgart, 1987: 143.
208. Gristina A. G., Christensen G. D., Simpson W. A., and Beachey E. "Microbial adherence in infection." In *Principles and Practice of Infectious Disease*, Ed. Mandell F. L., Jr., Bennett R. G. D. Wiley, New York, 1985: 6.
209. Bayston R. and Penny S. R. "Excessive production of mucoid substances in Staphylococcus SIIA: a possible factor in colonization of Holter shunts." *Dev. Med. Child. Neurol.*, 14:25, 1972.
210. Cao M. H., Holmes D. R., Gersh B. J., Maloney J. D., Meredith J., Pluth J. R., and Trusty J. "Permanent pacemaker infections, characteristics and management." *Am. J. Cardiol.*, 48:559, 1981.
211. Dankert J., Hogt A. H., and Feijen J. "Biomedical polymers: bacterial adhesion, colonization and infection." In *CRC Critical Reviews in Biocompatibility*, Ed. CRC Press, Boca Raton, FL, 1986: 219.
212. Mohammad S. F., Topham N. S., Burns G. L., and Olsen D. B. "Enhanced bacterial adhesion on surfaces pretreated with fibrinogen and fibronectin." *Trans. Am. Soc. Artif. Intern. Organs*, 34:573, 1988.
213. Switalski L. M., Speziale P., and Hook M. "Isolation and characterization of a putative collagen receptor from Staphylococcus aureus strain Cowan 1." *J. Biol. Chem.*, 264:21080, 1989.

214. Vaudaux P., Pittet D., Haeberli A., Huggler E., Nydegger U. E., Lew D. P., and Waldvogel F. A. "Host factors selectively increase staphylococcal adherence on inserted catheters: a role for fibronectin and fibrinogen or fibrin." *J. Infectious Dis.*, 160:865, 1989.
215. Cheung A. L. and Fischetti V. A. "The role of fibrinogen in staphylococcal adherence to catheters *in vitro*." *J. Infectious Dis.*, 161:1177, 1990.
216. Raja R. H., Raucci G., and Hook M. "Peptide analogs to a fibronectin receptor inhibit attachment of Staphylococcus aureus to fibronectin containing substrates." *Infect. Immun.*, 58:2593, 1990.
217. Stokes K., McVenes R., and Anderson J. M. "Polyurethane elastomer biostability." *J. Biomater. Appl.*, 9:321, 1995.
218. Cheung A. K., Parker C. J., Wilcox L. A., and Janatova J. "Activation of complement by haemodialysis membranes; polyacrylonitrile binds more C3a than Cuprophan." *Kidney Int.*, 37:1055, 1990.
219. Martinez-Martinez L., Pascual A., and Perea E. J. "Kinetics of adherence of mucoid and non-mucoid Pseudomonas aeruginosa to plastic catheters." *J. Med. Microbiol.*, 34:7, 1991.
220. Cierny G., Gouch L. and Mader J. *Adjunctive local antibiotics in the management of contaminated orthopaedic wounds.* American Academy Of Orthopaedic Surgeons Final Program of 53rd Meeting. New Orleans, LA, Feb. 20–25. 1986: 86.
221. Bakker D., van Blitterswijk C. A., Hesseling S. C., Daems W. T., Kuijpers W., and Grote J. J. "The behavior of alloplastic tympanic membranes in staphylococcus aureus-induced middle ear infection. I. Quantitative biocompatibility evaluation." *J. Biomed. Mater. Res.*, 24:669, 1990.
222. Price C. I., Horton J. W., and Baxter C. R. Topical liposomal delivery of antibiotics in soft tissue infection. J. Surg. Res., 49:174, 1990.
223. Golomb G. and Shpigelman A. "Prevention of bacterial colonization on polyurethane in vitro by incorporated antibacterial agent." *J. Biomed. Mater. Res.*, 25:937, 1991.
224. Sandham H. J., Brown J., Chan K. H., Phillips H. I., Burgess R. C., and Stokl A. J. "Clinical trial in adults of an antimicrobial varnish for reducing mutant streptococci." *J. Dental Res.*, 70:1401, 1991.

8 Degradation of Polyurethanes

I. INTRODUCTION

Polyurethanes are used in applications where the stability of the material is important. They were introduced in commercial long term medical applications in breast implants, catheters, and pacemaker lead insulation.[1] Much of the information on the degradation of polyurethanes has come as a consequence of observations of *in vivo* degradation of polyurethanes in breast implants and pacemaker leads.

It is now known that many polyurethanes degrade *in vivo*. This is the end result of a number of interrelated and diverse factors that include the polyurethane chemistry, mechanical properties, manufacturing and implantation techniques, and the complex biological environment of the implant site. Ultimately, degradation can lead to significant changes in the polymer mechanical properties, surface chemistry and structure leading to malfunction and implant failure. The major underlying causes of degradation in polyurethanes are hydrolysis and oxidation.[1]

II. MECHANISMS OF BIODEGRADATION

Biodegradation may occur by many different routes. Components responsible for the degradation of polymers in the body include water, salts, peroxides, and enzymes. Theoretically other molecules including vitamins, and free radicals also may catalyze degradation. If the polyurethane is hydrophobic, the degradation is usually limited to the surface of the material. However, if the polyurethane is hydrophilic, water will be present in the polymer bulk and degradation may occur throughout the material.[2]

Polymer degradation in chemically active media (for example plasma and tissue) generally includes the following processes: (1) Adsorption of medium on the polymer surface, (2) Diffusion and absorption of the medium into the bulk of the polymer, (3) Chemical reactions with the chemically unstable bonds in the polymer, and (4) Desorption and transport of the degradation products out of the polymer matrix and desorption of the degradation products from the polymer surface. Not all components of degradation will necessarily occur in every case. Generally, polyester based polyurethanes are subject to hydrolysis and polyether based polyurethanes are subject to oxidation.

A. Hydrolysis

Hydrolysis is one of the dominant mechanisms for polyurethane degradation in the aqueous environment of the body. Hydrolysis can essentially be considered as a "reversal of condensation".[3] Hydrolytically unstable bonds typically found in polyurethanes include ester linkages and hydrolysis also appears to be facilitated by polar groups in the side chain of the polymer backbone.[4,5] The urethane bonds appear to be more resistant to hydrolytic cleavage,[6] and are not considered susceptible to hydrolysis under normal implant conditions.[7] However, hydrolysis of this bond occurs at high temperatures in the presence of water. These conditions can occur during extrusion or injection molding. Relatively, the hydrolytic degradation of polyurethanes in pure water is low; however the presence of anions and cations has a strong catalytic effect.

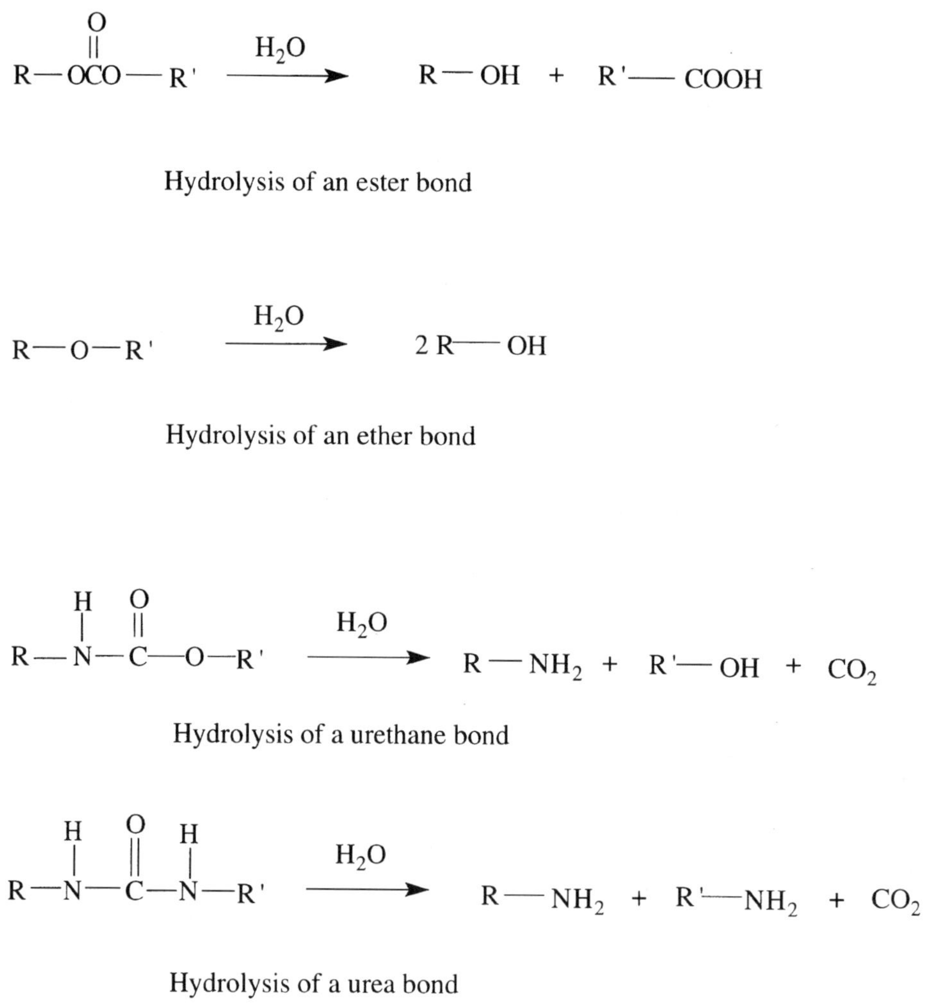

$$R-OCO-R' \xrightarrow{H_2O} R-OH + R'-COOH$$
(with C=O on the OCO group)

Hydrolysis of an ester bond

$$R-O-R' \xrightarrow{H_2O} 2\,R-OH$$

Hydrolysis of an ether bond

$$R-NH-CO-O-R' \xrightarrow{H_2O} R-NH_2 + R'-OH + CO_2$$

Hydrolysis of a urethane bond

$$R-NH-CO-NH-R' \xrightarrow{H_2O} R-NH_2 + R'-NH_2 + CO_2$$

Hydrolysis of a urea bond

FIGURE 1 Hydrolysis reactions of polyurethanes

The hydrolysis reactions for some of the bonds typically involved in polyurethane degradation are illustrated below in Figure 1.[8] The hydrolysis rate will depend not only on the reactivity of susceptible chemical bonds but also on the water concentration within the polyurethane. Both hydrolysis by pure water and catalysis by the presence of salts requires water in the polymer. Hydrophilic polymers are thus more susceptible to hydrolytic degradation than hydrophobic polymers.

Pavlova and Draganova have found that the diffusion properties of polyurethanes have a significant impact on the biodegradation and have correlated both diffusion coefficients and permeabilities with the rate of hydrolysis.[8] Defining a diffusion index D, a sorption index C and the permeability P of polymeric films, they found that biodegradation of urethane-acrylate adhesives occurs most rapidly when D and P are highest.

Because hydrolysis results in chain cleavage, the physical properties of the material can be affected through the reduction in molecular weight. However, the hydrolysis must be fairly extensive before this occurs. A sign of extensive hydrolysis is the presence of deep, usually random cracks on the surface of the material resulting from significant molecular weight reduction.

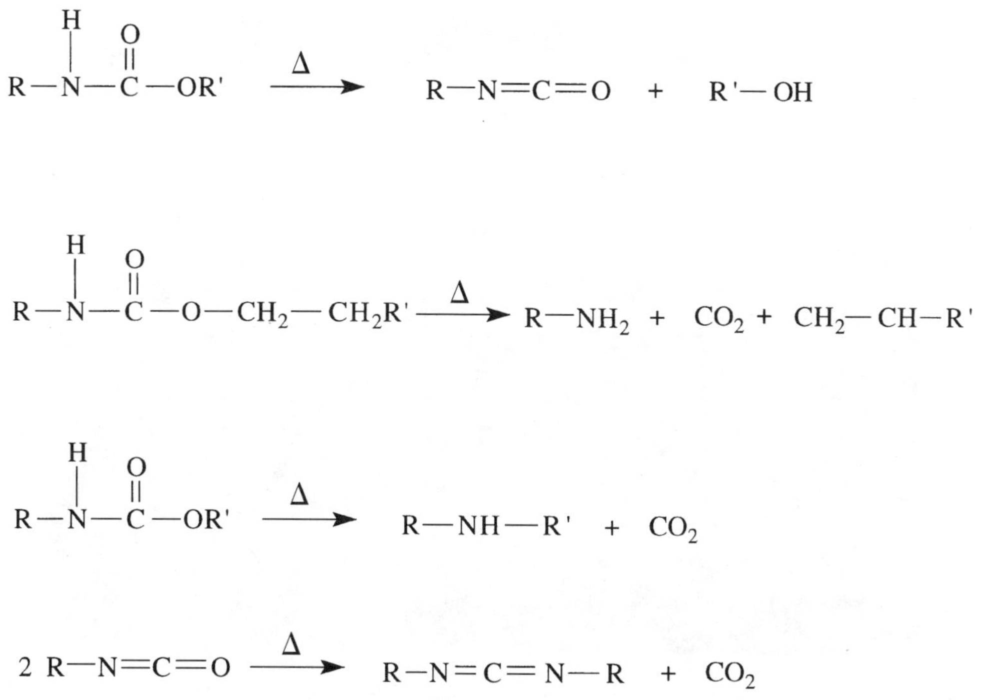

Degradation of Polyurethanes

$$R-\underset{\underset{H}{|}}{N}-\underset{\overset{O}{\|}}{C}-OR' \xrightarrow{\Delta} R-N=C=O + R'-OH$$

$$R-\underset{\underset{H}{|}}{N}-\underset{\overset{O}{\|}}{C}-O-CH_2-CH_2R' \xrightarrow{\Delta} R-NH_2 + CO_2 + CH_2-CH-R'$$

$$R-\underset{\underset{H}{|}}{N}-\underset{\overset{O}{\|}}{C}-OR' \xrightarrow{\Delta} R-NH-R' + CO_2$$

$$2\ R-N=C=O \xrightarrow{\Delta} R-N=C=N-R + CO_2$$

FIGURE 2 Thermal degradation reactions of polyurethanes.

B. OXIDATION

The degradation of polyether polyurethanes is more often associated with oxidative processes than with hydrolysis. There are several different mechanisms of oxidation including autoxidation, oxidation by peroxides, free radicals, enzymes and metal catalyzed oxidation (MO). It appears that oxidation occurs in the polyether soft segment at the α-methylene position. Free radicals also can degrade the polymer directly, abstracting a hydrogen atom from the methylene carbon in the polyether segment. Anions and cations of electrolytes found in biological media can catalyze the oxidation in a manner similar to the way they catalyze hydrolysis.[1]

1. Autoxidation

Heat can affect the physical properties of a polyurethane and can contribute to degradation. Most polymers including polyurethanes undergo a process of autoxidation which progresses at a negligibly slow rate. Heat and ultraviolet light can catalyze this reaction which results in more rapid degradation.[7,9] In the case of thermal degradation (frequently resulting from overheating during processing) the polyurethane will cleave at the urethane linkage between the isocyanate and the diol. In combination with water this can result in the formation of the amine of the isocyanate (i.e., TDA from TDI) compounds that have been shown to be carcinogenic in animal models. The high temperatures required for thermal degradation hypothetically could be associated with overheating during sterilization and processing of biomedical polyurethanes. Thermal degradation reactions are shown in Figure 2.

Autoxidation is considered thermal oxidation that takes place at elevated temperatures, approximately 150°C and is believed to take place by free-radical reaction.[7,10] The steps of initiation, propagation, and termination result in chain cleavage which can be self propagating once initiated. The initiator can be light, radiation, heat, strain, oxygen, etc.[7] Autoxidation is usually initiated by

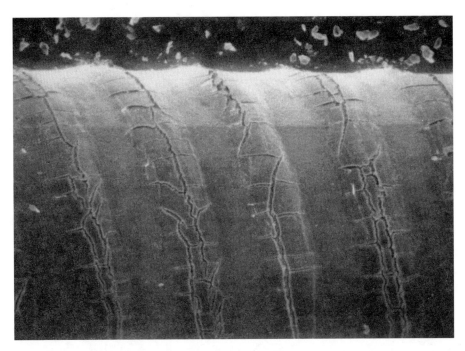

FIGURE 3 The beginnings of MO in the insulating sheath of a pacemaker lead. The polymer has oxidized where it contacts the MP35N conductor coil. Oxidation reduces molecular weight and affects the glass transition temperature, the degraded material shrinks when it dries out, producing cracked grooves. Courtesy Medtronic Inc.

the abstraction of a hydrogen but when the polymer is under stress, chain cleavage may be more important. The reactions are detailed in an excellent article by Stokes *et al.*[7] Once the initiation has occurred, further interactions with oxygen can produce hydroperoxides which are degraded during the propagation phase of oxidation. Species involved in the many reactions include carbonyl and hydroxyl groups such as ROO•, ROOR, RCO•, RO• and R•.[7] Low oxygen concentrations lead to relatively fast termination and with such species as ROOR', RR', and RCR' being formed. High oxygen concentrations will enhance the propagation step and result in greater degradation.

2. Metal Catalyzed Oxidation

Polyether polyurethanes are also sensitive to metal catalyzed oxidative degradation. This phenomenon, metal catalyzed oxidation (MO), first was described in the pacemaker literature (see Chapter 9). Stokes *et al.*[11] showed that the corrosion products from the metallic components from early generation pacemaker lead wire coils were strong catalysts for polyether polyurethane oxidation.

Several different mechanisms have been proposed for MO. Ions may be produced by reaction of the metal with radicals of hydrogen peroxide or superoxide, produced by macrophages and other phagocytic cells during inflammation. Phillips and Thoma have proposed that metal ions complex with the polyether soft segment of the polyurethane resulting in a conformational change and subsequent embrittlement of the material.[6,12] Metal ions often are found at sites of degradation, cobalt and molybdenum have been implicated as particularly vigorous promoters of MO.[13]

Stokes *et al.*[7] have shown that MO can occur in pacemaker leads in the absence of cell encapsulation i.e., without high concentrations of hydrogen peroxide or superoxide from cells. They suggest that MO also can occur by anaerobic processes as well as autoxidation. In the anaerobic mechanism, transition metals oxidize and initiate polymer oxidation through the abstraction of hydrogen.[7] It is likely that more than one mechanism can facilitate metal catalyzed oxidation given the complex biological environment. An example of the effects of MO on a pacemaker lead sheath are whown in Figure 3.

C. Chemical Degradation

Various chemicals also can contribute to the degradation of not only polyurethanes but other polymers. Organic and inorganic chemicals can affect polyurethane stability either by physical or chemical mechanisms. In certain fluids polyurethanes will swell but return to their original dimensions on drying. Alcohols, acids, ketones, and esters tend to cause swelling and degradation, especially at high temperatures. The mechanisms by which degradation occurs include hydrolysis, random chain scission, and aminolysis. Aliphatic hydrocarbons and esters are generally inert, but aromatic hydrocarbons are more active and promote swelling at room temperature and gradual breakdown at higher temperatures. Chemical exchange is a general term which includes such reactions as glycolysis, aminolysis, and transesterification. These reactions can result in changes in molecular weight and molecular-weight distribution.

Chlorinated solvents cause swelling and sometimes enhance degradation significantly, reducing the tensile and tear strength.[6,14] With most organic fluids, except solvents, short-term contact does not affect polyurethanes to any great extent. In biomedical applications only short-term contact may be necessary for cleaning or priming the polyurethane during the processing stages. The aqueous and biological environment of the body has a much greater influence on degradation, because it interacts with the polyurethane over very long time periods.

The exposure of aromatic polyurethanes to sunlight results in a loss of mechanical properties and discoloration.[6] The loss of mechanical properties includes embrittlement and loss of tensile strength. MDI based polyurethanes change from a light yellow (generally) to amber, and with greater exposure, dark brown via autooxidation. Aliphatic polyurethanes do not undergo this change. Aromatic polyurethanes may be stabilized with antioxidants and UV stabilizers.

D. Sterilization

Polyurethanes are generally considered resistant to the effects of high-energy radiation. At very high doses (above those used in sterilization) irradiation results in progressive degradation.[6] However, recent work has indicated that γ radiation may result in the release of MDA in MDI based potting materials. Shintani and Nakamura found a dose dependent relationship between release of MDA and radiation levels.[15] They did not find release during autoclave sterilization. Steam sterilization has been associated with formation of MDA and polyurethane resin suppliers caution against using this method for polyurethanes in medical applications.[16]

E. Biological Catalysis of Degradation

Cells and enzymes either produce oxidative and hydrolytic components or are themselves the agent of degradation. The basic mechanisms of hydrolysis and oxidation also can be the mechanisms of enzyme and cell associated polyurethane degradation. Many previously observed degradation phenomena, including calcification and environmental stress cracking have been found in association with cells and enzymes.

1. Enzymes

Cells release many active compounds that affect the degradation of a polyurethane *in vivo*. Both macrophages and neutrophils have been directly implicated in the degradation of polyurethanes.[17,18] Phagocytes, macrophages and neutrophils will attempt to engulf foreign material and "kill" or digest it through either an oxygen-dependent or oxygen-independent mechanism. In the oxygen-dependent mechanism, these cells release superoxide anions, hydrogen peroxide, hydroxyl radicals and a host of halogenating substances which are likely one of the main causes of oxidative degradation of polyurethanes.[7,19-22] The nonoxygen dependent mechanism appears to involve hydrolytic enzymes.

Enzymes are now known to be involved in both hydrolysis and oxidative degradation of polyurethanes, whether secreted from cells or from the blood.[3,18,23-27] A number of investigators have shown that enzymes alone can degrade many different polymers *in vitro*. In a group of studies, Smith et al.[3,23] investigated the degradation of numerous materials including polyurethanes, using several different enzyme systems. They investigated the effect of the enzymes esterase, papain, trypsin, and chymotrypsin on polyethylene terephthalate, nylon 66, and polymethyl methacrylate. The polymers were affected differently by the enzymes but their results indicated that degradation appeared to be both enzyme and material dependent. In a second study, published in the same journal, Smith et al.[23] specifically looked at polyurethane degradation in the presence of esterase, papain and lysosomal liver enzymes. They found that these enzymes caused the release of radiolabeled ^{14}C species from a polyetherurethane. Santerre et al.[26] also found that the degradation of materials appears to be enzyme and material specific. They compared the degradation of a polyester urea-urethane and a polyether urea-urethane using radiolabeled tracers in the presence of cholesterol esterase, collagenase, cathepsin B and xanthine oxidase. Interestingly, they found that the polyester was sensitive to cholesterol esterase as measured by release of radioactive substances but there was no significant change in weight for any of the materials in the presence of any of the enzymes.

Papain (a protease) and trypsin (a hydrolase) have been used in many investigations involving polyurethanes because they cleave peptide linkages. Takahara et al.[25] showed that in a papain solution a polyethyleneoxide based polyurethane was susceptible to degradation and Ratner et al.[28] showed that Pellethane 2363-80A and other polyurethanes were sensitive to several different enzymes including chymotrypsin and papain. Bouvier et al.[29] showed that Pellethane 2363-80A also is sensitive to trypsin. They found that incubation with the enzyme resulted in the release of low molecular weight materials, with cleavage occurring at the ether bond. Zhao et al.[19] showed that the mechanical properties of poly(ether urethane ureas) deteriorated after incubation with papain. Phua et al.[30] also found that papain and urease degraded Biomer but in different ways.

The mechanisms appear to differ according to the material and the enzyme. Several possible influences on the way in which enzymes interact are discussed under the section on the influence of polyurethane chemistry.

2. Cells

A large amount of both *in vitro* and *in vivo* work relating biodegradation of polyurethanes to the presence of cells has been undertaken in the last several years. Labow et al.[18] have implicated elastase activity with the degradation of polyurethane in the presence of neutrophils. The work done *in vitro* with neutrophils showed that it was possible to distinguish between the polymers tested based on their response to the white cells. The enzymes released by the neutrophils appeared to interact preferentially with the hard segment but the soft segment also was being hydrolyzed. The authors related the degradation by neutrophils to a similar pattern of degradation by elastase. Elastase is a specific marker of neutrophil activation so it is perhaps not surprising that this enzyme might be implicated in the interaction of the neutrophils with the biomaterial.[18] Cells also appear to be implicated in calcification, surface cracking and environmental stress cracking, all major pathways of degradation in polyurethanes.

Kaplan et al.[31] found that biomaterials activate neutrophils resulting in superoxide release. This activation appears to be attachment dependent and differs from that of cells in suspension. In addition, these investigators found that the mechanisms of biomaterial activation of the neutrophils were material dependent. Polymer structure also has been implicated in degradation connected with cells. It has been observed that the higher the porosity of the polyurethane, the greater the degradation rate.[32]

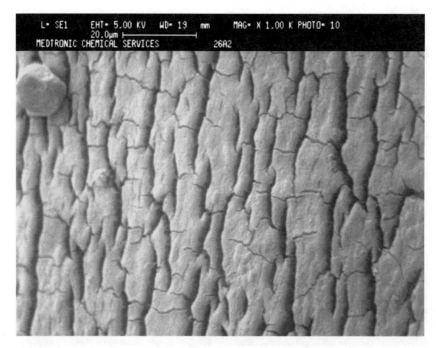

FIGURE 4 Pellethane 2363-80A with surface microcracking. An ATR–FTIR spectrum would show that this involves oxidation of the surface. Bulk analysis would show neither cracking nor oxidation. Courtesy of Medtronic Inc.

3. Surface Cracking

The term autoxidation also is used to describe the cause of cracking which occurs in a very shallow zone (less than 10 μm) at the surface of the material. It occurs in the absence of stress and this differentiates it from environmental stress cracking.[1] Explanted polyether polyurethanes frequently show shallow random cracks that do not appear to propagate.[1,7] An SEM of surface cracking of polyurethane is presented in Figure 4.

Using this definition, autoxidation does not result in significant changes in the polymer's mechanical properties. However, if a component of the material is located at the surface only, it could be lost from the surface due to autoxidation. Autoxidation and the resultant surface cracking appears to result from the foreign body response associated with biomaterials *in vivo*,[1,7,17,19,33-35] which is described in Chapter 7. Zhao *et al.*[19] found that macrophages adhered to the surface of the polyurethane, formed foreign body giant cells (FBGCs), and subsequently areas of surface cracking were found in association with the FBGC. The investigators found no cracking in the absence of adherent cells and were able to correlate surface cracking with areas of adherent cells. Surface cracking may be a pre-requisite for environmental stress cracking. Marchant *et al.*[33] found preferential adherence of macrophages to Biomer surfaces and associated these with pitting.

F. Environmental Stress Cracking

Environmental stress cracking (ESC) is a problem associated with polymers across their spectrum of applications. ESC of a material occurs under conditions that provide an active chemical agent and tensile stress.[13] The environment encountered *in vivo* implantation is a hostile one and thus provides a number of suitable agents. Stress may be inherent, due to the phase separated nature of polyurethanes, or may be applied to a device during manufacture, implantation, or through intracorporeal movement. The failure of pacemaker leads was believed to be caused by environmental

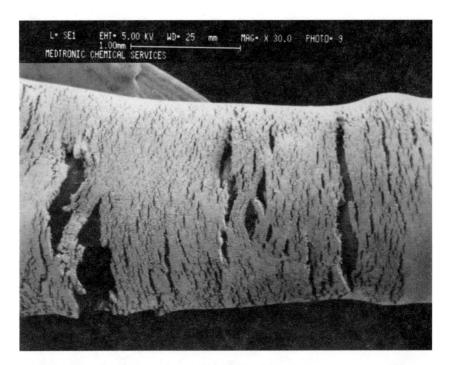

FIGURE 5 Surface microcracks have propagated through the bulk in response to residual strain (stress cracked). FTIR of the crack faces would probably show oxidation, but the bulk (between cracks) is not measurably degraded. Courtesy of Medtronic Inc.

stress cracking, and initiated many studies into ESC of implanted medical devices. It was suspected that the manufacturing method employed to produce lead insulation was introducing stress into the sheaths, which in turn contributed to lead failure. Alterations were made to the manufacturing process to reduce the stress in the material. Leads manufactured after this modification was implemented were much more successful. A discussion on the performance of pacemaker leads can be found in Chapter 9.

Environmental stress cracking is characterized by deep, ragged fractures within the polyurethane, often occurring perpendicular to the direction of stress.[1,7] In the more advanced case the polyurethane has three-dimensional cracks often referred to as mud-cracks. Tissue surrounding an implant which has environmental stress cracking is often well integrated into the material due to ingrowth into the cracks. As a phenomenon, it has been difficult to show ESC *in vitro*, and it appears to require tissue contact.[1] A SEM of a polyurethane that has undergone environmental stress cracking is shown in Figure 5.

Further studies of environmental stress cracking of polyurethanes in the biological environment have reported that cracks appear within six months of implantation although they do not propagate more than 20–30 μm within three years.[36] Fissures on the surface may be more interactive with platelets, phagocytes, enzymes, and tissue. Cracking also may lead to a reduction in the tensile strength of the polyurethane. Studies comparing the degree of surface cracking on explanted surfaces of Pellethane grades show that Pellethane 2363-55D which has a higher hard segment content is much less susceptible to surface cracking than Pellethane 2363-80A.[37]

It is now apparent the ESC is not just the result of stress, and requires cellular interaction or other chemical agents (possibly released from cells) to occur. Investigators have shown that unstressed polyurethanes show autooxidation and that stress simply propagates the surface cracks.[38] More recently Kao *et al.*[39] specifically investigated macrophage adhesion and FBGC formation on strained polyetherurethane urea elastomers. They found that the presence of additives (an antioxidant powder, Santowhite©) affected ESC. The kinetics of foreign body giant cell formation were also affected resulting in a decreased number of adherent macrophages, rate of FBGC formation and lower FBGC density. Interestingly, these researchers also found that the strain on the polyurethanes did not appear to directly modulate the adhesion of the macrophages and subsequent FBGC formation. The strained materials supported a faster rate of macrophage fusion but did not appear to influence the initial FBGC formation, density and size distribution in comparison with the unstrained controls. Wabers et al.[40] investigated sulfonated polyurethanes and also found a correlation with the presence of stabilizers and a reduction of surface cracking. The presence of the stabilizers reduced the cracking to a greater degree than the sulfonation of the hard segments.

Two different theories have been proposed to explain environmental stress cracking based on the above evidence. The first has been proposed by Sutherland et al., and involves HOCl and NO^3 release from PMNs. The other has been proposed by Stokes et al. and requires a four factor interaction associated with the foreign body response.[7] The evidence supports both theories. It has been proposed that polymorphonuclear leukocytes (PMNs) are the major player in the phenomenon through their activation and subsequent secretion of nitric oxide and oxidants.[41] Others propose a greater role for the foreign body response and the oxidants secreted by macrophages and foreign body giant cells.[7] The reader is referred to the two original papers by Sutherland et al.,[41] and Stokes et al.[7] for a more detailed description of the theories.

G. Impact of Polyurethane Structure on Biodegradation

Both *in vitro* and *in vivo* investigations have been employed to study the relation between the chemical structure of a polyurethane and its biodegradation. The nature of the soft segment, diisocyanate, and chain extender used all play a role in the biostability of the polyurethane.

1. Soft Segment

Ester groups are sensitive to both water hydrolysis and esterase activity. In their work, Smith et al.[3] found that enzymes will degrade both an aliphatic and an aromatic polyester and the soft segment chemistry of polyurethanes, specifically at the surface, has been implicated in both the enzymatic and oxidative degradation of the material.[42] This sensitivity to hydrolysis has resulted in polyester polyurethanes being used minimally in permanently implantable devices. It appears that polyester macroglycols were used in the foam covering of the Meme breast implant. The porous coating on the Meme breast implant, Microthane, a polyester foam, is believed to be made from a diol-terminated polyadipate soft segment. Its degradation has become the center of considerable ongoing debate.

There have been many studies published in recent years on the degradation of the Meme breast implant.[43–45] In retrospect it is not surprising that this material degraded to some degree. The foam, with its large surface area and porous structure, provides an avenue for water, enzymes and cells to contact the material and initiate bulk degradation. Several general reviews state that investigators have found the polyurethane coating separated from the implant surface and fragmented.[43–45] Clinically based studies using explanted specimens, X-rays, scanning electron microscopy, and histological evaluations have found physical evidence that the polyurethane has degraded into fragments.[43–45] Sinclair et al.[44] found that older implants had fewer foam particles in the fibrous capsule surrounding the implant than the younger specimens and the fragments were smaller. Interestingly, Szycher and Siciliano came to different conclusions, finding that the polyurethane embedded in the surrounding fibrous capsule formed a continuous sheet visible only after enzymatic digestion of the tissue capsule.[16]

Although polyester based polyurethanes have not been used extensively in permanently implantable devices, they have been used in biomaterials for temporary use including wound dressings and gastric bubbles. Dillion and Hughes investigated the degradation of what they suspected was an aromatic polyester polyurethane gastric bubble. They based their assumptions about its chemistry on ATR–IR characterization which indicated the presence of aromatic groups, ester peaks at 1168 and 1140 cm^{-1} and no urea group absorbances. They found that the gastric bubble, a device for use as temporary treatment for obesity, explanted after insertion into the gastric cavity, showed significant chemical and physical changes. Although the exact implantation times were not known, the investigators were able to determine a decrease in the number average molecular weight, Mn, using size exclusion chromatography. In addition, major changes were observed in the differential scanning calorimetry scan including decreases in T_g and a broadening of the T_m. Their results suggest that low molecular weight soft segment degradation products containing carboxylic acid or alcohol end groups were being produced during degradation. They had no evidence that the hard segment was degraded in this material.

In a detailed study on polyurethane adhesive dressings, Pavlova and Dragnova investigated the effect of the soft segment on the stability of polyurethane adhesive wound dressings.[8] They compared both polyester and polyether containing polyurethanes and found that the hydrolytic stability of polyurethanes based on their soft segment was in the order of: polycaprolactone polyol< polyethylene glycol < polyethylene adipate < branched polyester < polycarbonate < polyether polyol. These studies and many others have continued to confirm that the polyesters are susceptible to hydrolytic cleavage. Brandwood et al. used a series of polyurethanes based on soft segments with increasing numbers of CH_2 groups in the polyether macroglycol to investigate the effect of modifying the soft segment on stress cracking.[46] They found that the polyurethanes made with the novel soft segments showed less stress cracking than Pellethane 2363-55D and Tecoflex EG80A. This group also found that molecular weight of the polymers tested did not correlate well with SEM observations of stress cracking. Wu et al.[47] investigated the creep of a polyetherurethane urea in an $H_2O_2/COCl_2$ environment and found that the creep of the stressed material was dramatically accelerated in the oxidative environment. This suggests that oxidation may be an integral part of the stress cracking mechanism.

Takahara et al.[25] also showed that in a papain solution, a polyethyleneoxide based polyurethane was susceptible to degradation and that the degradation was due to the dissociation of the urethane linkage. In addition, the authors also found that lipid sorption contributed to the degradation of a polydimethylsiloxane based polyurethanes. Tingfei et al.[48] studied segmented and nonsegmented MDI-based polyurethane producing . Upon implanting these two polyurethanes subcutaneously in rats, they found varying degrees of degradation.

Recent research has focused on developing new soft segments that contain neither ester nor ether linkages in order to make "biostable" polyurethanes for medical applications. These include polycarbonate polyurethanes, polycarbonate urethane ureas, and polyaliphatic urethanes.

2. Hard Segment

The hard segment type and content will also influence the biodegradation of polyurethanes. The use of aromatic verses aliphatic isocyanates has been hotly debated over the past few years. Based on their fundamental chemistry, aromatic isocyanates should be more stable than aliphatic ones. Aromatic groups are stabilized by resonance involving the sharing of π-electrons by adjacent atoms. This strengthens the linkages between the atoms and results in higher bond strengths than found in the equivalent aliphatic linkages. These higher bond strengths mean that it is harder to degrade aromatic linkages. In addition, aromatic polyurethanes also have greater intermolecular bond strengths than cycloaliphatic polyurethanes because of their semicrystalline nature. Cycloaliphatic isocyanates do not crystallize due to the configurational isomers present.[1]

Using accelerated *in vitro* experiments, Stokes found that Pellethane 2363-55D, which contains an aromatic isocyanate, showed little stress cracking compared to the equivalent polyurethane made with an aliphatic isocyanate, Tecoflex EG-60D (Thermedics, Woburn, MA).[9] Tecoflex showed severe cracking in 19% of the test specimens. Szycher confirmed this work,[49] and Christ et al.[50]

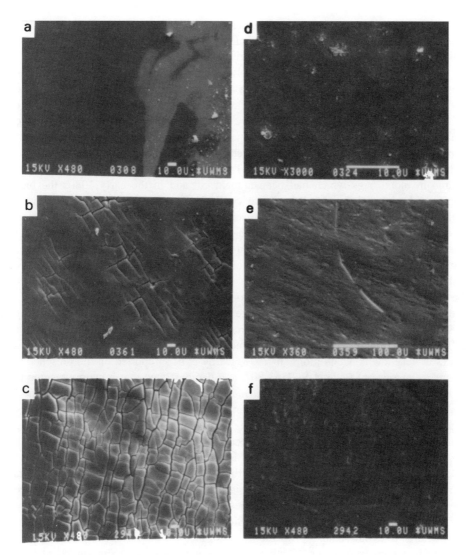

FIGURE 6 SEMs of explanted H_{12}MDI-based PEU. Unstrained (a) four weeks, (b) eight weeks, (c) 12 weeks. Strained (d) four weeks, (e) eight weeks, (f) 12 weeks. From Hergenrother R. W., Wabers H. D., and Cooper S. L., *Biomaterials,* 14(6):449, 1993. With permission.

also demonstrated that aliphatic polyurethanes experience severe stress cracking after short (as little as 30 days) subcutaneous exposure in rabbits. Hergenrother et al.[51] compared an aliphatic isocyanate (H_{12}MDI) based polyurethane with an aromatic based (MDI) polyurethane and also showed significantly greater surface cracking and molecular weight changes in the H_{12}MDI based material compared to the aromatic polyurethane, possibly due the inability of H_{12}MDI to form a crystalline hard segment. These are shown in Figure 6.

Polyurethanes which are polymerized using aromatic isocyanates have characteristics which tend to increase their inherent biodurability. They show better flex fatigue and reduced stress cracking in many applications, better wet tensile strength and better heat stability. Aliphatic polyurethanes absorb more water and frequently soften at or near body temperature. Blamey et al.[52] found this property an advantage for a hip joint where an aliphatic polyether urethane was found to maintain its fluid-film lubrication better than aromatic polyurethane materials. However, both the water absorption and the softening increase the potential for hydrolysis in these polymers by increasing the surface area in contact with water (and body fluids).[1] It is perhaps not surprising that investigators have shown enhanced biodegradation of polyurethanes based on aliphatic diisocyanates as compared to those from aromatic diisocyanates.

The degradation of the hard segment in polyurethanes is an area of controversy. Potentially carcinogenic compounds may be released when cleavage occurs at the urethane linkage of polyurethanes containing aromatic isocyanates, resulting in the formation of either 2,4-toluene diamine (TDA) or 4,4' methylene dianiline (MDA). There are really two issues under this topic. First, does an aromatic polyurethane degrade in such a manner that TDA or MDA, the potentially carcinogenic compounds are liberated and second, are these chemicals carcinogenic in humans.

In the late 1970s, a publication by Baxter–Travenol stated that a small amount of MDA had been found in blood bags which had been autoclaved, and in the early 1980s the biomedical community hotly debated the use of aromatic vs. aliphatic isocyanates in polyurethanes. By the end of the decade aromatics still were being used primarily because of their superior mechanical properties with the stipulation that they not be steam sterilized.[1] However, the issue became controversial again in 1988 with the publication of a study, by Pierre Blais, on the Meme breast implant. Using harsh conditions, Blais and his colleagues found that TDA could be produced from the implant.

The studies to investigate degradation of aromatic polyurethanes particularly from TDI based polyester urethane foam systems have been extensive. In earlier studies it was not clear whether the TDA that was found in aged samples occurred as a result of contamination from residual TDI or was from degradation of the hard segment.[53] Indeed, TDA is difficult to detect because it adsorbs to surfaces at very low concentrations. In 1978, Darby et al.[54] reported on the presence of MDA in the aqueous extracts of Pellethane 2363-80A and demonstrated that it had mutagenic potential assessed by test strains of *Salmonella typhimurium*. The extraction procedure was extremely harsh, involving exposure of the material to steam sterilization conditions for many hours, causing the Pellethane to undergo thermolysis. MDA also has been found in polyurethane plasma storage bags. Ulrich and Bonk also found that MDA was produced during one steam sterilization cycle at 120°C.[55] The FDA has reported three parts per billion of MDA in the plasma stored in these bags.[56,57] The manufacturer has withdrawn these materials from use although there has been no connection between the bags and cancer. At present, despite the fact that MDA has been produced under extreme conditions with MDI based polyurethanes, there does not appear to be any direct evidence that it is produced *in vivo*. Indeed Szycher and Siciliano state that "so long as care is exercised by the manufacturer to avoid steam sterilization, or extrude wet polyurethane pellets no MDA has been detected in these prostheses.[16] Only when these polyurethanes are subjected to extreme temperature conditions is MDA formed by thermohydrolytic degradation".

In 1993, Amin et al.[58] investigated the hydrolysis of the breast implant foam Microthane, under many different conditions, using HPLC. Microthane is highly hydrophilic (in excess of 70%) and cleavage was assumed to be at the ester linkages at physiological pH. Based on their results, Amin et al.[58] concluded that TDA found in *in vitro* and *ex vivo* extractions was an artifact of the high pH used to extract the samples.

More recently, Wang et al.[27] have identified several different degradation products produced by the degradation of a polyester urethane urea. The polymer was synthesized with toluene diisocyanate, a soft segment of polycaprolactone (m.w. 1250) and ethylene diamine as the chain extender. Two materials were synthesized, one with ^{14}C radiolabeled toluene diisocyanate and the other with radiolabeled ethylene diamine. These materials were then incubated in the presence of cholesterol esterase. These investigators found that approximately 20 different degradation products were formed but free TDA did not appear to be one of them.[27] The authors did find TDA derivatives substituted with end units of the polyester segment at the N and N'. The structure of the two major degradation products are shown in Figure 7 and the likely cleavage sites resulting in the two dominant products are shown in Figure 8.

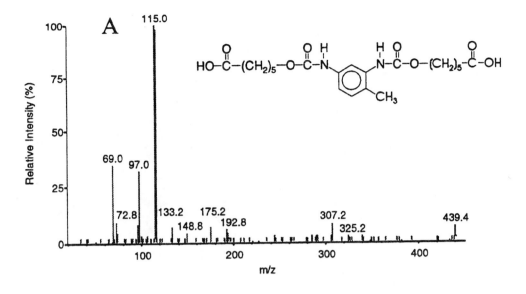

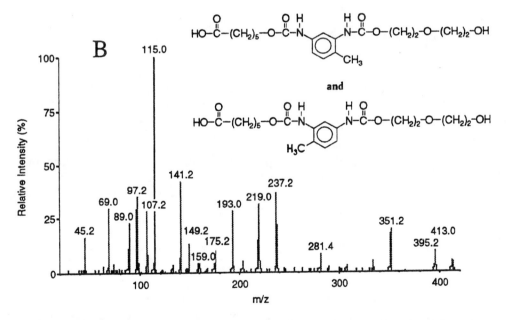

FIGURE 7 MS/MS spectra of molecular ions of the two major degradation products found from cleavage of radiolabeled polyurethanes containing TDI/PCL/ED. From; Wang, G.B., Santerre, J. P., and Labow, R. S. "Biodegradation of a poly(ester)urea-urethane by cholesterol esterase: Isolation and indentification of principal biodegradation products," *J. Biomed. Mater. Res.*, 35; 371, 1997. With permission.

However, Santerre and Labow found that hard segment content and the ability of the polyurethane to form hard segment domains has a significant impact on the degradation of the material by cholesterol esterase.[59] They investigated a series of segmented polyether-urea polyurethanes differing in their hard segment content only and investigated the relationship between hard segment domain formation and the hydrolysis of urea/urethane groups. The materials had significant differences

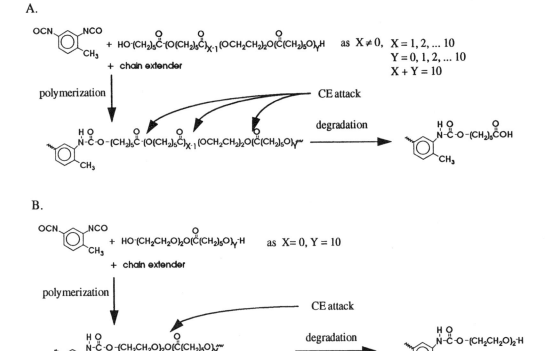

FIGURE 8 Generation of the principal degradation products when diglycol is in the middle of the PCL molecule (A) and at the end of the PCL molecule (B). From; Wang, G. B., Labow, R. S., and Santerre, J. P., "Biodegradation of a poly(ester)urea-Urethane by cholesterol esterase: Isolation and indentification of principal biodegradation products," *J. Biomed. Mater. Res.*, 35; 371, 1997. With permission.

in hard segment domain formation with the polyurethane containing the highest number of hydrolytically labile urea and urethane bonds exhibiting the most biostability. The authors hypothesize that hard segment microdomains may form a protective structure for the hydrolyzable hard segment linkages which are located within these microdomains.

H. OTHER MECHANISMS OF BIODEGRADATION

Takahara et al.[60] found that lipid sorption can contribute to the degradation of polydimethylsiloxane based polyurethanes. Darby and Kaplan, and Jayabalan and Shunmugakumar have found fungal growth and fungal degradation on polyurethanes.[54,61] Jayabalan and Shunmugakumar specifically designed polyurethanes resistant to fungal attack through the incorporation of crosslinks.

I. IMPLANT LOCATION

In addition to the chemical structure, the implant location also has a significant influence on polyurethane degradation. This is not surprising when one considers the diversity inherent in the enzymes and cell populations within different structures within the body. Christ et al.[50] found that polyetherurethanes implanted intraocularly and subcutaneously degraded to different extents although the type of degradation appear to be similar. The material implanted as a lens lost most of the optical resolving power within six months, showing surface pitting and cracking. The degradation of the same material was more extreme subcutaneously. Christi et al. suggested that the subcutaneous position could be used as an accelerated test for intraocular materials. However, the degradation mechanisms might be different given the great differences between the two sites.

III. TOXICITY AND CARCINOGENICITY

Clearly, biomaterials should not be toxic to the patient they are intended to benefit. Detailed toxicological studies of potential and current biomaterials, including polyurethanes, are now considered an extremely important part of a material development process. Unfortunately, there is no simple test which can be used to determine the overall toxicity of material and, importantly, it is difficult to take data from one material and extrapolate to another. There are three likely sources of toxic components from biomaterial; (1) leachable substances; (2) physical contact detrimental to cells; and (3) release of bioactive degradation products.

All the components of a polyurethane, the soft segment, hard segment, and chain extenders potentially could be toxic by themselves or as part of degradation products. Toxicity studies on various materials, including polyurethanes, have found cell death *in vitro* in the absence of serum in the medium but not in its presence.[62] Aromatic isocyanates, particularly TDI, are known to cause asthma,[63] and recently have been found to cause contact dermatitis.[64] Hexamethylene diisocyanate has been shown to cause occupational allergic contact dermatitis,[64] and HMDI also causes skin sensitivity in animals but does not appear to result in pulmonary sensitivity nor in antibody production.[65] These sensitivities are due to the monomeric materials and are not expected to be an issue in the polyurethanes used, for example, *in vivo* in an implant situation. Certainly, care must be taken to avoid exposure to the monomers in the laboratory or chemical plant when a polyurethane is being made in large quantities.

Bakker *et al.* found that polypropylene oxide degradation may be accompanied by the release of toxic substances, but that Estane degradation was not.[66] The authors found that macrophages surrounded alloplastic tympanic membrane materials including Estane and polypropylene oxide. They also found that the tissue reaction was different between the Estane and the other materials, and that it appeared to degrade in a time dependent manner.[67]

Many of the issues around the carcinogenicity of polyurethanes are a result of varying and inconsistent test methods between investigators, making comparisons difficult; and the use of animal models to correlate carcinogenicity in mice to carcinogenicity in humans. To date, there has been no published reports of cancer being linked to polyurethane implants or to the degradation of polyurethanes.[1] The most common isocyanates used in medical devices are either TDI or MDI. TIA and TDA, the two amine compounds which can be formed from TDI are thought to be formed using the path shown in Figure 9. There is little question that the two amine compounds TIA and TDA are carcinogenic in rodents, regarded to be tumor prone, and mutagenic in cell culture.[54,68–71]

Batich *et al.*[72] detected TDA in the extract of polyester polyurethane foam shells covered breast implants. Their extraction took place under extremely harsh conditions, 3.0 N NaOH heated overnight at 150°C. The controversy around polyurethane covered breast implants reached its height with the report that an implant recipient had free 2,4 toluenediamine (TDA) in her urine between 21 days and seven months after surgery.[73,74] In the last few years numerous investigations have been undertaken to determine if TDA itself is released from polyurethane implants under both extreme and physiologic conditions.[16,75-78] It now appears that very small amounts of TDA may be formed under physiologic conditions. However, no link to increased cancer rates is indicated. It has been more difficult to detect TDA under physiologic conditions and there are as many investigators who find do not find TDA as those that do. Most TDI which is metabolized by the body is in the form of TDI linked to low molecular weight segment oligomers. Very little molecular TDA is produced under physiological conditions.

Guidoin *et al.*[75] found that TDA could be released from Meme breast implants on exposure to mild hydrolytic conditions *in vitro* but that this could be significantly reduced by washing the

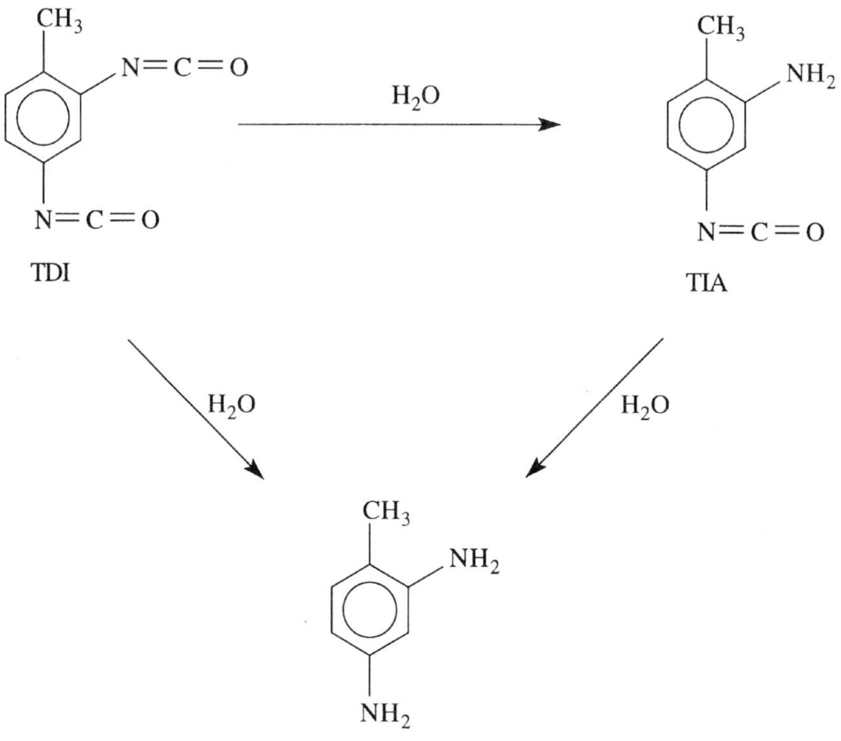

FIGURE 9 Conversion of Toluene Diisocyanate (TDI) and Toluene Isocyanate Amine (TIA) to Toluene Diamine (TDA). Redrawn From Benoit F. M., *J. Biomed. Mater. Res.*, 27:1341, 1993.

implant before testing, suggesting that the TDA was left from processing. They also found that the material degraded in 1 N sodium hydroxide. Szycher and Siciliano found that a maximum of 8.3 μg of TDA per gram of Surgitek polyurethane foam (8.3 parts per million) was produced in the first four days of exposure to a papain solution.[16] Based on standard risk assessment by the authors, the amount of TDA produced would result in a risk of developing cancer of one in four hundred million with one in a million considered insignificant.[16] Their results are shown in Figure 10. The Canadian Medical Association expert panel on the safety of polyurethane covered breast implants used the FDA assessment of estimated increase in lifetime risk of breast cancer at five cancers per 10 million women, each with two implants, for their recommendations to doctors.[79]

Brand investigated the potential carcinogenicity of several different materials including polyvinylchloride acetate (PVCA), Millipore filters, and polyurethane coated breast implants in a study with mice.[80] While the investigators found that there was a strong foreign body response with the polyurethane and Millipore large pore filters, they did not find any tumors in the mice. Some of the animals were studied for over 30 months. This was in comparison to PVCA plates and Millipore Filters (0.2 μ pore size)which had tumor incidence of 95% and of glass which had a tumor incidence of 70%. In this study the authors concluded that foreign body tumorgenesis or cancer caused by the presence of any implant polyurethane would be extremely rare because of the effect of the material on macrophages and fibroblasts.[80]

At present, there does not appear to be any link between the many MDI and TDI based polyurethane implants and cancer in humans.

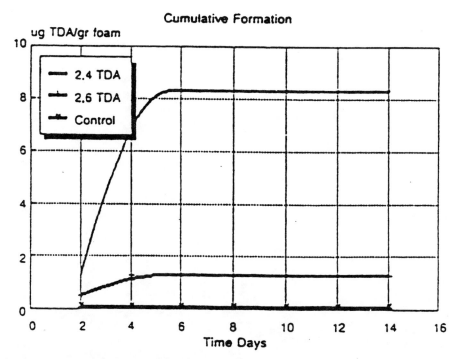

NOTE: CONTROL EXTRACTED (Meth Chlor).

FIGURE 10 Cumulative formation of TDA isomers following exposure of 150 mg samples of Surgitek foam (lot number 1529) to the enzyme papain. Following enzymatic digestion, 2,4 TDA was formed from the polyurethane foam, to a maximum level of 8.3 g TDA/gram of foam. As seen in this graph, the authors found that no more TDA was formed after day 4. In addition the authors note that all test forms were exhaustively purified with methylene chloride prior to enzymatic digestion. From: Szycher, M., and Siciliano, A.A., *J. Biomater. Applic.* 5:323-336, 1991, with permission.

IV. CALCIFICATION OF POLYURETHANES

The use of polyurethanes as a biomaterial is often limited by calcification.[81] Both *in vitro* and *in vivo* calcification of polyurethanes have been reported and it is associated with stiffening of polyurethanes, failure in flexure, and perforations.[82-86] Biomer, Mitrathane, and Pellethane have been reported to calcify both *in vivo* and *in vitro*.[81,87] Much of the effect of calcification on polyurethanes has been investigated in relation to cardiovascular devices.[82,88] Calcification is the deposition of calcium phosphates (chiefly hydroxyapatite) mineral in a material or tissue,[81,88] and is unusual in soft tissue. It has been associated with both biological materials chemically modified for implantation, and with synthetic materials.[88] The calcification appears to occur both in the material itself and in surrounding tissue associated with the biomaterial. It is not clear whether or not calcification requires cellular components. SEMS of calicified polyurethane are shown in Figure 11.

Calcification occurs in prosthetic heart valves, blood pumps,[82] contact lenses, total artificial hearts,[81,83] and some contraceptive devices.[88] The process of calcification is usually divided into two different types or stages.[83] In the first type, nucleation sites are formed through the adsorption of calcium onto the material surfaces in association with proteins, lipids or phospholipids.[83,87-88] These macromolecules are thought to bind calcium. In the second type, the calcium is associated with cell membranes that appear to be from injured, degenerated, or dead cells and crystal proliferation occurs.[83,88] Schoen *et al.*[88] further described these two types of calcification based on the site of mineral nucleation as either intrinsic or extrinsic. In the intrinsic case, the nucleation site is

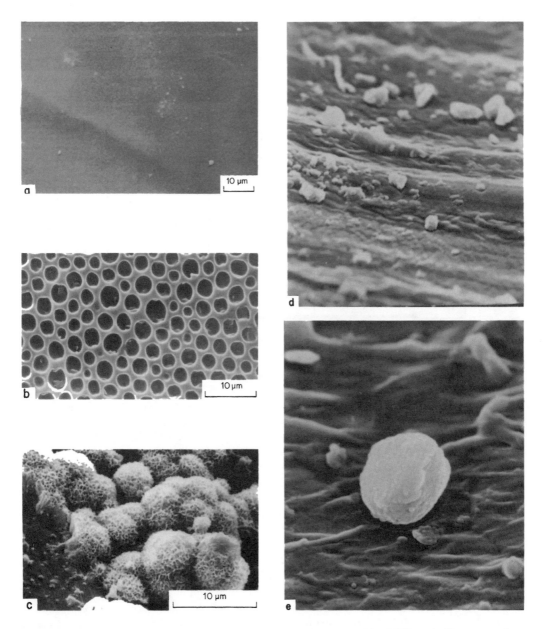

FIGURE 11 Scanning electron micrographs of (a) a plain polyurethane film (THF cast), (b) porous polyurethane film (20% w/w polyethylene glycol 3000 extracted), (c), (d), and (e) calcified plain polyurethane films after 30-day incubation in 9mM calcium phosphate solution, (c) film's surface, (d) and (e) cross-section view (magnification ×10000) From Golomb, G. and Wagner, D., Biomaterials, 12:400, 1991. With permission of Elsevier Inc.

within the biomaterial and in the extrinsic case, the site is associated with tissue, thrombus, blood elements or cellular debris. Intrinsic calcification is found only rarely in pacemaker leads.[7]

It is believed that the pathogenesis of polyurethane calcification is different from that of bioprosthetic heart valves. However, it is likely that the principal mineral phase component of calcification is most likely hydroxyapatite in both.[81] An additional mechanism has been proposed for polyurethanes which is based on the removal and complexation of calcium from body fluids on the surface of the polymer.[12] Urry suggested that calcification in atherosclerosis could be associated with hydrophobic sites in elastin, a highly hydrophobic extracellular matrix protein.[89] These sites could be responsible for attracting calcium. It is possible that the driving force for this alternative mechanism in polyurethanes is complex formation between calcium ions and the polyether soft segment of the polyurethane. As discussed in this chapter and Chapter 9, metal ions have been found to accelerate the degradation of pacemaker leads. There is evidence that the metal ions form complexes with the polyether soft segment. Phillips and Frauschti believe that the calcium is complexed with the soft segment, leading to increased surface concentration and ultimately surface calcification. From this point of view, calcification does not require cellular components. Other investigators also have found that polyurethanes may calcify in the absence of cells.[90,91]

These mechanisms of calcification are not understood completely. Factors which appear to influence calcification include age of the patient, the methods of preparation of the biomaterial, and mechanical stress and deformation. In blood pumps, investigators have found that calcification occurs along the areas of flexure, in association with the diaphragm and the pump housing.[82,88] In heart valves, calcification also appears to be associated with areas of mechanical stress. Hilbert *et al.*[87] implanted Biomer trileaflet valves in sheep in the mitral position and found the two types of calcification sites. Their work also indicated a relationship between surface modification of the polyurethane and calcification. Golomb and Wagner incubated polyurethane films in a calcium phosphate metastable solution,[92] and found that different polymer samples exhibited very different results; with thicker and more porous materials showing marked increases in calcification. Han *et al.*[93] have demonstrated that a highly anionic sulfonated polyurethane is resistant to calcification.

The stress-strain distribution within a material has been correlated with the location of calcification; however it is not clear if repeated flexing causes cell deposition on the surface of the material followed by calcification or if the mechanical changes are causing damage to the adjacent tissue resulting in calcification. It does appear, however that just elongation or straining of the polyurethane is not enough and that dynamic stresses may be required to produce the mineralization.[91]

It has been shown that *bis* phosphonate (2-hydroxy ethane *bis* phosphonic acid (HEBP), reduces calcification in polyurethanes.[81] The exact mechanism of inhibition of physiological and pathological calcification by HEBP is still incompletely understood. Some believe HEBP prevents calcification by steric chemoabsorption to calcium phosphate nuclei, leading to the inhibition of further crystal growth, whereas others have reported HEBP to behave as a detergent, reducing calcification by decreasing the number of available nucleation sites for hydroxyapatite. It also has been postulated that HEBP may act by inhibiting alkaline phosphatase. Pierce *et al.*[82] found that warfarin-sodium administration decreased the amount of calcification associated with the segmented polyurethane sac in a blood pump.

Calcification is a major limitation to the use of polyurethane heart value replacements and other cardiovascular devices. Research in this area continues in an effort to reduce the initiation and consequences of mineral deposition in devices. Calcification of polyurethane heart valves is discussed in more detail in Chapter 9.

V. BIODEGRADABLE POLYURETHANES

Some investigators have chosen to take advantage of the *in vivo* degradation of polyurethanes and purposely design these materials to degrade. This has frequently been achieved by incorporating polylactide or polyglycolic acid into the polyurethane. These degradable polyesters have been used extensively in other biomedical applications although their mechanical properties are not as diverse as those of polyurethanes. In the early 1980s polyurethane/polylactide blends as degradable materials for skin substitutes, vascular prostheses and nerve regeneration guides were developed.[94-95] However, while the material was degradable, in these cases the polyurethane portion of the blend was nondegradable and served only to provide favorable mechanical properties. Subsequent work by Bruin *et al.*[96] involved the synthesis of crosslinked polyurethane networks incorporating lactide or glycolide and ε-caprolactone joined by a lysine-based diisocyanate. These polymers displayed good elastomeric properties and were degraded within 26 weeks *in vitro* and 12 weeks *in vivo* (subcutaneous implantation in guinea pigs). However, these highly crosslinked polymers may not be processed by standard techniques such as solution casting or melt processing as is the case for typical linear, segmented polyurethanes.

Kobayashi *et al.* specifically took advantage of the hydrolysis of the polyurethane soft segment to develop a water curable and biodegradable prepolymer for use in a bioadhesive. These investigators found that by copolymerizing D,L-lactide or D,L-lactide-ε-caprolactone (50:50) with polyethylene glycol they obtained biodegradable polyesters that could be combined with isocyanates to cure *in situ* in the body. Through a series of *in vivo* and *in vitro* experiments they also concluded that the mechanism of degradation was hydrolysis. These materials degraded to small pieces within 16 weeks of subcutaneous implantation and were completely degraded at 12 months. More recently, poly(phosphoester urethanes) have been synthesized by Dahiyat *et al.*[97] for drug delivery applications. These polymers are relatively stiff, low tensile strength materials. It is thus possible to achieve rapid degradation with polyurethanes that combine hydrophilicity and hydrolyzable groups in the polyurethane backbone.

SUMMARY

Polyurethane implants degrade. How, to what extent, and with what impact is the subject of continued work by many investigators. It is clear that no material is perfect and in evaluating the use of biomaterials, particularly in long term implants, a choice needs to be made between the risks of not using the implant and using it. Because long term effects like degradation are not easily predicted and depend on the patient as well as the material, there will always be an inherent risk with any implant. However, with proper implant design and material selection, polyurethanes that are currently available can be selected for applications requiring many years of implant function.

The knowledge gained in the last several years about how polyurethanes degrade both *in vivo* and *in vitro* has resulted in a greater understanding of how the different systems within the body interact with foreign materials. The continued efforts in this area will ultimately aid researchers in designing better polyurethanes for many different applications.

REFERENCES

1. Pinchuk L. "A review of the biostability and carcinogenicity of polyurethanes in medicine and the new generation of 'biostable' polyurethanes." *J. Biomater. Sci., Polym. Ed.,* 6:225, 1994.
2. Sawhney A. S., Pathak C. P., and Hubbell J. A. "Bioerodible hydrogels based on photopolymerized poly(ethylene glycol)-co-poly(a-hydroxy acid) diacrylate macromers." *Macromolecules,* 26:581, 1993.
3. Smith R., Oliver C., and Williams D. F. "The enzymatic degradation of polymers *in vitro*." *J. Biomed. Mater. Res.,* 21:991, 1987.
4. Ossefort Z. T. and Testroet Z. T. "Hydrolytic stability of urethane elastomers." *Rubber Chem. Technol.,* 37:17, 1966.
5. Gahimer F. and Nieske F. "Hydrolytic stability of urethane and polyacrylate elastomers in the human environment." *J. Elast. Plast.,* 1:266, 1969.
6. Lelah M. D. and Cooper S. L. *Polyurethanes in Medicine.* CRC Press, Boca Raton, FL, 1986.
7. Stokes K., McVenes R., and Anderson J. M. "Polyurethane elastomer biostability." *J. Biomater. Appl.,* 9:321, 1995.
8. Pavlova M. and Draganova M. "Hydrolytic stability of polyurethane medical adhesive dressings." *Biomaterials,* 15:59, 1994.
9. Stokes K. B. "Polyether polyurethanes: biostable or not?" *J. Biomater. Appl.,* 3:228, 1988.
10. Hawkins W. L. *Polymer Stabilization.* Wiley–Interscience, New York, NY, 1972.
11. Stokes K., Berthelsen W.A., and Davis M. W. *Metal catalyzed oxidative degradation on implanted polyurethane devices.* ACS Division of Polymeric Materials: Science and Engineering,. 1985: 6.

12. Phillips R. and Thoma R. In *Polyurethanes in Biomedical Engineering, 3,* Ed. Planck H., Syre I., Dauner M., and Egbers G. Elsevier, 1989: 91.
13. Stokes K., Coury A., and Urbanski P. "Autooxidative degradation of implanted polyether polyurethane devices." *J. Biomater. Appl.,* 1:411, 1987.
14. Hepburn C. *Polyurethane elastomers.* (2nd Ed.): Elsevier Applied Science, London, 1992.
15. Shintani H. and Nakamura A. "Formation of 4,4'-methylenedianiline in polyurethane potting materials by either γ-ray or autoclave sterilization." *J. Biomed. Mater. Res.,* 25:1275, 1991.
16. Szycher M. and Siciliano A. A. "An assessment of 2,4,TDA formation of a polyurethane foam under simulated physiological conditions." *J. Biomater. Appl.,* 5:323, 1991.
17. Anderson J. M. "Inflammatory response to implants." *Trans. Am. Soc. Artif. Intern. Organs,* 34:101, 1988.
18. Labow R. S., Erfle D. J., and Santerre J. P. "Neutrophil-mediated degradation of segmented polyurethanes." *Biomaterials,* 16:51, 1995.
19. Zhao Q., Topham N., Anderson J. M., Hiltner A., Lodoen G., and Payet C. R. "Foreign-body giant cells and polyurethane biostability: *In vivo* correlation of cell adhesion and surface cracking." *J. Biomed. Mater. Res.,* 25:177, 1991.
20. Stokes K., Urbanski P. and Upton J. "The *in vivo* auto-oxidation of polyether polyurethane by metal ions." *J. Biomater. Sci., Polym. Ed.,* 1:207, 1990.
21. Szycher M. "Biostability of polyurethane elastomers: a critical review." In *Blood Compatible Materials and Devices,* Ed. Sharma C. P., Szycher M. Technomic, Lancaster, PA, 1991: 33.
22. Thoma R. J. and Phillips R. E. "Note: Studies of poly(ether)urethane pacemaker lead insulation oxidation." *J. Biomed. Mater. Res.,* 21:525, 1987.
23. Smith R., Williams D. F., and Oliver C. "The biodegradation of poly(ether urethanes)." *J. Biomed. Mater. Res.,* 21:1149, 1987.
24. Marchant R. E, Hiltner, A., Hamlin C., Rabinovitch A., Slobodkin R., and Anderson J.M. "*In vivo* biocompatibility studies: I. The cage implant system and a biodegradable hydogel. *J. Biomed. Mater. Res.,* 17:301, 1983.
25. Takahara A., Hergenrother R. W., Coury A. J., and Cooper S. L. "Effect of soft segment chemistry on the biostability of segmented polyurethanes. II. *In vitro* hydrolytic stability." *J. Biomed. Mater. Res.,* 26:801, 1992.
26. Santerre J. P., Labow R. S., and Adams G. A. "Enzyme-biomaterial interactions: Effect of biosystems on degradation of polyurethanes." *J. Biomed. Mater. Res.,* 27:97, 1993.
27. Wang G. B., Labow R. S., and Santerre J. P. "Biodegradation of a poly(ester)urea–urethane by cholesterol esterase. Isolation and indentification of principal biodegradation products." *J. Biomed. Mater. Res.* In press, 1997.
28. Ratner B. D., Gladhill K. W., and Horbett T. A. "Analysis of *in vitro* enzymatic and oxidative degradation of polyurethanes." *J. Biomed. Mater. Res.,* 22:509, 1988.
29. Bouvier M., Chawla A. S., and Hinberg I. "*In vitro* degradation of a poly(ether urethane) by trypsin." *J. Biomed. Mater. Res.,* 25:773, 1991.
30. Phua S. K., Castillo E., Anderson J. M., and Hiltner A. "Biodegradation of a polyurethane *in vitro*." *J. Biomed. Mater. Res.,* 21:231, 1987.
31. Kaplan S. S., Basford R. E., Jeong M. H., and Simmons R. L. "Mechanisms of biomaterial-induced superoxide release by neutrophils." *J. Biomed. Mater. Res.,* 28:377, 1994.
32. Marchant R. E., Zhao Q., Anderson J. M., and Hiltner A. "Degradation of a poly(ether urethane urea) elastomer: infra-red and XPS studies." *Polymer,* 28:2032, 1987.
33. Marchant R. E., Miller K. M., and Anderson J. M. "*In vivo* biocompatibility studies. V. *In vivo* leukocyte interactions with Biomer." *J. Biomed. Mater. Res.,* 18:1169, 1984.
34. Zhao Q. H., Anderson J. M., Hiltner A., Lodoen G. A., and Payet C. R. "Theoretical analysis on cell size distribution and kinetics of foreign-body giant cell formation *in vivo* on polyurethane elastomers." *J. Biomed. Mater. Res.,* 26:1019, 1992.
35. Anderson J. M. "Mechanisms of inflammation and infection with implanted devices." *Cardiovasc. Pathol.,* 2:33S, 1993.
36. Bluhm G., Larsen F. F., Nordlander R., and Pehrsson S. K. "Long-term comparison of the electrical characteristics of polyurethane and polyethylene insulated ventricular leads." *PACE,* 13:583, 1990.

37. Phillips R., Frey M., and Martin R. O. "Long-term performance of polyurethane pacing leads: mechanisms of design-related failures." *PACE,* 9:1166, 1986.
38. Pinchuk L., Martin J. B., Esquivel M. C., and MacGregor D. C. "The use of silicone/polyurethane graft polymers as a means of eliminating surface cracking of polyurethanes prostheses." *J. Biomater. Appl.,* 3:260, 1988.
39. Kao W. J., Zhao Q. H., Hiltner A., and Anderson J. M. "Theoretical analysis of *in vivo* macrophage adhesion and foreign body giant cell formation on polydimethylsiloxane, low density polyethylene, and polyetherurethanes." *J. Biomed. Mater. Res.,* 28:73, 1994.
40. Wabers H. D., McCoy T. J., Okkema A. T., Hergenrother R. W., Wolf M. F., and Cooper S. L. "Biostability and blood-contacting properties of sulfonate grafted polyurethane and Biomer." *J. Biomater. Sci., Polym. Ed.,* 4:107, 1992.
41. Sutherland K., Mahoney J. R., Coury A. J., and Eaton J. W. "Degradation of biomaterials by phagocyte-derived oxidants." *J. Clin. Inv.,* 92:2360, 1993.
42. Tyler B. J., Ratner B. D., Castner D. G., and Briggs D. "Variations between Biomer™ lots. 2. The effect of differences between lots on *in vitro* enzymatic and oxidative degradation of a commercial polyurethane." *J. Biomed. Mater. Res.,* 27:327, 1993.
43. Slade C. L. and Peterson H. D. "Disappearance of the polyurethane cover of the Ashley Natural Y prosthesis." *Plastic Reconstr. Surg.,* 70:379, 1982.
44. Sinclair T. M., Kerrigan C. L., and Buntie R. "Biodegradation of the polyurethane foam covering of breast implants." *Plastic Reconstr. Surg.,* 92:1003, 1993.
45. Steinbach B. G., Hardt N. S., and Abbitt P. L. "Mammography: breast implants — types, complications, and adjacent breast pathology." *Curr. Prob. Diagn. Radiol.,* 22:39, 1993.
46. Brandwood A., Meijs G. F., Gunatillake P. A., Noble K. R., Schindelm K., and Rizzardo E. "*In vivo* evaluation of polyurethanes based on novel macrodiols and MDI." *J. Biomater. Sci., Polym. Ed.,* 6:41, 1994.
47. Wu Y. K., Lodoen G. A., Anderson J. M., Baier E., and Hiltner A. "Creep in a poly(etherurethane urea) in an oxidative environment." *J. Biomed. Mater. Res.,* 28:515, 1994.
48. Tingfei X., Wenhua T., Xuehei L., Lejun Z., and Ishihara K. "Haemocompatibility of polymer having phospholipid polar groups evaluated by monoclonal antibody method." *Biomaterials,* 13:357, 1992.
49. Szycher M. "Biostability of polyurethane elastomers: A critical review." *J. Biomater. Appl.,* 3:297, 1988.
50. Christ F. R., Buchen S. Y., Fencil D. A., Knight P. M., Solomon K. D., and Apple D. J. "A comparative evaluation of the biostability of a poly(ether urethane) in the intraocular, intramuscular, and subcutaneous environments." *J. Biomed. Mater. Res.,* 26:607, 1992.
51. Hergenrother R. W., Wabers H. D., and Cooper S. L. "Effect of hard segment chemistry and strain on the stability of polyurethanes: *in vivo* biostability." *Biomaterials,* 14:449, 1993.
52. Blamey J., Rajan S., Unsworth A., and Dawber R. "Soft layered prostheses for arthritic hip joints: a study of materials degradation." *J. Biomed. Eng.,* 13:180, 1991.
53. Benoit F. M. "Degradation of polyurethane foams used in the Meme breast implant." *J. Biomed. Mater. Res.,* 27:1341, 1993.
54. Darby T. D., Johnson H. J., and Northup S. J. "An evaluation of a polyurethane for use as a medical grade plastic." *Toxicol. Appl. Pharmacol.,* 46:449, 1978.
55. Ulrich H. and Bonk H. W. "Emerging biomedical applications of polyurethane elastomers." *SPI, 27th Annual Conference,*. Bal Harbour, FL. 1982: 143.
56. FDA. *Devices and Diagnostic Letter,* 6:2, 1979.
57. FDA. *Devices and Diagnostic Letter,* 7:1, 1980.
58. Amin P., Wille J., Shah K., and Kydonieus A. "Analysis of the extractive and hydrolytic behaviour of Microthane poly(ester-urethane) foam by high pressure liquid chromatography." *J. Biomed. Mater. Res.,* 27:655, 1993.
59. Wang G. B., Santerre J. P., and Labow R. S. "Biodegradation of a poly(ester)urea-urethane by cholesterol esterase. Isolation and identification of principal biodegradation products." *J. Biomed. Mater. Res.,* 35:371, 1997.
60. Takahara A., Takahashi K., and Kajiyama T. "Effect of polyurethane surface chemistry on its lipid sorption behavior." *J. Biomater. Sci., Polym. Ed.,* 5:183, 1993.

61. Jayabalan M. and Shunmugakumar N. "Interactions of enzymes and fungi with crosslinked polyurethanes prepared for biomedical applications." *Med. Prog. Tech.,* 20:261, 1994.
62. Ertel S. I. and Kohn J. "Evaluation or a series of tyrosine-derived polycarbonates as degradable biomaterials." *J. Biomed. Mater. Res.,* 28:919, 1994.
63. Balboni A., Baricordi O. R., Fabri L. M., Gandini E., Ciaccia A., and Mapp C. E. "Association between toluene diisocyanate-induced asthma and DBQ1 markers: A possible role for aspartic acid at Position 57." *Eur. Respir. J.*:207, 1990.
64. Estlander T., Keskinen H., Jolanki R., and Kanerva L. "Occupational dermatitis from exposure to polyurethane chemicals." *Contact Dermatitis,* 27:161, 1992.
65. Karol M. H. and Magreni C. "Extensive skin sensitization with minimal antibody production in Guinea pigs as a result of exposure to Dicyclohexylmethane-4-4'diisocyanate." Toxicol. Appl. Pharmacol., 65:291, 1982.
66. Bakker D., van Blitterswijk C. A., Hesseling S. C., and Grote J. J. "Biocompatibility of a polyether urethane, polypropylene oxide, and a polyether polyester copolymer. A qualitative and quantitative study of three alloplastic tympanic membrane materials in the rat middle ear." *J. Biomed. Mater. Res.,* 24:489, 1990.
67. Bakker D., van Blitterswijk C. A., Hesseling S. C., Daems W. T., and Grote J. J. "Tissue/biomaterial interface characteristics of four elastomers. A transmission electron microscopical study." *J. Biomed. Mater. Res.,* 24:277, 1990.
68. Dunaif C. B., Stubenbord W. T., and Conway H. *Surg., Gyn. Obst.,* 117:454, 1963.
69. Schoental R. "Carcinogenic and chronic effects of 4,4-diamino-diphenyl methane, an epoxy resin hardener." *Nature,* 219:1162, 1968.
70. Sittig M. and Noyes. *Handbook of Toxic and Hazardous Materials.* Park Ridge, N.J., 1981. (Author: This reference is incomplete)
71. Hearing before the Subcommittee on Human Resources and Intergovernmental Relations. U.S. House of representatives, 1990.
72. Batich C., Williams J. and King R. "Toxic hydrolysis product from a biodegradable foam implant." *J. Biomed. Mater. Res.,* 23:311, 1989.
73. Chan S. C., Birdsell D. C., and Gradeen C. Y. "Urinary excretion of free toluenediamines in a patient with polyurethane-covered breast implants." *Clin. Chem.,* 37:2143, 1991.
74. Chan S. C., Birdsell D. C., and Gradeen C. Y. "Detection of toluenediamines in the urine of a patient with polyurethane-covered breast implants." *Clin. Chem.,* 37:756, 1991.
75. Guidoin R., Therrien M., Rolland C., and Roy C. "The polyurethane foam covering the Meme breast prosthesis: A biomedical breakthrough or a biomaterial tar baby?" *Ann. Plast. Surg.,* 28:342, 1992.
76. Dunn K. W., Hall P. N., and Khoo C. T. K. "Breast implant materials: sense and safety." *Brit. J. Plast. Surg.,* 45:315, 1992.
77. Bradley S. G., White K. L., Jr., McCay J. A., Brown R. D., Musgrove D. L., Wilson S., Stern M., Luster M. I., and Munson A. E. "Immunotoxicity of 180 day exposure to polydimethylsiloxane (silicone) fluid, gel and elastomer and polyurethane disks in female B6C3F1 mice." *Drug Chem. Toxicol.,* 17:221, 1994.
78. Bradley S. G., Munson A. E., McCay J. A., Brown R. D., Musgrove D. L., Wilson S., Stern M., Luster M. I., and White K. L., Jr. "Subchronic 10 day immunology of polydimethylsiloxane (silicone) fluid, gel and elastomer and polyurethane disks in female B6C3F1 mice." *Drug Chem. Toxicol.,* 17:175, 1994.
79. Boyes D. C., Adey C. K., Bailar J. *et al.* "Safety of polyurethane-covered breast implants." *Can. Med. Assoc. J.,* 145:1125, 1991.
80. Brand K. G. "Foam-covered mammary implants." *Plastic Reconstr. Surg.,* 15:533, 1988.
81. Joshi R. R., Frautschi J. R., Phillips R. E., and Levy R. J. "Phosphonated polyurethanes that resist calcification." *J. Appl. Biomater.,* 5:65, 1994.
82. Pierce W. S., Donachy J. H., Rosenberg G., and Baier R. E. "Calcification inside artificial hearts: Inhibition by warfarin-sodium." *Science* 1980 9 May:601.
83. Dostal M., Vasku J., Vasku J., Sotolova O., Vasku A., Dolezel S., and Hartmannova B. "Mineralization of polyurethane membranes in the total artificial heart (TAH): a retrospective study from long-term animal experiments." *Int. J. Artif. Organs,* 13:498, 1990.

84. Glasmacher B., Reul H., Rau G., Erckes C., and Wieland J. "*In vitro* investigation of the calcification behaviour of polyurethane biomaterials." In *Polyurethanes in Biomedical Engineering II,* Ed. Planck H., Syre I., Dauner M., Egbers G. Elsevier Science Publishers, Amsterdam, 1987: 151.
85. Lo H. B., Herold M., Reul H. *et al.* "A tricuspid polyurethane heart valve as an alternative to mechanical prostheses or bioprostheses." *Trans. Am. Soc. Artif. Intern. Organs,* 34:839, 1988.
86. Wouters L. H. G., Rousseau E. P. M., Van Steenhoven A. A., and German A. L. "An experimental set-up for the *in vitro* analysis of polyurethane calcification." In *Polyurethanes in Biomedical Engineering II,* Ed. Planck H., Syre I., Dauner M., Egbers G. Elsevier Science Publishers, Amsterdam, 1987: 169.
87. Hilbert S. L., Ferrans V. J., Tomita Y., Eidbo E. E., and Jones M. "Evaluation of explanted polyurethane trileaflet cardiac valve prostheses." *J. Thorac. Cardiovasc. Surg.,* 94:419, 1987.
88. Schoen F. J., Harasaki H., Kim K. M., Anderson C., and Levy R. J. "Biomaterial-associated calcification: pathology mechanisms and strategies for prevention." *J. Biomed. Mater. Res.,* 22:11, 1988.
89. Urry D. W. "Neutral sites for calcium binding to elastin and collagen: A charge neutralization theory for calcification and its relationship to atherosclerosis." *Proc. Natl. Acad. Sci., U.S.A.,* 68:810, 1971.
90. Shumakov V. I., Rosanova I. B., Vasin S. L., Salomatina L. A., and Sevastianov V. I. "Biomaterial calcification without direct material-cell interaction." *Trans. Am. Soc. Artif. Intern. Organs,* 36:181, 1990.
91. Golomb G. and Wagner D. "Development of a new *in vitro* model for studying implantable polyurethane calcification." *Biomaterials,* 12:397, 1991.
92. Golomb G. and Wagner D. "Evaluation of polyurethane calcification by a new *in vitro* model." *Biomaterials,* 12; 129, 1990.
93. Han D., K., Park K. D., Jeong S. Y., Kim Y. H., Kim U. Y., and Min B. G. "*In vivo* biostability and calcification-resistance of surface-modified PU-PEO-SO3." *J. Biomed. Mater. Res.,* 27:1063, 1993.
94. Eling B., Gogolewski S., and Pennings A. J. "Biodegradable materials of poly(L-lactic acid): Melt-spun and solution-spun fibres." *Polymer,* 23:1587, 1982.
95. Gogolewski S. and Pennings A. J. "An artificial skin based on biodegradable mixtures of polylactides and polyurethanes for full-thickness skin wound covering." *Makromol. Chem., Rapid Commun.,* 4:675, 1983.
96. Bruin P., Veenstra G. J., Nijenhuis A. J., and Pennings A. J. "Design and sytesis of biodegradable poly(ester-urethane) elastomer networks composed of non-toxic building blocks." *Makromolecular Chemistry, Rapid Communications,* 9:589, 1988.
97. Dahiyat B. I., Hostin E., Posadas E. M., and Leong K. W. "Synthesis and characterization of putrescine-based poly(phosphoester-urethanes)." *J. Biomater. Sci., Polym. Ed.,* 4:529, 1993.

9 Polyurethanes in Biomedical Applications

I. INTRODUCTION

The successful application of a medical device in the clinic not only depends on the properties of the biomaterial or biomaterials used to fabricate the device, but also on numerous other factors, including the manufacturing and processing history of the material, and the specific application in which the device is used. Furthermore, the clinical performance of a device is influenced by the surgical technique and conditions, as well as the health status of the recipient. A single material may be used to fabricate a whole device, such as a vascular prosthesis. It is more usual, however, to find devices fabricated from a number of materials, particularly in more complicated devices such as hemadialyzers and the total artificial heart.

As seen in the preceding chapters, polyurethanes have good mechanical properties and blood compatibility, which have made polyurethanes a popular choice of material for use in medical devices. Polyurethanes have very high flexural endurance compared to most elastomers, making them prime candidates for cardiovascular implants. Biomaterials in cardiovascular applications are subjected to repeated loading and unloading; 72 beats per minute will approach 200,000,000 cycles in five years. Hence, fatigue resistance is essential, as failure may have catastrophic results. Thrombosis remains the main deterrent to the use of polyurethanes as cardiovascular prostheses. Infection of implanted devices also is a serious problem. It has been estimated that approximately 45% of hospital infections are associated with implants and medical devices.[1] Unlike systemic infections, device-centered infections do not respond well to conventional antibiotic therapy. In many cases, removal of the offending implant is the only effective solution.

In the evaluation and development of medical devices, the choice of material is only one of the factors that must be considered. The potential to integrate a device into the biological environment is of increasing importance, whether to minimize hemorheological disturbance through selection of a material with specific mechanical properties e.g., with a heart valve or a vascular prosthesis, or integration of the device into the vascular and nervous systems, as with the development of artificial organs. Many papers on the clinical performance of medical devices do not give sufficient information on the composition and history of a material to be of value to the materials scientist. This makes the evaluation of medical devices on the basis of material alone very difficult. Many trials of devices with new materials or new geometries have been performed using animal models, which introduces inter-species differences. Within these constraints, the applications and performance of polyurethanes as medical devices have been reviewed and are discussed below, under topics of cardiovascular devices, artificial organs, tissue replacement and augmentation and other applications.

II. CARDIOVASCULAR APPLICATIONS

A. CATHETERS

Catheters are used widely in medicine, for therapeutic and diagnostic purposes. They are used for the delivery and removal of fluids, and for monitoring central venous pressure. They are also employed in more complex procedures such as the compression of plaques in coronary arteries

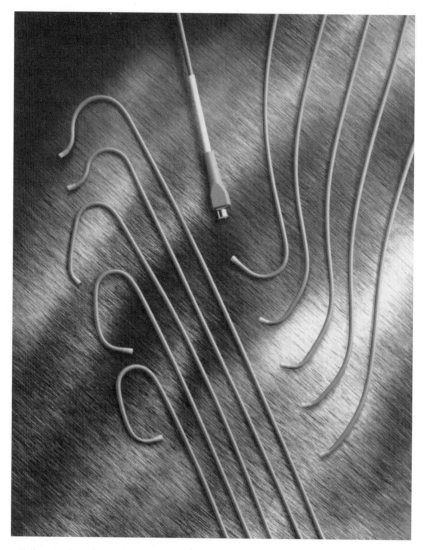

FIGURE 1 Cardiac guiding catheters made of polyurethanes of varying hardnesses. Courtesy of Medtronic Inc.

(angioplasty) and to obstruct blood flow to certain parts of the body. Catheters essentially form the outer insulating sheath of pacemaker leads (discussed in more detail in this chapter).

Among the properties required of a catheter are flexibility to allow easy insertion, and a low friction surface to minimize tissue trauma. Furthermore, they should be nonthrombogenic, nonkinking and not degrade in the biological environment. Catheters are fabricated from various polymeric materials, including polyethylene, plasticized polyvinylchloride (PVC), polytetrafluoroethylene, Nylon and silicone rubber, as well as from polyurethanes (Figure 1). Polyethylene catheters are relatively stiff, although they can be heat shaped to aid insertion. Nylon and Teflon materials also have been used to manufacture catheters, although they are stiff also. One of the drawbacks with these stiffer catheters is that they may perforate vessels on insertion and removal. PVC and silicone rubber catheters are more flexible, but need to have thicker walls, to avoid tearing. This limits the cross-sectional area of the lumen and hence blood flow. Plasticized PVC is the most common material for the manufacture of catheters. This may be attributable in part to its low cost, but it could also be because the flexibility of the material can be varied through the type and concentration of plasticizer used. Polydimethylsiloxane (PDMS) catheters are very flexible, which can make them difficult to insert. These catheters also may be more prone to breakage on removal. Generally, catheters also contain ground metals and metal oxides to impart radio-opacity.[2] Catheter performance is affected by surgical handling and technique, size and type of vessel, and duration of catheterization. The properties required of a catheter are determined by the application. For example, a catheter with a higher degree of thrombogenicity may perform better in arterial sites than in venous sites. Thrombus formation remains the primary reason for the loss of patency of catheters in the clinic.[3]

Factors that should be considered in evaluating the performance of catheters are the stiffness of the catheter, the roughness of the surface and the susceptibility to colonization by bacteria. Generally, catheter obstruction is more common in stiffer catheters. Costanzo et al.[4] have proposed two mechanisms through which catheters can induce thrombus formation and result in obstruction. The first is by inducing turbulent flow of the blood stream. The second mechanism is through the deposition of platelets and platelet aggregation, leading to fibrin deposition on the catheter surface. It also is thought that a stiffer indwelling catheter is more likely to lie against the vessel wall rather than float in the blood stream. Thus, stiffer catheters may create sites of blood stasis at the wall, and promote thrombus formation.[3] The primary advantages of polyurethane catheters include (1) superior blood compatibility, (2) improved stiffness for insertion and softening for catheter removal, (3) better combination of flow rate, stiffness and kink resistance, (4) wider applicability, and (5) reduced catheter assembly costs.[5] One of the earliest polyurethanes used for vascular catheters was Vialon, developed in the early 1980s. The unique feature of these materials was the controlled degree of softening after insertion. A range of polyurethanes with varying hardnesses provided an array of catheters with varying degrees of stiffness. Both heat and absorption of saline were shown to reversibly soften Vialon catheters at 37°C, which is believed to minimize the initiation of vascular wall damage and the potential for thrombus formation and phlebitis (venous inflammation).[6] Reduction in mural thrombosis extended the the service time of the inserted catheter.

Several researchers have suggested a link between the thrombogenicity of a catheter and the surface roughness. Catheters fabricated from Ducor© polyurethane have been problematic, due to their high thrombogenicity compared to other polyurethanes.[7-10] SEM studies showed that the surfaces of these catheters were very rough, leading to conclusion that the roughness contributed to the thrombogenicity. Other studies showed little difference between Ducor© and polyethylene with respect to roughness and thrombogenicity.[11-15] Hecker et al.[16] also have suggested a link between thrombogenicity and roughness of the catheter. The roughness of the catheters could have been due to the presence of radio-opaque particles. Assessment of the thrombogenicity of catheters often relies upon the visualization of thrombi after withdrawal from the site of implantation. It is possible that thrombi may be dislodged more easily from smooth catheters than rough ones during withdrawal.[3] Several studies have been performed on biologically modified catheters. Heparinized polyurethanes have been shown to reduce the degree of thrombus formation.[17,18] Kitamoto et al.[19] immobilized urokinase onto catheters and evaluated them clinically. They reported reduced levels of fibrin formation and platelet adhesion.

Infection is a major complication with cardiovascular devices, rivaling and perhaps intimately connected with thrombosis and inflammation.[20] Catheter related infection is the most common cause of life-threatening complication in infusion therapy.[21] Clinical infections are associated with 34-40% of venous catheters.[22] These infections usually start as local infections which can later become systemic. Lopez et al. investigated the adhesion *of Staphylococcus aureus, Staphylococcus epidermidis, Pseudomonas aeruginosa* and *Eschrischia coli* to catheters of PVC, polyurethane, Teflon, siliconized latex, and Vialon. They found that the polyurethane and Vialon had the lowest adhesion of staphylococcus and Teflon the lowest of *E.coli* and *P. aeruginosa*. Other catheter materials are also prone to infection and both slime and nonslime producing bacteria appear to adhere to polyvinyl chloride, Teflon®, Silastic® and polyurethane catheters in the absence of nutrients *in vitro* and proliferate on the catheters in the presence of nutrients.[23] Catheters are used in many different applications and results concerning the use of polyurethane dressings to protect against infection are varied, often because the protocols and materials vary, making comparisons difficult.

Balloon tip pulmonary artery catheters are widely used in the United States to treat patients with shock and disorders in oxygen transport. There are many ways in which these catheters can become contaminated and ultimately for bacteria to enter the bloodstream. Contamination may come from skin organisms introduced during insertion, from repositions, or from contamination of the hubs. Polyurethanes have been shown to have lower degrees of microbial colonization compared to other catheter materials.[24] Hydrogel coatings have been employed to reduce bacterial colonization.[25-27] Such a strategy also serves to reduce the friction of the catheter surface, reducing damage to the vessel wall, and thrombus formation.[28] Smith *et al.*[29] recently investigated the absorption of drugs by several Pellethane catheters. They reported a correlation between the octanol/water partition coefficient and the fraction of the drug absorbed by the catheters. Generally, hydrophobic drugs were absorbed by the catheter to a greater extent. Loss of the drug from solution to a Topecon catheter was significantly lower, probably due to the high proportion of hard segment in the material, leading to a decrease in void volume for drug diffusion within the polymer.

Other experimental catheters have been developed. Pierce *et al.*[30] fabricated a wire reinforced ventricular cannula from Biomer®. Kolobow and Zapol produced a nonkinking thin-walled steel-reinforced catheter by embedding a wire spring between two layers of Biomer polyurethane.[31] The internal diameter of the catheters ranged from 0.073 to 0.500 inches and wall thicknesses ranging from 0.010 to 0.012 inches. They found that the reinforced Lycra catheters allowed large blood flow with low pressure gradients, did not degrade after prolonged use, did not perforate or erode vessels, and were relatively nonthrombogenic.

B. Pacemaker Lead Insulation

Cardiac pacing is required to correct cardiac rhythmic disorders. The insulating material for a pacemaker lead needs to be tough and long-lasting, and provide stable insulation over a long period of time. The first transvenous cardiac pacing lead was introduced by Furman and Robinson in 1967.[32] Both silicone rubber and polyethylene were used as insulating materials, but an alternative material was sought as both of these materials evoke a fibrous endocardial reaction. In 1978, polyurethane was introduced as a lead insulator,[33] in an effort to supersede silicone rubber as the material of choice. Although silicone rubber is more flexible and has better thermal stability, it has poor mechanical properties, so that a thick insulating layer is required to withstand use. The tensile strength of polyurethane is approximately six times greater than that of silicone rubber; polyurethanes also possess better tear resistance, and these properties offered advantages over silicone rubber. Thus, thinner leads could be manufactured through the selection of polyurethane as the insulator, without compromising the handling properties. A reduction in lead diameter enhances insertion, and permits the introduction of more than one lead into a vein, for sequential pacing. Polyurethane also has a lower coefficient of friction compared to silicone rubber when in contact with blood; the smoothness also enhances the ease of insertion of the lead.[34,35] Figure 2 shows a polyurethane pacemaker lead.

Pellethane® has been the most widely used polyurethane in this application. Pellethane® can be thermally extruded into thin, smooth tubes, with the aid of processing additives.[36] Other polyurethanes that have been used as insulating material include Tecoflex® and Cardiothane®. Essentially, a pacemaker lead consists of conducting coil surrounded by an insulating sheath. Leads can be manufactured by one of two methods: a low stress method, or a high stress method. The low stress method involves the insertion of the metal coil into a tube of the insulating material of a slightly larger internal diameter than the diameter of the coil, to give a snug fit. The second method can be used to manufacture thinner leads. During this process, the polymer is fabricated into tubes of the finished lead diameter and swollen using solvent. The metal core is then inserted into the lumen. A close fitting insulating sheath is produced on evaporation of the solvent. The closeness

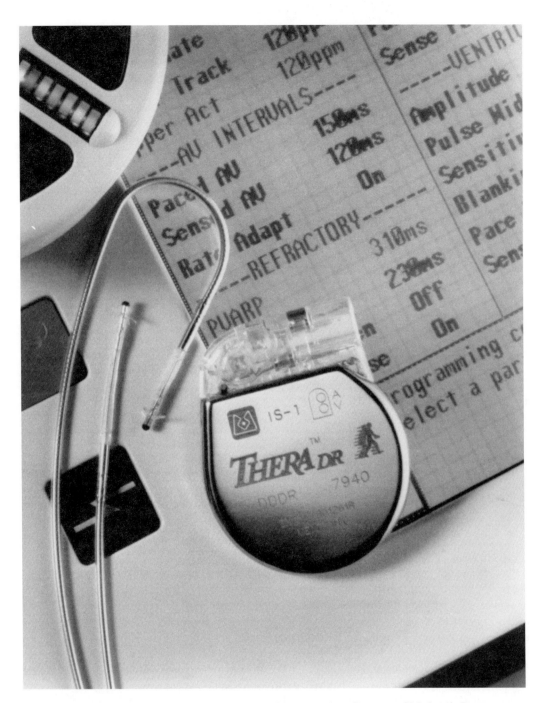

FIGURE 2 Polyurethane pacemaker lead and pacemaker. Courtesy of Medtronic Inc.

of the sheath with the metallic coil promotes transmission of stresses from the coil to the insulator. Constructions of unipolar and bipolar wires are shown in Figure 3. Bipolar systems require both internal and external insulation sheaths. On the whole, the first pacemaker leads were successful; however, there were incidences of failure in some of the earlier models, and closer examination of these reports suggested that most of the problems were associated with particular leads from certain manufacturers. The problems were extensive surface cracking, and failure of the lead, leading to

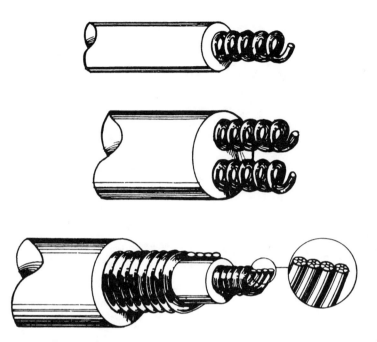

FIGURE 3 Typical lead conductor configurations. Top: unipolar — an insulated wire coil. Center: bi-polar — two wire coils in parallel, insulated with bilumen polymer tubing. Bottom: bipolar — two coaxial wire coils insulated with coaxial polymer tubing. From Stokes K., Urbanski P., and Upton J. *J. Biomat. Sci., Polymer Ed.*, 1:207, 1990. With permission.

leakage of the current; the problems of current leakage were characterized by reduced stimulation of the myocardium, muscle twitching and premature battery depletion. Many of these leads were insulated with Pellethane 2363-80A, which appeared to be degrading after implantation, and having a shorter lifetime than expected. This was the first clinical manifestation of polyurethane degradation.[37] Two distinct mechanisms of degradation of pacemaker lead insulation have since been proposed: environmental stress cracking and metal induced oxidation. The reader is directed to the previous sections on metal induced oxidation and environmental stress cracking in Chapter 8.

Environmental stress cracking (ESC) of a material occurs under conditions that provide an active chemical agent, and tensile stress. The failure of pacemaker leads was believed to be caused by environmental stress cracking. SEM studies by Scheuer-Leeser *et al.* showed that cracking occurred primarily at points of flexure of the lead, such as the J-curve of atrial leads, the distal tip of ventricular leads, and ligature sites.[34] A subsequent alteration in the manufacturing process was made, in order to reduce the residual stress in the material, and increase control over annealing, extrusion and molding procedures. Leads manufactured after this modification was implemented were much more successful. Protective sleeves were also introduced at points of ligature. In addition, a slightly harder polyurethane, Pellethane 2363-55D, was investigated and utilized. Both the 55D and 80A grades of Pellethane are synthesized from the same reagents, but Pellethane 2363-55D has a higher hard to soft segment ratio. Studies comparing the degree of surface cracking on explanted surfaces of Pellethane grades show that Pellethane 2363-55D is indeed less susceptible to surface cracking than Pellethane 2363-80A.[38] Further studies of environmental stress cracking of polyurethanes in the biological environment have reported that cracks may appear within six months of implantation although they do not propagate more than 20–30 μm within three years.[39] Cracking also may lead to a reduction in the tensile strength of the lead, although this is dependent on the extent of cracking and the thickness of the insulator. There also may be a fall in the impedance of a lead, although this is not believed to be clinically significant.[40] Severe cracking, however, may provide a breach in the insulating layer allowing permeation of fluid into the core, promoting oxidation of the metal wires. The metal ions may then promote degradation of the material from the inside.[41]

Metal induced oxidation (MO) is an auto-oxidative process, that may be initiated and propagated by certain metallic corrosion products.[42] The time between implantation and the onset of oxidative degradation is determined by the diffusivity of the species through the insulating layer. Free radicals can degrade the polymer directly; metal ions also may complex with the polyurethane, causing the surface to stiffen which may lead to cracking. Metal ions often are found at sites of degradation, and cobalt and molybdenum have been implicated as particularly vigorous promoters of MO.[43] During the development of polyurethane insulated pacemaker leads, there has been a transition from stainless steel coil wire through various alloys of platinum, copper and silver, to the more corrosion resistant MP35N, an alloy containing nickel and chromium, cobalt and molybdenum. In addition to enhanced resistance to corrosion, wires must possess fracture resistance and good flexibility. This also can be enhanced by using multifilar construction of the coil. Bipolar leads were observed to be more susceptible to metal induced oxidation than unipolar leads, due to the presence of two metal coils in the lead, breaches in the inner insulation and the presence of a higher number of joints in the device. The presence of processing additives may provide suitable oxidizing agents or promote oxidation by metal ions, although antioxidants required for processing may retard degradation. The metal core also may be oxidized under the electrochemical potential of the battery.

Observations of surface cracking on pacemaker leads created an awareness of surface cracking in catheters, and vascular grafts, and has stimulated much of the interest in the degradation mechanisms of polyurethanes. Recent reports of long-term studies of polyurethane-insulated leads indicate that a cumulative survival rate of over 99% after 10 years implantation can be anticipated for well designed leads.[44] Polyurethane performs at least as well as silicone rubber, if not better,[44-45] and their good blood compatibility may support their use in place of silicone rubber.[46] Such data support the contention that the earlier problems of failure were due to interactions between the polyurethane and the intravascular environment that were not anticipated, and are not indicative of an inherent problem that universally affects polyurethanes.

C. VASCULAR PROSTHESES

Synthetic vascular grafts are implanted into the body in order to replace damaged vessels, or to bypass blocked arteries and veins. Synthetic grafts are also employed as arterio–venous (A–V) shunts, in aortocoronary surgery and as a means of gaining vascular access in hemodialysis patients. Some of these applications require small diameter vascular prostheses that must remain patent, and not form clots that would obstruct blood flow, or embolize and cause damage downstream. Although synthetic vessel replacements are available, they are limited to replacement of large diameter vessels. To date, there is no satisfactory synthetic small diameter vascular prosthesis. The problem of surface thrombosis remains the greatest obstacle to the production of a successful small diameter vascular prosthesis. Polyurethanes are one of the strongest candidates for development, due to their high tensile strength, compliance, and relatively good blood compatibility. A review of the development of polyurethane vascular grafts was published recently.[47] One example of a polyurethane vascular prosthesis is shown in Figure 4.

Synthetic vascular grafts made from fabric were first introduced by Voorhees et al.[48] Later, Boretos and Pierce developed synthetic vascular grafts fabricated from the polyurethane, Lycra as this material retained its elastic characteristics well after repeated immersion in hot water.[49] At present, the grafts of choice for large diameter and small diameter vessels are synthetic and autologous respectively. Of the synthetic materials that have been used as graft materials, polyethylene terephthalate (PET), sold under the name Dacron®, and expanded polytetrafluoroethylene (e-PTFE), more commonly known by its trade name Gore-Tex®, predominate. These materials perform best in regions where there is high blood flow and low resistance to flow. At such sites, both of these materials exhibit long term patency. Both PET and e-PTFE are thrombogenic materials; their

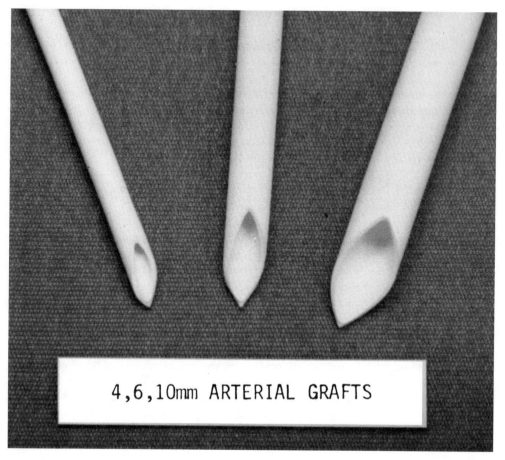

FIGURE 4 Vascular prostheses fabricated from BioSpan. Courtesy of the Polymer Technology Group.

use is limited to large diameter vessels, as at graft diameters of less than 6mm, the patency of these grafts made from these materials is less than 50%. For smaller grafts, autologous material is favored. Sections of blood vessel are removed from the patient, usually the saphenous vein in the leg. There are a number of advantages of using autografts, including the elimination of immunological problems associated with use of other tissues and materials. Disadvantages of using the saphenous vein include the limited supply of the material, the condition of which depends on the particular disease state of the patient. Removal of graft material also places further demands on the patient during surgery and recovery. Furthermore, venous grafts are prone to aneurysm formation once they are used at arterial pressures.[50] In applications such as extra-anatomic bypass and A–V shunts for vascular access, synthetic materials are preferred, because they are able to withstand higher external pressures.

Much of the research effort into the development of synthetic small diameter vascular prostheses has focused on the thromboresistance, porosity and the mechanical characteristics of candidate materials, which can all affect the long term patency of the graft and the development of a stable neointima. Additional features that are highly desirable in a synthetic small diameter vascular prosthesis include durability, resistance to infection and immediate availability.

Thromboresistance is required of a vascular prosthesis to retain graft patency so that thrombi do not form and occlude the vessel or embolize and lodge in a distal site. Polyurethanes are relatively thromboresistant compared to both PET and e-PTFE and this has driven the development of a small diameter vascular prosthesis from polyurethane. Within small diameter vessels, graft occlusion can

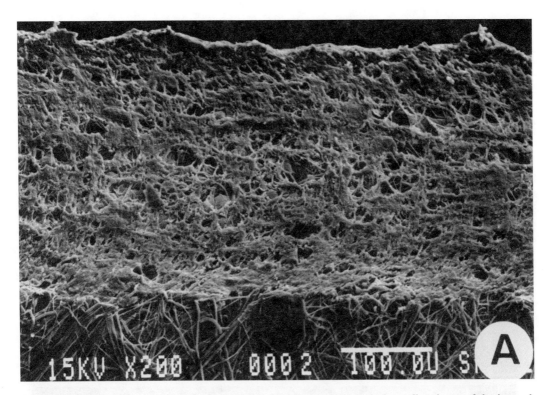

FIGURE 5 SEM photomicrographs showing longitudinal section thorugh the wall and part of the internal surface of three types of prostheses (A} Vascugraft, (B) Mitrathane, (C) Reinforced Goretex. Reprinted from *Biomaterials*, 15(7):483, Zhang Z., King M. W., Guidoin R., Therrien M., Pezelot M., Adnot A., Ukpabi P., and Vantal M. H., Copyright 1994, Elsevier Science Ltd. With permission.

occur before a stable neointima can develop. The thickness of the neointimal layer can affect the final internal diameter of the prosthesis.[51] If a material is of low thrombogenicity then formation of a thin fibrin layer may facilitate the growth of a thin neointima. This in turn may support the growth of an endothelial layer, the thromboresistant characteristics of which are desirable to retain the long term patency of the graft. Other approaches to increase the thromboresistance of polyurethane grafts include the grafting of heparin onto vascular prostheses. Van der Lei et al.[52] ionically bound heparin to polyurethane, which was then stabilized via treatment with glutaraldehyde. Ito et al.[53] compared the thromboresistance of ionically and covalently bound heparin *in vitro* and *in vivo*. Arnander found that immobilization of heparin fragments on the surface of vascular grafts extended the duration of graft patency in dogs from 3.5 days to 25.9 days, although all the grafts eventually failed.[54] All of these approaches met with limited success. Han et al.[55] modified the surface of a porous polyurethane graft made of Pellethane 2363-80AE with polyethylene oxide and sulfonate groups. They reported lower platelet adhesion and thrombus formation on the modified surfaces than on the control unmodified surfaces after implantation in dogs for 39 days. They also observed a lower extent of calcification on these surfaces.

The texture of the internal and external surfaces also is important. Cross-sectional SEMs of a number of different prostheses that have been fabricated from polyurethane are shown in Figures 5–9. The porosity of a vascular graft affects its patency and long-term healing. With respect to the internal luminal surface, porosity can greatly influence neointima formation, which has been discussed in Chapter 7. Ingrowth of endothelial cells on the inner surface of vascular grafts is desirable as the endothelium maintains the fluidity of the blood through the synthesis of many factors and proteins, providing a regulatory role beyond that achievable through the use of synthetic

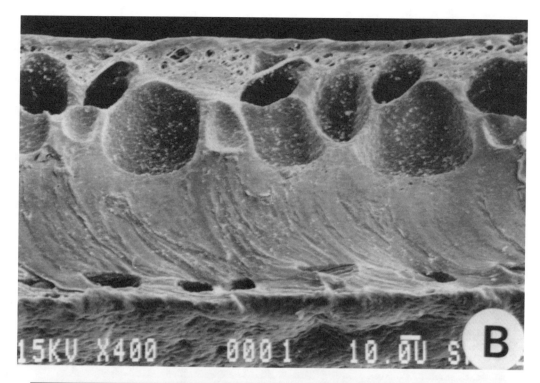

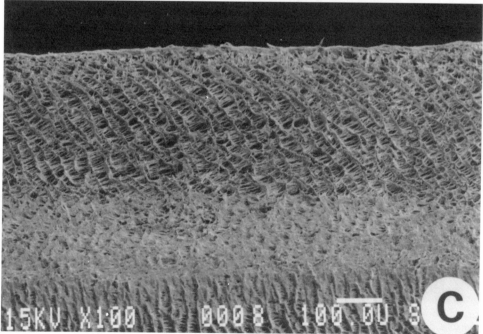

FIGURE 5 (continued)

materials. Rapid ingrowth of cellular material also may reduce the likelihood of infection. As discussed in the previous chapter, the degree of cellular ingrowth can be influenced by the texture of the surface, as well as the surface chemistry. Thus the fabrication method used to manufacture a graft becomes important. Studies by Wesolowski et al.[56] have demonstrated that tissue ingrowth

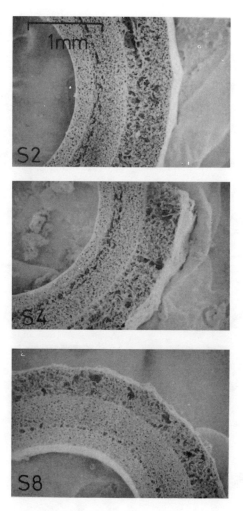

FIGURE 6 Scanning electron microphotograph of the cross sections of polyurethane grafts. From Hayashi, K., Takamizawa, K. Saito, T., Kira, K. Hiramatsu K., and Kondo, K., *J. Biomed. Mater. Res.* 23, A2: 229, 1989. With permission.

and neointima formation are enhanced on textured, porous surfaces, compared with smooth materials. Although rough surfaces can promote thrombus formation, textured surfaces may produce a thinner and more stable pseudoneointima. Since a neointima may be as thick as 1mm, and does not appear to depend on the size of the vessel,[57] development of such a lining can significantly reduce the effective vessel diameter. Thus control of the neointima thickness may be an important consideration in graft biocompatibility. The porosity also is important on the tissue contacting outer surface of the graft. The degree and type of tissue ingrowth can ultimately affect the compliance of the graft. Granular tissue is preferable to fibrous tissue, with respect to mechanical properties. Thus the pore size can be used to control the size of cell and type of ingrowth. Annis et al.[58] have developed a technique to produce porous grafts by the electrostatic spinning of polyurethane fibers. The porosity of the inner surface can be altered by the fiber diameter and the angle at which the fibers are spun. Cellular ingrowth was reported for a graft with a pore size of 10 μm. Hess et al.[59] evaluated a fibrous vascular graft in rats, and reported that neointima was supported on rough porous areas, whereas in areas where the fibers had fused and created a smooth surface, no cellular over-layer was observed. Further studies were performed and the formation of the new endothelial layer was examined.[60] At first the new endothelial cells were irregular in shape, but later became

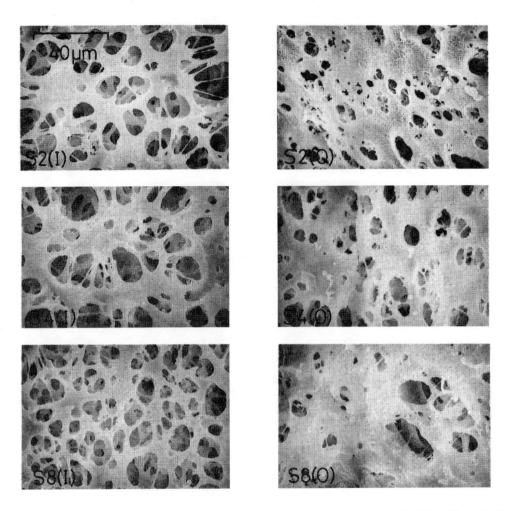

FIGURE 7 Morphology of inner (I) and *f* outer (O) surfaces of polyurethane grafts. From Hayashi, K., Takamizawa, K. Saito, T., Kira, K. Hiramatsu K., and Kondo, K., *J. Biomed. Mater. Res.* 23, A2: 229, 1989. Reproduced with permission.

regularly spindle-shaped, and aligned parallel to the direction of blood flow. The neointimal layer was comprised of myofibroblasts and smooth muscle cells and covered with endothelial cells. Beahan and Hull implanted fibrous polyurethane samples into rats for six months,[61] and reported that cellular ingrowth occurred via tissue ingrowth within the fibrous framework of the implant. More recently, Kogel et al.[62] have studied the endothelialization of e-PTFE and polyurethane of differing porosities in dogs. They reported significantly different patency rates between low and high porosity materials, those of high porosity achieving better tissue incorporation. There also was evidence of neointima formation. Thus it appears that there may be differences due to rheological characteristics of the blood flowing through the vessel, as well as differences due to the material from which the vessel is prepared. Okoshi et al.[63] implanted microporous vascular grafts in rats, and reported that the degree of endothelialization was influenced by the amount of penetrating micropores in polyurethane-polydimethylsiloxane grafts. The patency of the grafts after three months was acceptable.

Graduated and compartmentalized prostheses also have been developed to achieve the required blood response, tissue response and graft compliance.[64] These grafts were blended from polyurethane and polylactide with different porosities on the inside and outside walls. These were then

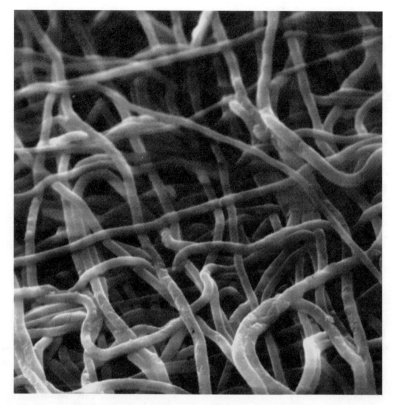

FIGURE 8 SEM of fibrous polyurethane vascular graft. Courtesy of T. V. How.

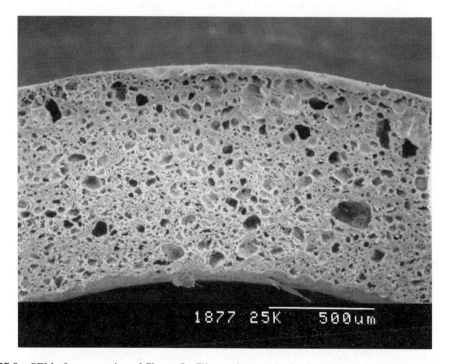

FIGURE 9 SEM of cross section of Chronoflex™ vascular prosthesis. Courtesy of CardioTech International.

implanted into rats and excised after a certain time. After three weeks, the inside of the vessel was coated with a thin neointima. After four months, little of the original polyurethane remained, and the mechanical properties of the conduit matched those of the aorta. The degradation rate of the polyurethane can be controlled by the molecular weight of the polymer, so that the vessel does not degrade before adequate tissue has been regenerated to transport the blood. Further studies on these degradable prostheses have been performed by Wildevuur *et al.*[65] who examined the degradation. They reported that the fragmentation rate of the prostheses was dependent on the mechanical characteristics of the polymer blends, whether or not either of the components was biodegradable. It is possible that these smaller fragments could become encapsulated by multinucleated cells, and degraded. Further studies are required in order to examine this.

Although many studies *in vivo* have shown that complete tissue ingrowth may occur in some animal models such as rats and dogs, complete neointima formation has not been observed in humans. Endothelial cell seeding of vascular prostheses has been performed to try and promote neointima formation after implantation and complete endothelialization of the luminal surface. Grafts have been coated with extracellular matrix components in order to promote attachment and proliferation of endothelial cells.[66,67] An improvement in the extent of endothelialization has been observed in animal models.

The compliance of the material also is believed to be a critical factor in the success of a material for small diameter vessels. There is confusion in the literature about the terms compliance and distensibility. The compliance of the material is the strain or elongation response to an applied stress, and is the reciprocal of Young's Modulus. Hence, it is an intrinsic property of the material. The distensibility of a material is a measure of the capacity of the vessel to increase in volume under a given internal pressure, or the extent of dilation of tubing, and unlike the compliance, it is dependent on the geometry of the sample. In the literature, compliance is often used interchangeably with the term distensibility. Ideally, a material for small diameter vascular prostheses should match the viscoelastic nature of the vessel wall as closely as possible. Natural arteries show an increase in diameter of about 10% when pressurized to 150 mm Hg (normal arterial pressure). In comparison, PET and e-PTFE grafts distend by about 1% under these conditions. Polyurethane has been shown to distend by about 6%,[58] and a polyurethane-polylactide prosthesis showed mechanical properties similar to rat abdominal aorta up to an elongation of 50%.[68] Arterial substitutes need to have matched mechanical properties. i.e., be strong and resilient. A mismatch of mechanical properties at the anastomosis (the junction between the natural artery and the graft) may lead to turbulent blood flow, which may in turn reach levels that result in thrombus formation or destruction of formed blood elements. The distensibility of the graft itself also may affect the blood compatibility. The compliance of the graft may affect the time course of thrombosis and embolism, by influencing the degree of thrombus adhesion. Material compliance mismatch also may produce an increased wave velocity leading to an increase in wave reflection and energy loss.

Some early studies of the effect of compliance on the patency of vascular grafts were performed using grafts where the polymer chemistry differed in addition to the compliance of the graft. Further studies between compliance and patency have been reported,[69,70] Lyman *et al.*[71,72] compared polyurethane grafts where the compliances (distensibilities) of the grafts were altered through sample geometry. The results showed that the distensibility of the graft can influence the biocompatibility through the degree of anastomotic hyperplasia. Anastomotic hyperplasia is the proliferation of tissue that occurs at the junction between the natural and the substitute vessel. In addition to the factors stated previously, it is believed that the mismatch in compliance between the synthetic graft and the natural vessel may cause sufficient trauma to the natural vessel to disrupt the endothelium, which will in turn initiate thrombosis and stimulate intimal hypertrophy (extensive tissue growth of the intima). Other possible mechanisms for anastomotic hyperplasia include the rigidity of synthetic grafts, which increases the amplitude of the pressure wave at the proximal anastomosis, increasing the stresses at the wall, which will in turn increase cell proliferation. It also is possible that the mismatch of mechanical properties between the replacement graft and the natural artery may provoke tissue reactions, leading to anastomotic hyperplasia. The degree of hyperplasia also may be dependent on the anastomotic technique used in surgery.[71,73] Prostheses retrieved from animals also have shown thrombus formation at the anastomosis.[72]

In recent years, a very detailed study on the development of a polyesterurethane small diameter vascular prosthesis has been reported in the literature.[74-78] This series of papers is noteworthy, as they detail the development of the graft, from fabrication through clinical trials. The grafts are characterized for physical and chemical properties, using techniques such as ESCA, contact angle measurements and tensile testing. The authors reported good reproducibility of the polyurethane synthesis, and performed experiments to evaluate the degree of phase separation before and after incubation in buffer. Degradation studies were performed *in vitro*, as well as after clinical implantation. Throughout the study, comparative tests were performed on a Mitrathane prothesis and a Goretex (e-PTFE) graft. Clinical trials did not show improved performance over the clinically-dominant e-PTFE graft in a below-knee application, and development on the graft has ceased.[79]

Current research acknowledges the possibility that the fabrication of a device can be used to influence the biological performance. Different manufacturing and fabrication techniques are being investigated in order to improve the re-endothelialization of prostheses through textural modifications, and the compliance of grafts through other fabrication techniques.[80,81] Recently, Nakayama and Matsuda have applied excimer laser ablation techniques to fabricate porous vascular grafts from Cardiomat polyurethane.[82]

Other features required of vascular prostheses are suturability, and ease of surgical handling. Furthermore, the graft should not kink when going around bends or traversing joints, and should not collapse under longitudinal extension. Grafts also may experience high stresses at suture points, which may lead to tearing.[83] Polyurethane materials can retain sutures well without tearing, or causing leakage around the needle holes. Polyurethanes also possess suitable mechanical characteristics that prevent the graft kinking when traversing joints without the need for crimping, which increases the luminal roughness. Grafts must also be evaluated for burst strength. Vascular grafts must withstand high physiological pressure, to prevent aneurysm formation.

D. Heart Valves

The natural heart valves are essentially unidirectional check valves which allow blood flow in one direction. Two valves, the mitral and the tricuspid, are located between the atrium and the ventricle, and open during diastole (filling of the ventricle). Two other valves, aortic and pulmonary, open during systole and allow blood to be ejected into the systemic and pulmonary circulation respectively. Replacement valves are required to replace those damaged due to valvular disease and congenital malformation. The development of synthetic prosthetic heart valves also is crucial to the development of the total artificial heart. Artificial heart valves have been in use since 1960. Replacement valves can be classified into two types — mechanical and tissue. There are several designs of mechanical valves, and these generally fall into one of three categories; ball valves, caged disk valves, and tilting disk valves. Tissue valves are chemically treated xenografts. There are still a number of problems associated with the design and performance of prosthetic heart valves including:

1. Trauma to formed elements in areas of turbulent flow. This includes hemolysis, which occurs during valve opening and closing.
2. High transvalvular pressure gradients across the valve, which are related to the degree of alteration in the central flow pattern. Regurgitation of the blood must be kept to a minimum.
3. Noise.
4. The imposition of unnatural constraints on the heart, by use of a rigid base to support the valve.
5. Thrombosis, which generally occurs in stagnant zones.

6. Calcification, which can limit the lifetime and performance of the valve.
7. Durability.
8. The need for the long term administration of anticoagulants. This is particularly true for mechanical valves.

The main limitation on the use of mechanical valves is the need for the long-term administration of anticoagulants. The greatest limitation on the lifetime of bioprostheses is the durability and calcification of the tissue. Polyurethanes have been used to manufacture prosthetic heart valves not only for their mechanical properties, but also for their blood compatibility, which may reduce the need for large quantities of anticoagulant and long term therapy. A number of polyurethane heart valves have been designed and tested. The most common configuration of polyurethane heart valves is the trileaflet valve, the designs of which closely resemble the natural trileaflet aortic heart valve, although bileaflet valves have been developed also. Russell et al.[84] fabricated seamless tri-leaflet valves from Avcothane-51. On the basis of in vitro and in vivo endurance studies, they concluded that with respect to material fabrication and handling, surface smoothness and rigorously clean fabrication procedures were necessary to minimize thromboembolytic complications. The importance of surface quality in influencing the degree of thrombogenicity of polyurethane heart valves also has been noted by other researchers.[85,86] Jansen et al.[87] have evaluated polyurethane trileaflet valves, prepared by dip-coating a valve in a half-open configuration, rather than a closed valve configuration. They reported good hydrodynamics, with low shear stresses distal to the valve. Many of the prototype valves have been prepared by multiple dipping of a mold into a solution of low polyurethane concentration. The main problem with this technique is that there is inadequate control of the leaflet thickness. Mackay et al.[88] recently reported a new procedure to prepare polyurethane tri-leaflet heart valves in a one-step coating process, achieving good uniformity of the valve leaflets.

A number of researchers have been studying and modeling the flow characteristics of fluid through trileaflet heart valves. A selection of trileaflet polyurethane heart valves is shown in Figures 10 and 11. The retention of the flow characteristics of the normal functioning heart is desired to minimize trauma to the blood cells, and reduce thrombus formation. Chandran et al.[89-91] have analyzed flow characteristics and stresses applied during the use of prosthetic heart valves. Analysis of a polyurethane trileaflet valve showed that the stress distribution is dependent on factors such as the stent height and rigidity as well as the thickness of the leaflets that comprise the valve. Increases in the transvalvular pressure gradient across a trileaflet polyurethane valve also has been reported by Herold et al.[92] Thicker leaflets are also associated with higher energy losses, but reduction of the leaflet thickness to reduce energy losses will also reduce fatigue resistance of the valves. The flow characteristics of fluid passing through the trileaflet polyurethane heart valve are considered to be similar to those obtained with bioprosthetic tissue heart valves.[93] In vitro studies also have shown less regurgitation of fluid with a polyurethane trileaflet heart valve compared to mechanical disc valves.[94,95]

One of the most persistent chronic problems with tissue and polymeric heart valves is their propensity to calcify.[96-98] Mineral deposition on heart valves causes the material to stiffen. This renders the valves stenotic and regurgitant, compromising the hemodynamic performance and durability. Calcification is most common in prosthetic aortic and mitral valves.[99] Calcification of polyurethanes has been discussed in some detail in the previous chapter. Examinations of heart valves retrieved after implantation have shown that the deposition of calcium phosphate on polyurethane leaflet heart valves occurs at sites where cellular matter and thrombotic debris are present on the surface. An additional mechanism for calcification of polyurethanes that has been proposed is the complexation of calcium ions with the polyether soft segment. Wisman et al.[100] reported the calcification of a polyurethane trileaflet valve implanted in calves. Hilbert et al.[101] implanted Biomer heart valves in the mitral position in sheep for up to 21 weeks and reported calcification. They observed two types of calcification on explanted devices. First, they observed calcification at the

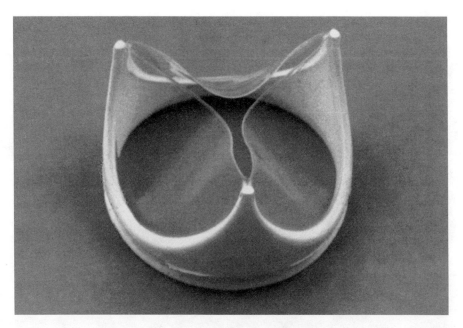

FIGURE 10 J-3 flexible leaflet polyurethane heart valve. From Jansen J., Willeke S., Reiners B., Harbott P., Reul H., and Rau G. *Int. J. Artif. Organs,* 14:655, 1991. Reproduced with permission.

interface between the polyurethane leaflet and the microthrombi and the fibrous sheath that were on the surface. They also noticed mineral deposits associated with degenerated cells within the fibrous sheath and thrombotic material.

Calcification of bioprosthetic heart valves also may be associated with areas of high stress.[102,103] The presence of residual stresses in a material after manufacture has been proposed as a contributor to calcification of polyurethanes.[101] High mechanical stresses may damage the structural integrity of the leaflet tissue, creating sites for initiation of mineral deposition at points of stress concentration and surface defects. It is possible that high fluid dynamic stresses may promote calcification.[104] Lo et al.[92] evaluated trileaflet polyurethane valves manufactured by dip coating 4 different polyurethanes; Cardiomat, Mitrathane and two prototype materials. Valves were implanted in the mitral position in calves. The polyurethanes performed well, with the investigators reporting that some of the polyurethane materials remained relatively free of mineralization for 250 days or more, whereas tissue valves generally calcified within 30–75 days. Other researchers also have reported that polyurethane heart valves show lower degrees of calcification than heart valves prepared from bovine pericardium, both *in vitro* and *in vivo*.[105] Removal of low molecular weight components from polyurethanes has been shown to reduce the degree of calcification.[105,106]

A number of researchers have chemically modified polyurethanes in order to improve the blood compatibility and reduce calcification. Han et al.[55] modified the surface of a Sinkhole graft valve and vascular prosthesis, fabricated from Pellethane and modified with polyethylene oxide and sulfonate groups. These were then implanted into canines for 39 days. These valves exhibited reduced levels of calcification in both devices after removal, when compared with unmodified polyurethane. They reported lower calcification on the vascular graft when compared with the heart valve, suggesting that the flow conditions and the stresses in the device environment may be contributory factors to calcification. They also reported lower platelet adhesion and thrombus formation on the modified surfaces, implying improved blood compatibility. Results from an *in vitro* study by Joshi et al. on a modified polyurethane with covalently attached phosphonate groups suggest that this approach may reduce calcification.[107]

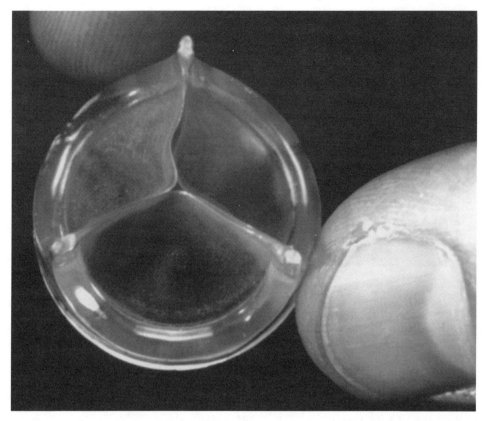

FIGURE 11 Trileaflet polyurethane valve. Reprinted from *Biomaterials,* 17:1857, MacKay T. G., Wheatley D. J., Bernacca G. M., Fisher A. C., and Hindle C. S., Copyright 1996, Elsevier Science Ltd. With permisison.

Moulopoulos *et al.*[108] have described the design and construction of catheter mounted aortic valves based on balloon and umbrella designs, manufactured from Estane 5710FI, and attached to a catheter system. Testing in dogs indicated that the prostheses operated efficiently, reducing aortic regurgitation to almost zero. The limitations of the valve included the possibility of rupture and difficulty in flow regulation. No thrombus formation was observed on the valve in the short-term (4 hours), but clots were reported to have formed within seven days.

Valves with polyurethane components also have been investigated. Gerring *et al.*[85] used Biomer in the fabrication of valve cusps for use in Oxford aortic/pulmonary valve prostheses. The Biomer valves compared well with silicone analogs. Kay *et al.*[109] evaluated a polyurethane-coated Teflon valve. This was reported to reduce incidence of thrombosis, thromboembolism and tissue overgrowth.

E. Cardiac Assist Devices

Cardiac assist devices are employed in situations where assistance is required in either pumping the blood, or preventing regurgitation of the blood. Other devices such as the total artificial heart are employed when assistance with both pumping and oxygenation are necessary. The main methods for assisting the heart are the use of left ventricular assist devices (LVADs), and intra-aortic balloon pumps (IABPs). The use of polyurethanes in these applications is reviewed below. Other methods of cardiac assist which have used polyurethanes include mechanical massage support, venoarterial bypass devices, and dynamic aortic patches.[110–111] The LVAD and IABP are considered to be transient devices; the TAH and the VAD may be classed as interim devices and considered for longer periods of implantation e.g., as a bridge to transplantation of a suitable donor organ.[112] The

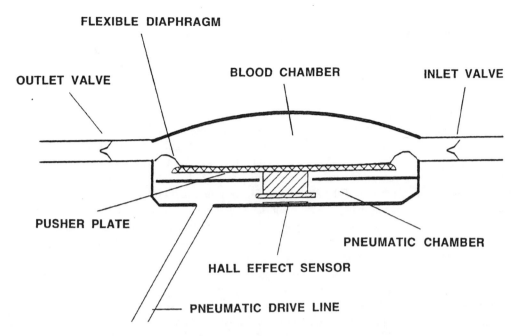

FIGURE 12 Cross-section of a Ventricular Assist Device. From Coumbe A., Salih V., and Graham T. R. *Am. J. Cardiovasc. Pathol.*, 4:302, 1993. Reproduced with permission.

use of synthetic materials in cardiovascular applications may lead to an increased incidence of stroke in human subjects due to embolic episodes. The propensity of implanted polyurethanes to calcify remains a chronic problem, in applications such as heart valves, and artificial blood pumps.[96-98]

1. Left Ventricular Assist Devices (LVADs)

Bypass of the left side of the heart is one of the most common methods of heart assist. Infarction of the left ventricle is a common cause of death and disability since the left ventricle accounts for 80% of the heart's work. Thus, there is a need for a Left Ventricular Assist Device (LVAD) that could serve permanently. During bypass of the left heart, the blood is drained from the left side and pumped into the systemic circulation using either extracorporeal or implanted devices. Polyurethanes are used in the fabrication of blood pump diaphragms because of their excellent flexure and wear properties. However, in many studies of LVADs, the emphasis has been on the design of the device rather than the performance of the components. Figure 12 shows an example of an external temporary LVAD with a polyurethane bladder.[113]

A number of polyurethanes have been used in the construction of ventricular assist devices. Snow et al.[114] used a Biomer flexing surface in an intrathoracic variable volume device. After 6 months implantation, the Biomer chamber had developed thick tissue capsules and exhibited persistent acute tissue reaction at the interface. Capsule formation was attributed to the continuous cycling of the chamber. McGee et al.[115] used a Biomer/butyl rubber/Biomer composite diaphragm in an electrically actuated intra-abdominally positioned blood pump (E-type blood pump). Polyurethanes are water permeable, and if used in the electrically actuated E-type systems, polyurethane diaphragms may transfer water into the actuator mechanism a rate of up to two ml/day. This can affect the performance of the actuator and may eventually lead to system failure.[116] Butyl rubber has low moisture transmission, so a trilaminar composite diaphragm, consisting of outer surface of Biomer with a central butyl rubber layer, was fabricated. Silicate particles coated with a mixture of epoxy and ethylene diamine were added during milling of the butyl rubber to create amine terminated surfaces and facilitate bonding between the two elastomers. MDI was added as a coupling agent to covalently bond to the butyl rubber filler and the urethane linkages in the Biomer. This composite diaphragm reduced water permeation through the membrane while simultaneously retaining most of the mechanical flexure properties of the original Biomer diaphragm.

Avcothane-51, a polyurethane with a polydimethylsiloxane component also has been used in LVADs. Engelman et al.[117] used Avcothane in the construction of the bladder and balloon valves of a totally implantable, pneumatically activated LVAD. In short term tests (up to eight hours) neither thromboembolism nor thrombosis was seen. Bernstein et al.[118] coated inflow and outflow catheters and the epoxy pump housing of a compact centrifugal pump for extracorporeal left ventricular bypass with Avcothane-51. In this configuration Avcothane-51 was bonded to all the blood-contacting surfaces. About half of the animal trials failed due to mechanical construction faults, or insufficient adhesion of the Avcothane-51 elastomer and clot formation.

Other polyurethanes that have been used in LVADs include Estane,[118] and polyurethane-polyvinyl chloride-graphite coatings.[119-120] Hayashi et al.[121] used two different polyurethanes, Toyobo TM3 and Toyobo TM5, to manufacture LVADs. The polyurethane components were fabricated by dip coating. These were then implanted into goats for up to 72 days. They reported a decrease in the tensile strength and ultimate elongation, and a slight increase in the elastic modulus of the polyurethanes after implantation. Removal of residual oligomers from the materials improved the mechanical stability of the polyurethanes during implantation. Weiss et al.[122] have used a segmented polyurethane to fabricate the blood sac of a totally implantable LVAD (Penn State LVAD). The sac was fabricated by dip-casting, to avoid the creation of seams. The presence of seams and other discontinuities may promote thrombogenesis.[123] The device was then implanted into calves for up to 244 days. Lack of thromboembolic complications was reported.

Ventricular assist devices have been implanted into human subjects.[124] A total of three VADs were implanted for up to 43 days. Retrieved samples underwent mechanical and SEM examination. They found that the mechanical strength of the polyurethanes increased after implantation. The blood contacting side of the VAD was covered with a biofilm, containing cells and cellular debris on the surface. They also reported no calcification, no changes in the microstructure of the surfaces and no evidence of microbial colonization of the materials.

Farras et al.[125] have modified a polyurethane of MDI, ED and PTMO, by adding low levels (1–5%) of a surface-active high molecular weight additive. This additive was to modify the surface by migration from the bulk to the surface. The mechanical properties were reported to be similar to Biomer. Blood sacs were fabricated from this polyurethane and Biomer sacs were used as controls. Sacs were implanted into calves for four weeks and examined after retrieval. All of the Biomer sacs had white thrombi on the surface; three of the four Biomer controls also had red thrombi. The surface modified polyurethanes showed no thrombus formation on the surface after retrieval. There were also fewer renal infarcts in the animals that had the modified polyurethane rather than Biomer sacs.

A few researchers have approached the improvement of biocompatibility of ventricular assist devices by using textured surfaces for the blood-contacting side of the pump. The use of smooth surfaces can lead to thromboembolic complications in VADs as the continual flexing of the surface may create surface defects that promote thrombus formation. Dasse et al.[126] examined textured VADs implanted into human subjects. After six weeks, there were no deleterious thromboembolic episodes, suggesting that textured blood contacting surfaces decreased the likelihood of thromboembolic events. The textured polyurethane was reported to promote neointima formation in a Thermedics pneumatically driven ventricular assist device. Cells were present in the lumenal pseudoneointima of the VAD. These cells were believed to be of blood origin, because of the speed at which they appeared. Coumbe et al.[127] implanted LVADs into calves. Their results implied that smooth surfaces in VADs can lead to thromboembolic complications owing to the continual flexing of the surface. The presence of a textured surface appeared to reduce thromboembolism, possibly by anchoring fibrin and hence allowing the formation of a stable neointima.

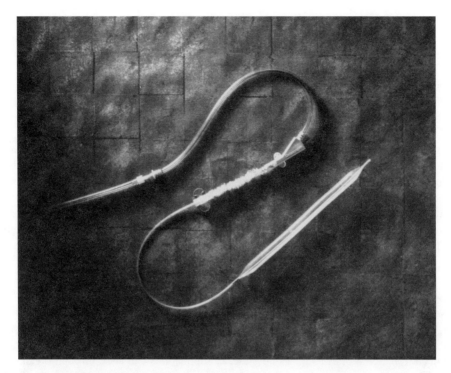

FIGURE 13 The intra-aortic balloon pump is the most frequently used cardiac assist device. It is typically fabricated from different grades of polyurethane polymers to impart abrasion and fatigue resistance to the membrane and insertability and kink resistance to the catheter. Courtesy of Datascope.

Biological modification of polyurethane surfaces also has been attempted to improve the blood compatibility of the inner surfaces of ventricular assist devices. Bernhard et al.[56,128] examined electrically actuated devices with collagen lined blood pumps that were implanted into calves. The collagen lining was achieved by seeding the surfaces with fetal bovine fibroblasts prior to implantation. There were fewer thromboembolic episodes in the collagen lined devices than in the unlined controls. The collagen lined devices also functioned for a longer time than the controls. Studies with textured fibril surfaces were also performed, and they reported the development of a thinner fibrin layer on the fibril surfaces than on the smooth controls. They also reported a drop in the compliance of the polyurethane after implantation.

2. Intra-aortic Balloon Pumps

Intra-aortic balloon pumps (IABPs) are used to facilitate arterioarterial pumping, and are the most commonly used method of circulatory assist (Figure 13). Generally, intra-aortic balloon pumps are employed for a period of the order of a few days, although a few patients have been supported for longer periods, up to one year. The IABP is a series-type of assist device. Intra-aortic balloon pumps consist of an elastomeric balloon that is pneumatically driven and controlled to raise central aortic pressure soon after left ventricular ejection and aortic valve closure. This reduces the workload of the heart. Moulopoulos was the first person to report the use of an intra-aortic balloon pump for counterpulsation.[129] The development, fabrication, and mechanical characterization of polyurethane IABPs have been summarized by Brash et al.[110]

Avcothane®-51 has been used in a number of IABPs.[130-133] Extensive studies have shown that the Avcothane®-51 IABPs did not appear to interfere with the metabolism of the host animal, and that no significant thromboembolic or hemolytic events occurred.[130] SEM examination of retrieved devices showed adhesion of a few platelets on the surface. Intracardiac polyurethane balloon pumps also have been developed for use in the mitral orifice, to reduce acute mitral regurgitation.[134]

IABPs can be inserted percutaneously via the femoral artery into the descending aorta, or placed directly into the aorta. The material used to fabricate a balloon pump needs to be pliable to allow insertion, but not distensible, ensuring the correct volume and geometry on inflation.[135] The biggest complication associated with intraaortic balloon pumps is lower limb ischemia, occurring in 11–18% of the 70,000 patients that receive an IABP.[136] Furthermore, IABPs are frequently employed in diseased vessels, that may be atheroschlerotic. Atheroschlerotic plaques may calcify, and the presence of hard spicules on the contacting surface of the pump may puncture the balloon.[135] This is a relatively uncommon complication, occurring in 0.12–1.3% of patients.[137] The consequences of balloon puncture are minimized by ensuring that the maximum air pressure in the balloon does not exceed the blood pressure. Recently, Myers et al.[136] reported the fracture of the internal lumen of a Percor polyurethane IABP. Examination of the retrieved device showed one fracture in the lumen and two other areas of stress fatigue. The authors noted that fractures of this nature are extremely rare.

III. ARTIFICIAL ORGANS

The development of artificial organs in medicine is necessary to perform the functions of organs that are diseased and no longer function adequately. Although the transplantation of organs from a donor is possible, there is limited scope for organ transplantation due to their limited availability and the need to match tissues as far as possible. Complications can arise through organ rejection, or through the use of immunosuppressive drugs that are required to prevent rejection of the transplanted organ. The use of artificial organs manufactured from synthetic biomaterials is associated with a number of other problems, including the need for anticoagulant therapy. These also have their own physiological side effects, particularly in the long-term.

A. Artificial Heart

Development of a totally implantable artificial heart (TAH) remains one of the greatest challenges in biomedical engineering. The development of such an artificial organ relies upon advances in four areas: biomaterials, pump design, transportable power source development and compatibility with the autonomous nervous system. Although development of the TAH has included application as a permanently implanted device, problems with thrombus formation and embolization has limited its use as a bridge to transplantation, until a suitable donor organ can be found. Short term use to take over the pumping action of an ailing heart also is feasible, allowing the cardiac tissue to rest until it can resume function again. The development of a total artificial heart relies heavily upon the development of suitable pumps and valves, which have been discussed above.

It is imperative that a totally implantable artificial heart works constantly without failure. Infection of the TAH is a serious problem and, unlike other medical devices, such a problem cannot be resolved by removal of the implant. Rheological characteristics are also crucial, with respect to the flow characteristics of the blood stream, and the possibility of trauma to the blood cells. In this section we shall focus on the biomaterial aspects of artificial heart development, by examining the performance of polyurethanes in this application. The main properties that are required of a material in an artificial heart are good blood compatibility on the inside surface, good tissue compatibility at the outer surface, and infection resistance on the skin-air interface. Good flexural properties and mechanical strength are critical to performance.

Polyurethane VC was used in the first artificial heart constructed from polyurethane.[138] This polyurethane also was implanted subcutaneously, and in the cardiovascular system. Investigations showed that the tensile strength decreased drastically after three years and its use was discontinued.[139] Boretos and Pierce reported the use of Biomer in an artificial heart in 1967.[140] They later investigated the *in vivo* performance of a Biomer coated LVAD, for possible artificial heart use.[141] They reported a good degree of blood compatibility and good physical stability. They also reported low lipid adsorption, which offered an advantage over similar devices manufactured from silicone rubber. Solution grade Biomer has since been used as a bladder material in a number of different artificial hearts. Other polyurethane materials that have been used in the artificial heart are Tecoflex, Avcothane, and Pellethane.

Additional material-related problems that need to be resolved to advance the development of a TAH, and other implants, are infection,[142] calcification and biodegradation. Calcification has already been discussed in some detail in the previous chapter and in earlier sections of this chapter. Calcification or mineralization occurs on flexing surfaces and can cause catastrophic failure through material stiffening, flexural failure and perforation of the membrane.[143-146] Calcification has been associated with micro defects on the surface and thrombus formation that may be initiated at such sites. Warfarin-sodium has been shown to inhibit calcification,[147] suggesting that a vitamin K dependent, protein carboxylation process may be contributing to the deposition of calcium phosphate on implanted surfaces.

Degradation of implanted polyurethane also has been reported. Lemm *et al.*[148-149] reported that the average molecular weight of Biomer decreased by 50% after exposure to enzymes and 20% following subcutaneous implantation for six months. Hunter *et al.*[150] reported the opposite, and observed an increase in molecular weight in polyurethanes implanted in calves for seven months. Other studies of degradation of polyurethanes have shown no change in chemical structure as determined by mass spectrometry.[151] Surface cracking of implanted materials also is of concern in development of the artificial heart and heart valves.[152] Surface cracking may promote thrombus formation, calcification and degradation. One strategy to solve this problem has been to use blends of silicone rubber and polyurethane, and interpenetrating networks (IPNs) of silicone rubber and polyurethane.[153]

B. Hemodialysis

The functions of the kidney include the removal of excess water and solutes, and toxic substances from the blood, and hormonal regulation. Intermittent dialysis utilizing an extracorporeal device is a substitute for kidney function, although at best, current dialytic therapy with cellulosic or synthetic membranes can only achieve clearance of some solutes.

The artificial kidney as known today originated from the work of Willem Kolff during the 1940s. Blood is circulated extracorporeally across a semipermeable membrane, while dialysate, a physiologically balanced salt solution flows on the other side of the membrane and solutes are removed from the blood by diffusion. The most widely used hemodialysis membrane is manufactured from a material virtually identical to that originally used by Kolff: regenerated cellulose. Cellulose membranes operate primarily as a sieve; the size of solute that can pass through the membrane is determined by the pore size. Clearance of middle to high molecular weight solutes may not be adequate, leading to long term complications such as amyloidosis and carpal tunnel syndrome. Despite the administration of anticoagulant in hemodialytic procedures, thrombus formation in the hemodialyser may occur, leading to loss of blood components and reducing the efficiency of the dialyser, ultimately compromising the quality of treatment. Filters are used on-line to prevent microemboli from entering the circulatory system.

Polyurethanes are presently used in hollow fiber dialysers, as a potting medium for embedding the fibers in the outer casing. When dialysis units are sterilized using ethylene oxide, the polyurethane may absorb the gas and subsequently release the compound. Ethylene oxide has been implicated in hypersensitivity reactions in hemodialysis patients.[154-156] The amount of ethylene oxide that a patient receives can be reduced by allowing the dialyser unit to degas for a period of time before use, so that residual ethylene oxide can diffuse from the material, and by rinsing the device prior to use.[157]

Effort also has been directed towards the design of a polyurethane membrane, with improved solute clearance and blood compatibility compared to regenerated cellulose. Lyman and Loo synthesized a series of membranes from MDI, 1400 and 2950 m.w. PEO and aliphatic, alicyclic and aromatic diols.[158] *In vitro* studies showed that relatively small changes in the hard segment noticeably affected the transport of glucose and some amino acids. A nonlinear relationship between molecular weight and half-time rate of transfer implied that there were specific interactions between the solutes and the hydrophilic hard segment, imparting a degree of selectivity to the membrane. The effect of processing parameters on the permeability of polyurethane membranes has been studied by Jayasree and Sharma.[159] Porous polyurethane films were prepared by precipitation of the material from a methanol-water mixture, and precipitation onto glass from water. The permeability of the membrane to urea, creatinine and uric acid were affected by the method of precipitation. Sterilization by either glutaraldehyde or autoclaving reduced the permeability of the membrane, through a reduction in pore size as determined by microscopy. A blended membrane of polyurethane and polymethylmethacrylate had increased solute permeability compared to the polyurethane membranes.

Polyurethanes also can be cast into hollow fibers for use in hemodialysis. The low glass transition temperature and high elasticity of polyurethanes make spinning difficult, but a wet spinning process has been sucessful.[160]

C. Artificial Lung/Blood Oxygenation

Extracorporeal blood oxygenation is required to perform the oxygenation task of the lung and removal of carbon dioxide during cardiopulmonary surgery. The main types of oxygenator are bubble, membrane, film and disc.

Polyurethanes are also being considered for blood oxygenation applications, due to their hemocompatibility. Knight and Lyman have developed a composite membrane for extracorporeal membrane oxygenation, and evaluated its performance with respect to oxygen and carbon dioxide permeability and blood compatibility. The polyurethane was synthesized from MDI, PPG and ED. A thin layer of polyurethane was cast onto hydrophilic and hydrophobic supports. The permeability of the membrane to carbon dioxide was shown to be dependent on the support used; hydrophilic supports were liable to swell leading to a reduction in pore size, and hence gas permeability. Gas permeability characteristics of the polyurethane on hydrophobic supports were similar to silicone rubber. The hemocompatibility as measured by protein adsorption and platelet deposition was most favorable on the polyurethane, when compared to the silicone rubber, poly(propylene) and poly(tetrafluoroethylene).

Polyurethanes also have been used in the heat exchanger component of oxygenators, such as the Shiley S-100.[161] The presence of a layer of polymer may compromise thermal transfer.

D. Hemoperfusion

Hemoperfusion is an extracorporeal detoxification process where waste products are removed by sorption, rather than diffusion. Hemoperfusion has been applied to treat long term hemodialysis patients, as the removal of middle molecular weight solutes is superior to conventional hemodialysis. Kawanishi *et al*.[162] have used a charcoal-embedded polyurethane film to remove bilirubin and other middle to high molecular weight solutes; the levels of removal exceeded those achieved in hemodiafiltration, a procedure where higher molecular weight solutes are removed by filtration, in conjunction with hemodialysis.

The same charcoal embedded polyurethane also has been used in hepatic failure, to remove proteinaceous components from the circulatory system. Results in a canine model were encouraging, achieving 70% removal of bilirubin and 90% of bile acid. Subsequent studies with jaundiced patients attained maximal removal of 23% of bilirubin and 31% of bile acid. Removal was improved when 3 columns were used as opposed to one, to 43% and 55% removal respectively.[163]

E. ARTIFICIAL PANCREAS

In the broadening scope of artificial organs, polyurethanes also have been incorporated into designs for an artificial pancreas. Approaches focus towards the utilization of polyurethanes to encapsulate or support Islets of Langerhans. Fast diffusion of insulin and glucose through the substrate to the immobilized cells is of importance, as is mechanical strength.

Zondervan et al.[164] crosslinked an aliphatic polyurethane with dicumyl peroxide in order to retard degradation of the polymer following implantation. A porous material was fabricated by salt leaching. Results with encapsulated Islets of Langerhans showed a good insulin response to glucose, although the speed of response was slower than that of free cells. A pore size of 0.3–0.7 μm offered protection against the invasion of granulocytes. Ward et al.[165] have fabricated polyurethanes into hollow fibers by a dip casting method. The polymer was synthesized from an aromatic, diamine-extended hard segment, and an alkylene oxide soft segment. *In vitro* culture of pancreatic cells was maintained after six months. Seeded tubes were implanted in mice; a low level of rejection was observed. The surrounding tissue was vascularized, nonfibrous, and not strongly attached to the implant. The membrane was permeable to glucose and insulin, but not immunoglobulins. The permeability characteristics were believed to be governed by activated diffusion.

F. BLOOD TUBING

In recent years there has been a growing interest in the biocompatibility of blood tubing. Blood lines are an essential feature of extracorporeal circuits; plasticized polyvinyl chloride (PVC) is the predominant material in this application. In order to attain the required flexibility, plasticizers are incorporated into the PVC, and may constitute up to 40% of the finished product. Diethylhexylphthalate (DEHP) the most common plasticizer for medical grade PVC. The toxicology of DEHP has been widely studied, although the blood compatibility of PVC has not. It has been shown that plasticizers can migrate from tubing into the blood stream and enter the body. Further complications arise from the spallation of small particles from the inner surface of blood tubing, due to the repeated flexure of sections of the tubing in peristaltic roller pumps.

Pivipol (Bellco SpA) is a co-extruded PVC/polyurethane tubing, with polyurethane forming the inner blood-contacting surface. Such a strategy has been shown to improve the blood compatibility by reduction in C3a generation compared to PVC tubing.[166] A different study on the same material showed that particle spallation from the co-extruded tubing was increased, although the size of particles generated was smaller.[167] It is possible that the pump design may influence spallation as well as the type of tubing used. Pump design also may influence plasticizer migration.[168] It has been demonstrated that coating plasticized PVC tubing with polyurethane is not an effective method to reduce plasticizer migration,[169] although other studies do not support this finding.[168] Ljunggren reported that the release of plasticizer from polyurethane coated tubing was comparable with release from uncoated tubing, and higher than the uncoated material after storage for three months.[169] The inconsistency between this study and a later one by Hoenich et al. could be attributed to the test method; plasticizer migration was shown to be reduced overall from a polyurethane/PVC co-extruded tube when used as a blood line, rather than as a pump insert.[168]

G. BLOOD FILTERS

Blood filters are required to remove platelet and leukocyte aggregates, microemboli and fibrinopeptide debris after blood storage, extracorporeal circulation or exsanguination. Debris of the order of 15 μm needs to be removed before the blood enters systemic circulation, yet the filter must neither hinder the passage of cells, nor induce cell lysis. Further requirements of a blood filter are that it should be capable of handling large volumes of blood without clogging up. Depth type filters have long passages and trap microaggregates by adhesion. Screen types work by sieving.

The Fenwal 4C 2417 is a depth filter.[170] The upper filter is manufactured from nylon mesh, and screens out the larger debris. The upper section of the filter elements consist of a portion of polyurethane sponge with pore sizes ranging from 500–200 μm. The lower section is made from a nylon mesh screen. The polyurethane sponge removes particles by both adhesion and screening mechanisms. Significant reduction in platelet counts occur during use, which is true for other depth-type filters.

The Bentley series of polyurethane foam filters are essentially depth filters. Three filters are available for dialysis, oxygenation and filtering stored blood. The Bentley 427 comprises three layers of polyurethane foam of decreasing pore size. Adhesion of particles smaller than the smallest pore was observed, implying that adhesion to the filter surface was the underlying mechanism for removal of small particles, whereas the larger particles were removed by entrapment. Bruil *et al.* have recently investigated the application of polyurethane filters for leukocyte removal. The optimal pore size was 11–19 μm. Both adhesion and trapping mechanisms contributed to the removal of cells.[171] Studies by the same workers have supported a hypothesis that morphological factors such as configuration, roughness, tortuosity, and porosity have a greater effect on a filter's performance than physicochemical properties.[172]

IV. TISSUE REPLACEMENT AND AUGMENTATION

Polyurethanes are versatile materials that can be made with diverse properties. They have therefore been used in a large number of different applications including breast implant devices and implants in dentistry, urology, cardiology and wound dressings.

A. Breast Implants

The topic of breast implants has been extremely controversial over the last number of years and it is still not entirely clear how these implants affect the body. Several epidemiological stuides suggest that the effect is minimal or that there is no increase in illness beyond that found in control subjects. The literature is divided on the benefits and complications associated with breast implants in general, and polyurethane implants specifically. In 1993, approximately 1.5 million women in the United States had breast implants, 20% of which were for reconstruction principally after radical mastectomies.[173] In the late 1950s, Pangman described a composite breast implant that utilized a polyurethane foam.[174] His later work led to the development of the Natural-Y prostheses,[175] the forerunner of the Meme implant. Smooth walled silicone gel breast implants were first introduced in the early 1960s, followed in the 1970s and 1980s by implants covered by polyurethane foam.[175] The materials used in breast implants must have mechanical properties which mimic the human breast. They need to be soft and deformable while maintaining the appropriate shape.

All breast implants, coated with polyurethane or not, are subject to potential problems.[176] These include infection (< 1%), hematoma (1-4%), skin necrosis (rare), surgical removal of implant or fibrous capsule surrounding implant (4-20%), sensory changes in the nipple/areolar complex (1-10%), breast asymmetry (1-10%), and capsular contracture (30-40% for smooth implants, 2-10% for polyurethane covered).[176] In addition there is a possibility that tumor detection by mammography might be hindered and gel bleed and implant rupture may occur.

The smooth walled implants, although successful for many patients, were not without problems. These included formation of a capsule around the implant and its subsequent contracture, calcification, thinning of the skin, hardness, and implant rupture with the formation of silicone granulomas[177,178] Infections were not common.[179] Capsule contracture appeared to be the largest issue, [179,180] and indeed one author states that a survey of the Plastic and Reconstructive Surgery Cumulative Index between 1977-1983 contained 140 references on this subject.[181] Polyurethane covered implants were introduced to eliminate the contracture problems, and there is clinical evidence that the polyurethane covered implants were successful at *delaying* the incidence of capsule formation,[178,182-183] and contracture.[177,181,184-188]

The positive impact on contracture in comparison to the smooth implants appears to have been limited to short term clinical findings (less than 6 years). In a 19 year study, the authors found that after the initial low incidence of contracture in the first five–six years, the rate approached that for smooth implants over five–10 years, and decreased after year 15.[189] Other complications associated with polyurethane implants including difficulty in removing infected fragments, prolonged foreign body reactions including granulomas,[190,191] late pain,[182,191] breast deformities,[192] and skin lesions.[193] In addition, degradation of the foam coating, and separation of the foam from the silicone implant were other issues that had to be faced.[194]

The controversy around polyurethane breast implants reached its height with the report that a patient had free 2,4 toluenediamine (TDA) in her urine between 21 days and seven months after surgery.[195-196] Although the link between polyurethane hydrolysis products such as TDA and cancer in humans is unproven (see Chapter 8), the polyurethane coated implants are no longer available for use in Canada or the United States.

B. Wound Dressings

Polyurethanes are used extensively in wound healing applications, particularly for occlusive and semiocclusive (barrier dressings). The skin is made up of the epidermis and the dermis.[197-201] The epidermis is composed of many layers of epithelial cells (keratinocytes). It provides a barrier to water loss, invasion by foreign organisms, and physical and chemical threats. The dermis, underneath is composed of extracellular matrix and provides the elasticity, strength, and blood vessels of the skin. Wound healing in the skin is a complex process requiring the co-ordination of events in the capillaries, epidermis, dermis and basement membrane of the skin. In normal wound healing, keratinocytes begin to migrate over a wound within a few hours.[201] Within a day, cells that are on the outer edges of the wound start to divide, and between these new cells and the migrating cells a neo-epithelium is formed. Wound dressings must encourage the various stages of wound healing while minimizing contracture or scar formation.

1. Types of wounds

Wounds can be divided into acute and chronic, and partial thickness and full thickness. Acute wounds heal rapidly. Chronic wounds are considered to be wounds of long duration that fail to heal within a reasonable time period,[202,203] although the definition of reasonable varies depending on the wound, site, and patient. Chronic wounds may involve the epidermis (erosion) only or with increasing severity, both the epidermal and dermal layers (ulcer).[203] At present, wound. dressings for chronic leg ulcers are frequently occlusive and impregnated with different agents. These agents include glycerine, zinc, dermis, collagen and a host of others. The progress of chronic wounds towards healing is frequently inconsistent. Excellent media for bacteria, chronic wounds are commonly associated with peripheral vascular disease and arterial insufficiency although the etiology of these wounds is not well understood.[202,203]

Chronic venous leg ulcers resulted in more than 1.3 million outpatient visits in the United States between 1990 and 1992 and in Scandinavia the cost of treatment of this subclass of chronic wounds alone cost over $25 million U.S. dollars in 1985.[202] Researchers in the United States estimate that the costs in that country are an order of magnitude larger based on population demographics and health care costs.[202] Despite considerable research, the multitude of present clinical procedures, including different types of wound dressings, are meeting with limited success in healing chronic wounds.[202] Although there is an extensive literature available on chronic wounds, particularly venous leg ulcers, there is no consensus on the treatment of these wounds.[202,203]

Burns are divided generally divided into two categories: partial thickness and full thickness depending on the depth of wound. Partial thickness wounds were previously called first degree and second degree burns and are now divided into superficial and deep partial thickness wounds. A superficial wound is one which heals within three weeks. Deep partial thickness wounds often are the most difficult to both define and treat, and are frequently the most painful, often healing with severe scars.[204-206] In a full thickness burn re-epithelialization cannot occur spontaneously because both the epidermis and dermis have been destroyed.

Wound dressings are designed to produce the optimum conditions for healing. The type of dressing used will involve the type of skin wound, its depth, its cause, and the stage in wound healing. Wound dressings initially need to isolate the wound from the surroundings particularly from fluid loss and sources of possible infection. Because of their good barrier properties and oxygen permeability, polyurethanes are frequently used in wound dressings. Research has indicated that semipermeable dressings, many of which are polyurethanes, enhance would healing.[199,201] The permeability to water is particularly important so that exudate from the wound does not build up under the covering or that wound desiccation does not occur.

There are different types of dressings but polyurethanes are most frequently used as occlusive or semiocclusive dressings and are the most common type of occlusive dressing.[204] In addition, polyurethanes are frequently used as backing materials in composite or combination dressings. The characteristics of some types of dressings are described in Figure 14:[199]

Some of the polyurethanes used commercailly in wound dressings are given in Table 1, along with many other wound dressing systems.

2. Occlusive and semiocclusive dressings

Work on occlusive wound dressings actually began with the observation that a blister healed faster if left unbroken and in 1962 Winter showed that covering a wound with a polyethylene film significantly decreased the time it took to epithelialize the wound.[207,208] Following this original work, research was conducted to determine the effect of occlusive dressings on the healing of wounds particularly whether or not a moist environment contributed to enhanced healing. Polyurethanes were used in many of these studies.[208–211] It is now generally believed that for many wound types, a moist environment helps healing. Leipzig et al.[210] found that Opsite® (Smith and Nephew) along with another nonpolyurethane occlusive dressing (DuoDerm, Squibb Corp) increased the rate of epidermal resurfacing and increased collagen production in full thickness wounds in comparison to air dried wounds. Other authors have had similar findings.[212] Some of the more water impermeable polyurethane dressings have shown a tendency to accumulate fluid under the material when used in burn applications.[213] However, there has been some success with the polyurethanes in partial thickness wounds.[213] It is now generally believed that the moist healing environment is beneficial for wound healing. The moist environment is provided when the vapor transmission rate through the dressing is lower that the moisture produced within the wound by the underlying tissue. Moist wounds heal 40% faster than wounds which are exposed to the air.[208]

In addition to increasing the epithelization, occlusive dressings have been shown to minimize pain and can affect the formation of granulation tissue ultimately resulting in less scar formation.[211–212,214] They also have been shown effective in the treatment of ulcers.[208, 215–216] Opsite® also has been used to close the wound (without sutures) after pacemaker implantation.[217] Some polyurethanes have vapor permeability close to skin while others are more occlusive.[218–219] The polyurethanes such as Tegaderm and Opsite are now used extensively as occlusive or semiocclusive dressings.

One of the drawbacks of the occlusive or semiocclusive dressings is that significant fluid accumulation can occur under them, particularly in the first few days of use.[220] This may require

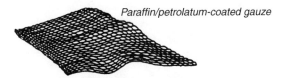

A. Nonadherent, nonabsorbent dressing

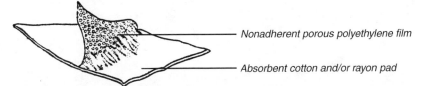

B. Nonadherent, absorbent dressing

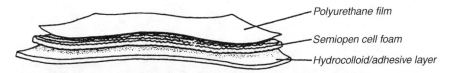

C. Nonadherent, absorbent hydrocolloid occlusive dressing

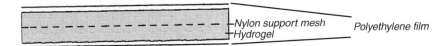

D. Nonadherent, absorbent hydrogel occlusive dressing

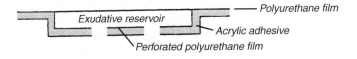

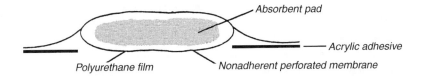

E. Nonadherent, absorbent composite occlusive dressing

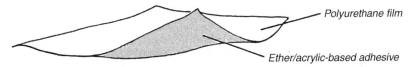

F. Semiocclusive, nonabsorbent transparent film dressing

FIGURE 14 Dressing construction and design. From Wiseman, D.M., Rovee, D.T., and Alvar.

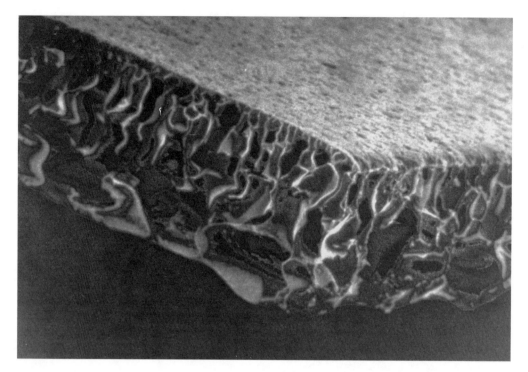

FIGURE 15 SEM of microporous polyurethane semi occlusive wound dressing (Spyroflex®). Courtesy of PolyMedica Industries, Inc.

aspiration of the wound, cause leakage, or infection.[221] In addition, occlusive and semiocclusive dressings sometimes stick to the normal skin around the wound and damage it.[221,222] Different polyurethanes have been synthesized to alter vapor and drug permeability through the membrane in order to eliminate the effects of exudate build-up and possible infection underneath the dressing.[221,223] Jonkman et al.[218,219] used salt cast Tecoflex EG-80A (a cycloaliphatic polyetherurethane) to produce a wound dressing, and more recently, Bruin et al.[224] combined this material with an Estane® underlayer to produce a pliable and a highly vapor permeable material. The authors showed improved wound healing of partial thickness wounds compared with uncovered controls and OpSite® covered wounds.

In burn care the conversion of an open wound to a closed wound as soon as possible is extremely important. Standard treatment is the use of split thickness skin grafts. Some of the characteristics of good wound dressings for burns are adherence to the wound (but not damaging to the surrounding skin), prevention of fluid and heat loss, and protection against both mechanical injury and infection.[213] Polyurethanes have been recommended for usage over donor sites and partial thickness wounds,[225-227] and Opsite® was used in a study that showed that it modified the cellular response in wound healing. There was a decrease in the number of inflammatory cells and an increase in the number of proliferative cells.[228] Opsite® (Smith & Nephew, Pinetown S.A.) also has been used for postoperative care of donor site skin grafts and has been proposed as a backer membrane.[229] The membrane then becomes the wound dressing over the graft.

Omiderm® is a polyurethane membrane (Jobskin; Jobst Institute Inc., Toledo, OH) which becomes pliable and adherent when wet. Designed as a burn dressing, it can be meshed or nonmeshed.[205-206] It is transparent and allows for inspection of the wound.[220] Omiderm® also has been used for burn treatment for both post skin graft, and meshed spit thickness skin grafts. Its other applications include use in plastic surgery for the treatment of free flaps,[230] and as a covering under ECG electrodes to protect the skin of low birth weight infants.[231,232]

TABLE 1
Commercially available dressings

Dressing type	Name and manufacturer	Description
Hydrogel dressings	Geliperm (Geistlich-Pharma/Fougera)	Hydrogel of polyacrylamide and agar (96% water); moist sheet, dry material, and gel; tape required for fixation
	Vigilon (Bard)	Crosslinked polyethylene oxide hydrogel (95% water) between two polyethylene films; nonadherent, gas-permeable; both film layers can be removed to enhance evaporation but may not exclude bacteria; tape required for fixation
	Other hydrogel dressings include Bard Absorption Dressing (Bard), Cutinova Gelfilm (Beiersdorf), and Elastogel (Southwest Technologies)	
Semiocclusive/ occlusive, nonabsorbent	Bioclusive (Johnson & Johnson Medical, Inc.)	Transparent polyurethane film with acrylic adhesive
	Blisterfilm (Chesebrough Pond's)	Polyurethane film with perimeter adhesive for atraumatic removal
	Opsite (Smith and Nephew)	Polyurethane film with polyether adhesive
	Tegaderm (3M)	Polyurethane film, acrylic adhesive
	Other products in this category include Acuderm (Acme United), Co Film (Chesebrough-Pond's) Ensure-It (Deseret) Opraflex (Professional Medical Products), Pharmaseal Transparent Dressing (Pharmaseal), Polyskin (Kendall), Uniflex (Howmedica-Pfizer), and Visulin (Beghin Say)	
Biological dressings	Biobrane (Woodroof Laboratories)	Silicone-nylon/collagen bilayer composite; depending on chosen porosity can be used on heavily or lightly exudative wounds
	E. Z. Derm (Genetic Labs)	Porcine xenograft, crosslinked collagen, stable at room temperature; contains silver as antimicrobial; recommended for use as a short-term dressing (i.e., daily changes) until adherence, when it may be allowed to slough off spontaneously
Medicated dressings	Bactigras (Smith and Nephew)	Chlorhexidine tulle gras
	Inadine (Johnson & Johnson Patient Care, Ltd., United Kingdom)	Rayon dressing impregnated with 10% povidone iodine ointment
	Actisorb (Johnson & Johnson Patient Care, Ltd., United Kingdom)	Nylon faced odor, and exudate activated charcoal cloth absorbent dressing
	Actisorb Plus (Johnson & Johnson Patient Care, Ltd., United Kingdom	Activated charcoal cloth containing an antibacterial silver salt
	Odor Absorbent Dressing (Hollister)	Tea-bag–like structure containing activated charcoal deodorant
	Scarlet Red Dressing (Chesebrough-Pond's)	Lanolin/olive oil/petrolatum impregnated gauze, containing scarlet red
	Tegaderm Plus (3M)	Contains idophor

TABLE 1 (continued)
Commercially available dressings

Dressing type	Name and manufacturer	Description
	Xeroform (Chesebrough-Pond's)	Absorbent gauze impregnated with bismuth tribromophenate in petrolatum base
Hemostats, absorbable	Collagen hemostats include Avitene (Alcon), Helistat (Helitrex) Hemopad (Astra), Instat (Johnson & Johnson Medical, Inc.) Oxycell (Parke-Davis) (Oxidised cellulose), Surgicel, and NuKnit (Johnson & Johnson Medical, Inc.) (Oxidised regenerated cellulose).	
Powders and pastes	A number of absorbent powders or pastes are available that are poured into the wound, absorb exudate, are somewhat occlusive, and may later be irrigated from the wound. These include Bard Absorption Dressing (Bard), Comfeel Granules (Coloplast), Debrisan Wound Cleaning Beads and Debrisan Wound Cleaning Paste (Johnson & Johnson Medical, Inc.), Duoderm Granules (Squibb), and Intact (Bard).	
Adherent, absorbent, nonocclusive		Many absorbent woven and nonwoven gauze products are available. Gauzes are based on cotton and/or rayon (regenerated cellulose)
Nonadherent, nonabsorbent, nonocclusive	Adaptic (Johnson & Johnson Medical, Inc.)	Knitted cellulose acetate impregnated with petrolatum emulsion
	Aquaphor (Beiersdorf)	Impregnated gauze
	Jelonet (Smith and Nephew)	Paraffin tulle gras gauze
	N-Terface (Winfield)	Polyethylene-based mesh
	Transite (Smith and Nephew)	Fenestrated film
	Vaseline (Chesebrough-Pond's)	Petrolatum gauze
Nonadherent, absorbent, nonocclusive	Melolin (Smith and Nephew)	Nonadherent perforated poly(ethylene terephtalate) film backed by absorbent cellulosic/acrylic layer
	NA Dressing (Johnson & Johnson Patient Care, Ltd., United Kingdom)	Knitted cellulose acetate fabric
	Release (Johnson & Johnson Medical, Inc.)	Lightly absorbent rayon pad sandwiched between porous polyethylene film
	Scherisorb (Schering)	Pourable nonadherent hydrogel, removable by irrigation; mild to moderate exudation only
	Silicone NA Dressing (Johnson & Johnson Patient Care, Ltd., United Kindgom)	Knitted cellulose acetate fabric with silicone coating
	Sorbsan (Steriseal)	Calcium alginate material; soluble gel forms on absorption of exudate; mild to moderate exudation
	Telfa (Kendall)	Cotton sandwiched between perforated nonadherent poly(ethylene terephtalate) sheets
	Other products in this category include Coraderm (Armour), Lyofoam (Ultra), Primaderm (Calgon), and Synthaderm (Dermalock)	

TABLE 1 (continued)
Commercially available dressings

Dressing type	Name and manufacturer	Description
Nonadherent, absorbent, occlusive/ semiocclusive		
Hydrocolloid dressings	Comfeel Ulcus (Coloplast)	Absorbent carboxymethylcellulose/adhesive layer backed by a polyurethane film; requires fixture with tape; also available as powder and paste containing guar, xanthan, and carboxymethylcellulose
	Duoderm (Granuflex in United Kingdom, Squibb)	Hydrocolloid layer composed of gelatin, pectin, sodium carboxymethylcellulose, and adhesive polyisobutylene; truly occlusive to gases and bacteria; backed by hydrophobic foam
	Johnson & Johnson Ulcer Dressing (Johnson & Johnson Medical, Inc.)	Hydrocolloid layer containing carboxymethylcellulose, karaya gum, silica, and polyisobutylene, backed by PVC foam sheet
	Other hydrocolloid dressings include Biofilm (Biotrol), Intact (Bard), Intrasite (Smith and Nephew), Restore (Hollister), and Ultec (Sherwood)	
Composite dressings	Tegaderm Pouch Dressing (3M)	Inner fenestrated film; exudate accumulates in pouch formed by outer film layer, which transmits water vapor only at high levels; not strictly an "absorbent" dressing, although it has the same effect, i.e., displaces wound exudate away from wound
	Viasorb (Sherwood)	Cotton polyester pad contained within a polyurethane sleeve; wound surface is slit fenestrated
	Other composite dressings include Lyofoam (Ultra) and Transigen (Smith and Nephew)	

From: Wahl and Wahl. "Inflammation." In *Wound healing:Biochemical and Clinical Aspects*. Cohen, K., Dieglemann R. F. and Lindblad W. J.,W.B. Saunders Co., Philadelphia, PA, 1991.

Polyurethane foam in a thin sheet, Delta-Tape, has been used to cover split thickness skin grafts.[233] The skin grafts were intact under the polyurethane and it appeared that the skin healed well. However, not all the evidence for use of polyurethanes as burn coverings is positive. One study showed that a polyurethane dressing had a greater healing time and more scarring in the treatment of partial thickness outpatient wounds in comparison to treatment with the conventional impregnated gauze dressing.[234] Interestingly, although partial burns have been extensively studied for a number of years, the best method of treatment is still not clear. In one investigation, Eldad et al.[206] found that Omiderm®, Xeroform® and Mettalin® all yielded the same healing results for partial thickness wounds (thermal injury) in pigs, and that the control and treatment groups were the same after 12 days.

Polyurethanes (Blisterfilm®) have been used successful to treat peritoneal exit sites. Compared to cotton gauze they had fewer infections and held the catheter securely.[235] Polyurethanes promote healing in donor sites in the elderly compared with gauze.[236] Polyurethanes have been used in combination with many other materials. Epiguard® is a polyurethane foam laminated to a sheet of microporous polypropylene which has been used as a temporary skin substitute.[213]

Ulcers, as described above, are different in their healing characteristics from burns or many other injuries. In the case of pressure ulcers, moisture increases damage to skin due to heat, friction and pressure, and therefore is believed to increase the potential for pressure ulcers.[237] Oleske et al.[237] concluded that there was a role to be played in the short term treatment of pressure ulcers by occlusive polyurethane dressings in protecting against infection but that their long term use is limited.

3. Wound dressings and infection

Polyurethanes are used for wound dressings primarily to prevent infection and as many of the bacterial strains become resistant to antibiotics, the antibacterial nature of wound dressings becomes more important. In contrast to the more traditional gauze dressing, polyurethanes permit continuous inspection of the wound, frequently are found to be more comfortable by the patient, and allow the patient to bathe.[238] In a detailed study of pulmonary catheters, Maki et al.[238] found that gauze had a lower rate of cutaneous colonization under the dressing at the time of catheter removal than did two polyurethane dressings, and that a more permeable polyurethane had lower numbers of colony forming units than the conventional polyurethane. However, neither of the polyurethane dressings represented an increased risk for device related infection compared with the gauze and the authors concluded that both were safe for use with pulmonary artery catheters.

Film type dressings (occlusive and semiocclusive materials) many of which are polyurethanes, used to cover surgical wounds and donor sites have been associated with reduced infection levels.[239-243] However, the evidence is not totally supportive of the use of polyurethane dressings. There is a relationship between the vapor permeability of the dressing and the bacterial protection provided. Behar et al.[223] found that Omiderm, a high vapor permeability polyurethane dressing was less effective than Opsite and Biobrane at preventing infection. Craven et al.[244] showed in a clinical study that Teflon catheters tips and their peripheral intravenous insertion sites had a greater number of infections when covered by a polyurethane dressing than when covered by dry gauze, particularly in summer months.

Comparing four dressing regimens for peripheral catheters, Maki and Ringer found that the different types of dressings used, gauze, a polyurethane dressing and a iodophor transparent dressing were comparable in their ability to prevent infection.[21] These authors were attempting to determine the most cost effective methods for treating catheter sites. They found that the most significant risk factors for infection were contamination of the catheter hub, moisture under the dressing, and prolonged catheterization. Although the polyurethane dressing showed slightly higher moisture build up under it, it did not show a statistically significant difference in infection rate. The authors recommended that it is not cost effective to redress peripheral venous catheters for most patients and for most patients either the sterile gauze or the polyurethane dressing, left on until the catheter was removed, was adequate. This clinical study involved 2088 cases. Aly et al.[245] had similar findings when they compared three polyurethane wound dressings, Op-Site, Tegaderm, and Uniflex, with gauze dressings as did Hoffmann et al.[246] when they also compared a polyurethane with a gauze dressing.

C. FACIAL RECONSTRUCTION

Materials used in facial reconstruction or as a facial prothesis must be strong yet pliable enough to respond to facial movement. Lewis and Castleberry recommend that the material show a tensile strength between 1000 to 2000 psi, an elongation at break of 400 to 800%, no water adsorption and a hardness of 25 to 35 Shore A scale.[241] The material should be easily processible, have adequate mechanical and physical properties and possess stable color. An idea cure time is one–two hours.

There appears to be four general classes of materials that are used or have been used for facial reconstruction: silicones, polyvinyls, polymethylmethacrylates and polyurethanes.[241-243] The polyurethanes are the most recent of the group. Ultraviolet light is one of the environmental factors which has the biggest impact on facial implants and can shorten the life of most facial prosthetic devices. Aromatic polyurethanes tend not to be used because of poor color stability and allergic reactions,[243] particularly in the presence of ultraviolet light. Although polyurethanes are used they do not appear to be used extensively in this application. Better resistance to UV radiation will be required before wider application in this area will be found, despite their flexibility and other desirable physical properties. Polyurethanes with cycloaliphatic hard segments are possible candidates for this application.

D. Adhesives

Surgical adhesives must seal a wound with minimal damage to the wound and they must also be easy to use in the operating theatre. Surgical adhesives have become important in a large number of surgical procedures.[247] However, polyurethanes have met with limited use in surgery because of the generally high curing temperature required (150°C), and their degradation. They have been most successful in dentistry and a polyurethane liner has been used in restorations, where their toughness and flexibility are of value, and the curing time and temperature are not as great a concern.[247] Polyurethanes adhesives are also used for bonding filling materials to dentin and cement.[156]

V. OTHER APPLICATIONS

A. Artificial ducts

Artificial ducts are replacements for tubular organs. Polyurethanes have been used not only for cardiovascular catheters but for ureteral catheters as well.[248] Urethral catheters are used to drain the bladder and can be for either short or long term use. They need to be flexible, and nonirritating to the urethral mucosa. There is a wide choice of different catheters, the polyurethanes being considered relatively stiff compared to the others that are available. It is well known that catheters in general cause problems and it is estimated that approximately 90% of patients with internal catheters suffer discomfort.[249] Polyurethanes are no exception and are known to cause mild edema, epithelial erosion and ulcerations,[248] and have been associated with encrustation, migration, and breakage.[250] However, these results appeared to be associated with indwelling times greater than 6 weeks. Some polyurethane failures have been associated with obstruction.[251]

An overview of four different indwelling ureteral catheters, including a polyurethane, concluded that there was no difference in problems between all four types.[249] One investigator reported coating natural rubber latex with a polyurethane hydrogel to combine the excellent properties of both.[252] Others have investigated the use of polyurethanes to drain bile in obstructive jaundice and found that the encrustation rate of the polyurrethane was four times lower than for Teflon.[253] The major complication with any catheter is infection. The prevalence of infection with polyurethane catheters is discussed in more detail earlier in this chapter, and in Chapter 7. Keane et al.[254] found that ureteric stents made from polyurethanes formed a profuse biofilm (28%:11 out of 40 patients) and encrustation was found on 58% of the stents. They did not find a link between the biofilm formation and the encrustation but did observe that both appeared to increase with the length of time that the stent was implanted. The bacteria associated with the biofilm included *Enterococcus faecalis* and the encrustation of the stents was not associated with calcium in the urine but was with urolithiasis. In this study, the polyurethanes became infected despite antibiotic treatment.

B. CONTRACEPTIVES

Vaginal sponges were investigated in the 1970s along with foaming tablets, and suppositories as methods of contraception that avoided the side effects of IUDs and oral contraception.[255] In addition, these were also nonprescription. In the early 1980, vaginal sponges made of polyurethane were in preclinical trials with a volunteer group in Mexico,[256] and the Collatex sponge then went on to multicentred trials through the International Fertility Research Program.[255-256] The Collatex sponge contained a spermicide and was made of a hydrophilic polyurethane. Both the sponge and the spermicide were seen as effect barriers against pregnancy. The largest reason for not using the sponge was cited as discomfort for the woman's partner during intercourse. The sponge was later marketed in the United States as the Today sponge and in 1985 was considered a reasonably safe and acceptable method of contraception,[257] and in 1988 it was tested as a delivery system for another spermicide.[258]

Estane has been used in other intravaginal devices,[259] and more recently a condom designed for women used polyurethanes.[260] This device is made up of a polyurethane sheath and two flexible polyurethane rings similar to diaphragms with one ring inside the sheath and the other outside. This device appeared successful in eliminating leakage of human immunodeficiency virus and cytomegalovirus.[260]

Polyurethanes also have been candidate materials for a male condom. Subjects in a recent study comparing a brand of polyurethane condom with latex condom reported that the polyurethane device possessed some favorable aesthetic qualities.[261] Polyurethanes are less susceptible to deterioration in storage than latex.

C. CONTROLLED DRUG DELIVERY

Polyurethanes have not found general use in controlled drug delivery. Many of the polymeric materials now being used or under investigation for controlled drug release are biodegradable. The formation of potentially toxic compounds during the degradation of the polyurethane has been limiting.[262] However, polyurethanes are still being considered for some applications.

Recently, disulfiram, an antialcohol drug was implanted subcutaneously in rats using a biodegradable TDI based polyether polyurethane as the carrier.[263] The authors reported good biocompatibility. Polyurethanes also have been used in hollow fibers for delivery of drugs,[264,265] and in matrices to release drugs.[266] A poly(ethylene)-oxide urethane hydrogel has recently been proposed for controlled drug release.[267]

Investigators have looked at biocompatible blood contacting polyurethanes and analyzed their potential to release drugs from catheters, stents and plaster.[268,269] Ikeda et al. investigated a polyurethane with a PEO-PTMO-PEO soft segment they had developed as a controlled release material. They found that the release increased with PEO content.[268] Similarly, Lambert et al. coated stents with Tecoflex® (Thermedics) and used the polyurethane membrane as a local drug delivery system.[269] Polyurethane microspheres loaded with tantalum have been suggested for use in particulate embolizations,[270] and polyurethanes have actually been synthesized from drugs. Bithionol, an antibacterial agent was incorporated into the polyurethane backbone.[271]

D. PENILE PROSTHESIS

The first penile implant was described in 1973,[272] and in 1983, Merrill introduced the Mentor inflatable penile prosthesis made of polyurethane. The original Scott prosthesis consists of a pump, a reservoir, and penile cylinders. In the Mentor penile prosthesis, all three components are made of Bioflex polyurethane. Clinical trials on 30 patients showed success, however other investigators found complications including spontaneous inflation, kinking of the tubing, and cylinder rupture.[273]

E. MISCELLANEOUS

Polyurethanes have been used experimentally in hollow fiber form for pituitary organ culture,[274] and to encapsulate islets of Langerhans in a microporous structure.[164] Several groups have investigated their potential as components in sensors including glucose sensors,[275-277] and as ion selective membranes in potentiometric sensors.[278] They have been suggested as possible materials to replace ligaments,[279] and to repair meniscal lesions.[280,281] In addition, because of their diverse properties they also have be investigated for or are in use as: nerve guides,[282] artificial corneas and intraocular lens,[283,284] invertebral discs,[285] sutures,[286] nipple prosthesis,[287] repair of cartilage defects,[288] as foam casts,[289] as tympanic membranes,[290] and as tracheal prostheses.[291]

Polyurethanes are also used to support or assist in medical imaging and surgery. Polyurethane resin was used to make a customized form to support the head of the patient during PET,CT or NMR.[292] and to make "belly boards" to enhance CT scanning of pelvic malignancies.[293] Urologists use a guidewire manufactured from a nitinol core, covered in a polyurethane jacket and a hydrophilic coating.[294]

REFERENCES

1. Arciola C. R., Radin L., Alvergna P., Cenni E., and Pizzaferrato A. "Heparin surface treatment of polymethyl methacrylate alters adhesion of Staphylococcus strain: utility of bacterial fatty acid analysis." *Biomaterials*, 14:1611, 1993.
2. Friedman D. W., Orland P. J. and Greco R. S. "History of Biomaterials." In *Implantation Biology — The Host Responses and Biomedical Devices*, Ed. Greco R. S. CRC Press, Boca Raton, FL, 1994: 1.
3. Hecker J. F. "Thrombus formation of intravascular catheters and cannulas." In *Blood Compatibility*, Ed. Willlaims D. F. CRC Press, Boca Raton, FL, 1987:79.
4. Costanzo J. D., Sastre B., Choux R., and Kasparian M. "Mechanism of thrombogenesis during total parenteral nutrition: role of catheter composition." *J. Parenteral Enteral Nutr.*, 12:190, 1988.
5. Zdrahala R. J., Solomon D. D., Lentz D. J., and McGary C. W., "Thermoplastic polyurethanes. Materials for vascular catheters." In *Polyurethanes in Biomedical Engineering II*. Ed. Planck H., Syre I., Dauner M., and Egbers G. Amsterdam: Elsevier Science Publishers, 1987:1.
6. Zdrahala R. J. and McGary C. W. "Thermoplastic polyurethanes softening in 37°C saline." *Mat. Res. Soc. Symp. Proc.*, 55:407, 1986.
7. Wilner G. D., Casarella W. J., Baier R., and Fenoglio C. M. "Thrombogenicity of angiographic catheters." *Circ. Res.*, 43:424, 1978.
8. Thomsen H. K., Kjeldsen K., and Hansen J. F. "Thrombogenic properties of arterial catheters: a scanning electron microscopic examination of the surface structure." *Cathet. Cardiovasc. Diagn.*, 3:351, 1977.
9. Nachnani G. H., Lessin L. S., Motomiya T., and Jensen W. N. "Scanning electron microscopy of thrombogenesis on vascular catheter materials." *Med. Intel.*, 286:139, 1972.
10. Bourassa M. G., Cantin M., Sandborn E. B., and Pederson E. "Scanning electron microscopy of surface irregularities and thrombogenesis of polyurethane and polyethylene coronary catheters." *Circulation*, 53:922, 1976.
11. Durst S., Leslie J., Moore R., and Amplatz K. "A comparison of the thrombogenicity of commercially available catheters." *Radiol.*, 113:599, 1974.
12. Rashid A., Hiltner F. J., Fester A., Javier R. P., and Samet P. "Thromboembolism associated with pigtail catheters." *Cathet. Cardiovasc. Diagn.*, 1:183, 1975.
13. Nejad M. S., Klaper M. A., Steggerda F. R., and Gianturco C. "Clotting on the outer surfaces of vascular catheters." *Radiol.*, 91:248, 1968.
14. Judkins M. P., Mitchell W. A., Simmons C. R., and Gander M. P. "Vascular catheters, smooth and rough." *N. Engl. J. Med.*, 287; 1100, 1972.
15. Triolo P. M. and Andrade J. D. "Surface modification and evaluation of some commonly used catheter materials. I. Surface properties." *J. Biomed. Mater. Res.*, 17:129, 1983.

16. Hecker J. F. and Scandrett L. A. "Roughness and thrombogenicity of the outer surfaces of intravascular catheters." *J. Biomed. Mater. Res.,* 19:381, 1985.
17. Nichols A. B., Owen J., Grossman B. A., Marcella J. J., Fleisher L. N., and Lee M. M. L. "Effect of heparin bonding on catheter-induced fibrin formation and platelet activation." *Circulation,* 70:843, 1984.
18. Dewanjee M. K., Rowland S. M., Kapadvanjwala M. et al. "The dynamics of platelet thrombus formation rate, thrombus retention time, and rate of embolization on a control and heparin bonded polyurethane angio-catheter." *Trans. Am. Soc. Artif. Intern. Organs,* 36:M745, 1990.
19. Kitamoto Y., Fukui H., Iwabuchi K., Taguma Y., Monma H., Ishizaki M., Takahashi H., Nakayama M., and Sekino H. "A femoral vein catheter with immobilized urokinase (UKFC) as an antithrombotic blood access." *Trans. Am. Soc. Artif. Intern. Organs,* 33:136, 1987.
20. Stokes K., McVenes R., and Anderson J. M. "Polyurethane elastomer biostability." *J. Biomater. Appl.,* 9:321, 1995.
21. Maki D. G. and Ringer M. "Evaluation of dressing regimens for prevention of infection with peripheral intravenous catheters." *J. Am. Med. Assoc.,* 258:2396, 1987.
22. Bambauer R., Mesters P., and Piroung K. J. "Raster-electron-microscopic investigations in large-bore catheters for extracorporeal detoxification." *Int. J. Artif. Organs,* 13:667, 1990.
23. Franson T. R., Sheth N. K., Menon L., and Sohnle P. G. "Persistent *in vitro* survival of coagulase-negative staphylococci adherent to intravascular catheters in the absence of conventional nutrients." *J. Clin. Microbiol.,* 24:559, 1986.
24. Martinez-Martinez L., Pascual A., and Perez E. J. "Effect of three plastic catheters on survival and growth of Pseudomonas aeruginosa." *J. Hospital Infec.,* 16:311, 1990.
25. Borow M. and Crowley J. G. "Evaluation of central venous catheter thrombogenicity." *Acta Anaesthesiol. Scand.,* Suppl. 81:59, 1985.
26. Kristinsson K. G. "Adherence of staphylococci to intravascular catheters." *J. Med. Microbiol.,* 28:249, 1989.
27. Markowitz D. M. and Denny D. F. "Enterostomy catheter exchange using new polymer-coated guide wire: technical note." *Gastrointest. Radiol.,* 15:64, 1990.
28. Noishiki Y., Yamane Y., Takahashi M., Kawamani O., Futami Y., Nishikawa T., Noguchi N., Nagaoka S., and Mori Y. "Prevention of thrombosis-related complications in cardiac catheterization and angiography using a heparinized catheter." *Trans. Am. Soc. Artif. Intern. Organs,* 33:359, 1987.
29. Smith J. C., Davies M. C., Melia C. D., Denyer S. P., and Derrick M. R. "Uptake of drugs by catheters: the influence of the drug on sorption by polyurethane catheters." *Biomaterials,* 17:1469, 1996.
30. Pierce W. S., O'Bannon W., Donachy J. H., Pennock J. L., and Waldhausen J. A. "A new technique for insertion of a large-bore cannula into the left ventricle of the calf." *J. Surg. Res.,* 17:24, 1974.
31. Kolobow T. and Zapol W. "A new thin-walled nonkinking catheter for peripheral vascular cannulation." *Surgery,* 68:625, 1970.
32. Furman S. and Escher D. J. W. "Retained endocardial pacemaker electrodes." *J. Thorac. Cardiovasc. Surg.,* 55:727, 1967.
33. Stokes K. and Cobian K. "Polyether polyurethanes for implantable pacemaker leads." *Biomaterials,* 3:225, 1982.
34. Scheuer-Leeser M., Irnich W., and Kreuzer J. "Polyurethane leads: facts and controversy." *PACE,* 6:454, 1983.
35. Harthorne J. W. "Pacemaker leads." *Int. J. Cardiol.,* 6:423, 1984.
36. Bruck S. D. and Mueller E. P. "Materials aspects of implantable cardiac pacemaker leads." *Med. Prog. Tech.,* 13:149, 1988.
37. Szycher M. "Biostability of polyurethane elastomers: a critical review." In *Blood Compatible Materials and Devices,* Ed. Sharma C. P., Szycher M. Technomic, Lancaster, PA, 1991: 33.
38. Meijs G. F., McCarthy S. J., Rizzardo E., Chen Y.-C., Chatelier R. C., Brandwood A., and Schindelm K. "Degradation of medical-grade polyurethane elastomers: the effect of hydrogen peroxide *in vitro.*" *J. Biomed. Mater. Res.,* 27:345, 1993.
39. Phillips R., Frey M. and Martin R. O. "Long-term performance of polyurethane pacing leads: mechanisms of design-related failures." *PACE,* 9:1166, 1986.
40. Bluhm G., Larsen F. F., Nordlander R., and Pehrsson S. K. "Long-term comparison of the electrical characteristics of polyurethane and polyethylene insulated ventricular leads." *PACE,* 13:583, 1990.

41. Thoma R. J. and Phillips R. E. "Note: Studies of poly(ether)urethane pacemaker lead insulation oxidation." *J. Biomed. Mater. Res.*, 21:525, 1987.
42. Stokes K., Urbanski P., and Upton J. "The *in vivo* auto-oxidation of polyether polyurethane by metal ions." *J. Biomater. Sci., Polym. Ed.*, 1:207, 1990.
43. Stokes K., Coury A., and Urbanski P. "Autooxidative degradation of implanted polyether polyurethane devices." *J. Biomater. Appl.*, 1:411, 1987.
44. Furman S., Benedek Z. M., and Registry T. I. L. "Survival of implantable pacemaker leads." *PACE*, 13:1910, 1990.
45. Mugica J., Daubert J. C., Lazarus B., Henry L., Duconge R., and Lespinasse P. "Is polyurethane lead insulation still controversial?" *PACE*, 15:1967, 1992.
46. Palatianos G. M., Dewanjee M. K., Panatsopoulos G., Kapadvanjwala M., Novak S., and Sfakianakis G. N. "Comparative thrombogenicity of pacemaker leads." *PACE*, 17:141, 1994.
47. Zdrahala R. J. "Small caliber vascular grafts. Part II. Polyurethanes revisited." *J. Biomater. Appl.*, 11:37, 1996.
48. Voorhees A. B., Jaretzki A., and Blakemore A. H. "The use of tubes constructed from Vinyon N cloth in bridging arterial defects." *Ann. Surg.*, 135:332, 1952.
49. Boretos J. W. and Pierce W. S. "Segmented polyurethane: a polyether polymer. An initial evaluation for biomedical applications." *J. Biomed. Mater. Res.*, 2:121, 1968.
50. Kowligi R. R., Maltzahn W. W. V., and Eberhart R. C. "Fabrication and characterization of small diameter vascular prostheses." *J. Biomed. Mater. Res.*, 22:245, 1988.
51. Nojiri C., Senshu K., and Okano T. "Nonthrombogenic polymer vascular prosthesis." *Artif. Organs*, 19:32, 1995.
52. Lei B. V. D., Bartels H. L., Dijk F., and Wildevuur C. R. H. "The thrombogenic characteristics of small caliber polyurethane vascular prostheses after heparin bonding." *Trans. Am. Soc. Artif. Intern. Organs*, 31:107, 1985.
53. Ito Y., Imanishi Y., and Sisido M. "*In vitro* platelet adhesion and *in vivo* antithrombogenicity of heparinized polyetherurethaneureas." *Biomaterials*, 9:235, 1988.
54. Arnander C. "Enhanced patency of small-diameter tubings after surface immobilization of heparin fragments. A study in the dog." *J. Biomed. Mater. Res.*, 23:285, 1989.
55. Han D. K., Lee K. B., Park K. D., Kim C. S., Jeong S. Y., Kim Y. H., Kim H. M., and Min B. G. "*In vivo* canine studies of a Sinkhole valve and vascular graft coated with biocompatible PU-PEO-SO3." *ASAIO J.*, 39:M537, 1993.
56. Bernhard W. F., Colo N. A., Wesolowski J. S., Szycher M., Fishbein M. C., Parkman R., Franzblau C. C., and Haudenschild C. C. "Development of collagenous linings on impermeable prosthetic surfaces." *J. Thorac. Cardiovasc. Surg.*, 79:552, 1980.
57. Kambic H. E. "Polyurethane small artery substitutes." *Trans. Am. Soc. Artif. Intern. Organs*, 22:1047, 1988.
58. Annis D., Bornat A., Edwards R. O., Higham A., Loveday B., and Wilson J. "An elastomeric vascular prosthesis." *Trans. Am. Soc. Artif. Intern. Organs*, 24:209, 1978.
59. Hess F., Jerusalem C., and Braun B. "A fibrous polyurethane microvascular prothesis. Morphological evaluation of the neo-intima." *J. Cardiovasc. Surg.*, 24:509, 1983.
60. Hess F., Jerusalem C., Braun B., and Grande P. "Three years experience with experimental implantation of fibrous polyurethane microvascular prostheses in the rat aorta." *Microsurg.*, 6:155, 1985.
61. Beahan P. and Hull D. "A study of the interface between a fibrous polyurethane arterial prosthesis and natural tissue." *J. Biomed. Mater. Res.*, 16:827, 1982.
62. Kogel H., Vollmar J. F., and Proschek P. "New prostheses for venous substitution." *J. Cardiovasc. Surg.*, 32:330, 1991.
63. Okoshi T., Soldani G., Goddard M., and Galletti P. M. "Penetrating micropores increase patency and achieve extensive endothelialization in small diameter polymer skin coated vascular grafts." *Trans. Am. Soc. Artif. Intern. Organs*, 42:M398, 1996.
64. Gogolewski S. and Galletti G. "Degradable, microporous vascular prosthesis from segmented polyurethane." *Colloid Polym. Sci.*, 264:854, 1986.
65. Hinrichs W. L. J., Kuit J., Feil H., Wildevuur C. R. H., and Feijen J. "*In vivo* fragmentation of microporous polyurethane- and copolyesterether elastomer-based vacular prostheses." *Biomaterials*, 13:585, 1992.

66. Lee Y., Park D. K., Kim Y. B., Seo J. W., Lee K. B., and Min B. "Endothelial cell seeding onto the extracellular matrix of fibroblasts for the development of a small diameter polyurethane vessel." *ASAIO J.*, 39:M740, 1993.
67. Miwa H., Matsuda T., Tani N., Kondo K., and Iida F. "An *in vitro* endothelialized compliant vascular graft minimizes anastomotic hyperplasia." *ASAIO J.*, 39:M501, 1993.
68. Gogolewski S., Pennings A. J., Lommen E., Wildevuur C. R. H., and Niewenhuis P. "Growth of a neo artery induced by a biodegradable polymeric vascular prosthesis." *Makromol. Chem., Rapid Commun.*, 4:213, 1983.
69. Kidson I. G. and Abbott W. M. "Low compliance and arterial graft occlusion." *Circulation*, 58 Suppl 1:I, 1978.
70. Wilson G. J., MacGregor D. C., Klement P., Lee J. M., Nido P. J. d., Wong E. W. C., and Leidner J. "Anisotropic polyurethane nonwoven conduits: a new approach to the design of a vascular prosthesis." *Trans. Am. Soc. Artif. Intern. Organs*, 29:260, 1983.
71. Lyman D. J., Albo D., Jackson R., and Knutson K. "Development of small diameter vascular graft prostheses." *Trans. Am. Soc. Artif. Intern. Organs*, 23:253, 1977.
72. Lyman D. J., Fazzio F. J., Voorhees H., Robinson G., and Albo D. "Compliance as a factor affecting the patency of a copolyurethane vascular graft." *J. Biomed. Mater. Res.*, 12:337, 1978.
73. Robinson P. H., Lei B. V. D., Schakenraad J. M., Jongebloed W. J., Hoppen H. J., Pennings A. J., and Nieuwenhuis P. "Patency and healing of polymeric microvenous prostheses implanted into the rat femoral vein by means of the sleeve anastomotic technique." *J. Reconstr. Microsurg.*, 6:287, 1990.
74. Guidoin R., Sigot M., King M., and Sigot-Luizard M. "Biocompatibility of the Vascugraft® evaluation of a novel polyester urethane vascular substitute by an organotypic culture technique." Biomaterials, 13:281, 1992.
75. Zhang Z., King M. W., Guidoin R., Therrien M., Pezelot M., Adnot A., Ukpabi P., and Vantal M. H. "Morphological, physical and chemical evaluation of the Vascugraft arterial prosthesis: comparison of a novel polyurethane device with other microporous structures." *Biomaterials*, 15:483, 1994.
76. Zhang Z., Guidoin R., King M. W., How T. V., Marois Y., and Laroche G. "Removing fresh tissue from explanted polyurethane prostheses: which approach facilitates physico-chemical analysis." *Biomaterials*, 16:369, 1995.
77. Zhang Y., Bjursten L. M., Freif-Larsson C., Kober M., and Wesslen B. "Tissue response to commerical silicone and polyurethane elastomers after different sterilization procedures." *Biomaterials*, 17:2265, 1996.
78. Zhang Z., King M. W., Marois Y., and Guidoin R. "*In vivo* performance of the polyesterurethane Vascugraft prosthesis implanted as a thoraco-abdominal bypass in dogs: an exploratory study." *Biomaterials*, 15:1099, 1994.
79. Zhang Z., Marois Y., Guidoin R. C., Bull P., Marois M., How T. V., Laroche G., and King M. W. "Vascugraft polyurethane arterial prosthesis as femoro-peroneal bypasses in humans: pathological, structural and chemical analyses of four excised grafts." *Biomaterials*, 18:113, 1997.
80. Lee J. M. and Wilson G. J. "Anisotropic tensile viscoelastic properties of vascular graft materials tested at low strain." *Biomaterials*, 7:423, 1986.
81. Underwood C. J., Tait W. F., and Charlesworth D. "Design considerations for a small bore vascular prosthesis." *Int. J. Artif. Organs*, 11:272, 1988.
82. Nakayama Y. and Matsuda T. "Surface microarchitectural design in biomedical applications: preparation of microporous polymer surfaces by an excimer laser ablation technique." *J. Biomed. Mater. Res.*, 29:1295, 1995.
83. Kinley C. E., Paasche P. E., MacDonald A. S., and Marble A. E. "Stress at vascular anastomosis in relation to host artery: synthetic graft diameter." *Surgery*, 75:28, 1974.
84. Russell F. B., Lederman D. M., Singh P. I., Cumming R. D., Morgan R. A., Levine F. H., Austen W. G., and Buckley M. J. "Development of seamless trileaflet valves." *Trans. Am. Soc. Artif. Intern. Organs*, 26:66, 1980.
85. Gerring E. L., Bellhouse B. J., Bellhouse F. H., and Haworth W. S. "Long-term animal trials of the Oxford aortic/pulmonary valve prosthesis without anticoagulants." *Trans. Am. Soc. Artif. Intern. Organs*, 20:703, 1974.
86. Sawyer P. N., Stanczewski B., Srinivasan S., Stempack J. G., and Kammlott G. W. "Implantation characteristics of metal-backed polymer-coated heart valves: biophysical scanning and transmission electron microscopic studies." *Trans. Am. Soc. Artif. Intern. Organs*, 20:692, 1974.

87. Jansen J., Willeke S., Reiners B., Harbott P., Reul H., and Rau G. "New J-3 flexible-leaflet polyurethane heart valve prosthesis with improved hydrodynamic performance." *Int. J. Artif. Organs*, 14:655, 1991.
88. MacKay T. G., Wheatley D. J., Bernacca G. M., Fisher A. C., and Hindle C. S. "New polyurethane heart valve prothesis: design, manufacture and evaluation." *Biomaterials*, 17:1857, 1996.
89. Schoephoerster R. and Chandran K. B. "Effect of systolic flow rate on the prediction of effective prosthetic valve flow area." *J. Biomechanics*, 22:705, 1989.
90. Dellsperger K. C. and Chandran K. B. "Prosthetic Heart Valves." In *Blood Compatible Materials and Devices*, Ed. Sharma C. P., Szycher M. Technomic, Lancaster, PA, 1991: 153.
91. Chandran K. B., Kim S. H., and Han G. "Stress distribution on the cusps of a polyurethane trileaflet heart valve prosthesis in the closed position." *J. Biomechanics*, 24:385, 1991.
92. Herold M., Lo H. B., Reul H. et al.. "The Hemholtz Institute tri-leaflet polyurethane heart valve prosthesis: design manufacturing and first *in vitro* and *in vivo* results." In *Polyurethanes in Biomedical Engineering II*. Ed. Planck H., Syre I., Dauner M., and Egbers G. Amsterdam, Netherlands: Elsevier Science Publishers, 1987:231.
93. Chandran K. B., Schoephoerster R. T., Wurzel D., Hansen G., Yu L. S., Pantalos G., and Kolff W. J. "Hemodynamic comparisons of polyurethane trileaflet and bioprosthetic heart valves." *Trans. Am. Soc. Artif. Intern. Organs*, 35:132, 1989.
94. Yu L. S., Yuan B., Bishop D. et al. "New polyurethane valves in new soft artificial hearts." *Trans. Am. Soc. Artif. Intern. Organs*, 35:301, 1989.
95. Leat M. E. and Fisher J. "Comparative study of the function of the Abiomed polyurethane heart valve for use in left ventricular assist devices." *J. Biomed. Eng.*, 15:516, 1993.
96. Rose A. G., Forman R., and Bowen R. M. "Calcification of glutaraldehyde-fixed porcine xenograft." *Thorax*, 33:11, 1978.
97. Silver M. M., Pollock J., and Bowen R. M. "Calcification in porcine xenograft valves in children." *Am. J. Cardiol.*, 45:685, 1980.
98. Bruck S. D. "Possible causes for the calcification of glutaraldehyde-treated tissue heart valves and blood contacting elastomers during prolonged use in medical devices." *Biomaterials*, 2:14, 1981.
99. Dunn J. M. "Porcine valve durability in children." *Ann. Thorac. Surg.*, 32:357, 1981.
100. Wisman C. B., Pierce W. S., Donachy J. H., Pae W. E., Myers J. L., and Prophet G. A. "A polyurethane trileaflet cardiac valve prosthesis: *in vitro* and *in vivo* studies." *Trans. Am. Soc. Artif. Intern. Organs*, 28:164, 1982.
101. Hilbert S. L., Ferrans V. J., Tomita Y., Eidbo E. E., and Jones M. "Evaluation of explanted polyurethane trileaflet cardiac valve prostheses." *J. Thorac. Cardiovasc. Surg.*, 94:419, 1987.
102. Thubrikar M. J., Piepgrass W. C., Shanner T. W., and Nolan S. P. "Stress analysis of porcine bioprosthetic heart valves." *J. Biomed. Mater. Res.*, 16:811, 1982.
103. Thubrikar M. J., Deck J. D., Aouad J., and Nolan S. P. "Role of mechanical stress in calcification of aortic bioprosthetic heart valves." *J. Thorac. Cardiovasc. Surg.*, 86:115, 1983.
104. Einav S., Stolero D., Avidor J. M., Elad D., and Talbot L. "Wall shear stress distribution along the cusp of a trileaflet prosthetic valve." *J. Biomed. Eng.*, 12:13, 1990.
105. Fisher A. C., Bernacca G. M., Mackay T. G., Dmitri W. R., Wilkinson R., and Wheatley D. J. "Calcification modelling in artificial heart valves." *Int. J. Artif. Organs*, 15:284, 1992.
106. Bernacca G. M., Mackay T. G., Wilkinson R., and Wheatley D. J. "Calcification and fatigue failure in a polyurethane heart valve." *Biomaterials*, 16:279, 1995.
107. Joshi R. R., Frautschi J. R., R. E. Phillips J., and Levy R. J. "Phosphonated polyurethanes that resist calcification." *J. Appl. Biomater.*, 5:65, 1994.
108. Moulopoulos S. D., Anthopoulos L., Stamatelopoulos S., and Stefadouros M. "Catheter-mounted aortic valves." *Ann. Thorac. Surg.*, 11:423, 1971.
109. Kay E. B. "Early years in artificial heart valve development." *Ann. Thorac. Surg.*, 48:S24, 1989.
110. Brash J. L., Fritzinger B. K., and Bruck S. D. "Development of block copolyether-urethane intra-aortic balloons and other medical devices." *J. Biomed. Mater. Res.*, 7:313, 1973.
111. Anstadt G. L., Rawlings C. A., Krahwinkel D. T., Casey H. W., and Schiff P. "Prolonged circulatory support by direct mechanical ventricular assistance for two or three days of ventricular fibrillation." *Trans. Am. Soc. Artif. Intern. Organs*, 17:174, 1971.
112. Kambic H. E. and Nose Y. "Biomaterials for blood pumps." In *Blood Compatible Materials and Devices*, Ed. Sharma C. P., Szycher M. Technomic, Lancaster, PA, 1991: 141.

113. Poirier V. "Fabrication and testing of flocked blood pump bladders." In *Synthetic Biomedical Polymers — Concepts and Applications*, Ed. Szycher M, Robinson W. J. Technomic, Westport, CT, 1980: 73.
114. Snow J., Harasaki H., Kasick J., Whalen R., Kiraly R., and Nosé Y. "Promising results with a new textured surface intrathoracic variable volume device for LVAS." *Trans. Am. Soc. Artif. Intern. Organs*, 27:485, 1981.
115. McGee M. G., Szycher M., Turner S. A., Clay W., Trono R., Davis G. L., and Norman J. C. "Use of a composite Biomer/butyl rubber/Biomer material to prevent transdiaphragmatic ater permeation during long-term electrically actuated left ventricular device (LVAD) pumping." *Trans. Am. Soc. Artif. Intern. Organs*, 26:299, 1980.
116. Holub D. A., McGee M. G., Edelman S. K. et al. "Development and evaluation of a long-term, low profile intracorporeal (abdominal) left ventricular assist device (The E-type LVAD)." NHLBI, NIH, Bethesda, MD, 1979.
117. Engelman R. M., Nyilas E., Lackner H., and Godwin S. J. "Left ventricular bypass without anticoagulation." *J. Thorac. Cardiovasc. Surg.*, 62:851, 1971.
118. Bernstein E. F., Cosentino L. C., Reich S., Stasz P., Levine I. D., Scott D. R., Dorman F. D., and Blackshear P. L. "A compact, low hemolysis, non-thrombogenic system for non-thoracotomy prolonged left ventricular bypass." *Trans. Am. Soc. Artif. Intern. Organs*, 20:643, 1974.
119. Serres E. J., German J. C., Wakabayashi A., Conolly J. E., Hirai J., and Mukherjee N. D. "Open chest pulsatile left-heart bypass without anticoagulation." *Arch. Surg.*, 101:18, 1970.
120. Wakabayashi A., Yim D., and Dietrik W. "Left ventricular bypass: a new nonthrombogenic device with homograft aortic valves." *Am. J. Cardiol.*, 25:450, 1970.
121. Hayashi K., Matsuda T., Takano H., Umezu M., Taenaka Y., and Nakamura T. "Effects of implantation on the mechanical properties of the polyurethane diaphragm of left ventricle assist devices." *Biomaterials*, 6:82, 1985.
122. Weiss W. J., Gosenberg G., Snyder A. J., J. Donachy S., Reibson J., Kawaguchi O., Sapirstein J. S., Pae W. E., and Pierce W. S. "A completely implanted Left Ventricle Assist Device. Chronic *in vivo* testing." *ASAIO J.*, 39:M427, 1993.
123. Chimoskey J. E., O'Bannon W., Cant J. R., Walker F. W., Eskin S. G., Noon G. P., and DeBakey M. E. "Recent experience with the Baylor left ventricular bypass pump." *Biomater., Med. Dev., Artif. Organs*, 5:361, 1977.
124. Bedini R., Chistolini P., Angelis G. D., Formisano G., and Caiazza S. "VAD Biomer blood sacs: mechanical tests and ultrastructural observations." *Med. Prog. Tech.*, 19:83, 1993.
125. Farrar D. J., Litwak P., Lawson J. H., Ward R. S., White K. A., Robinson A. J., Rodvien R., and Hill J. D. "*In vivo* evaluations of a new thromboresistant polyurethane for artificial heart blood pumps." *J. Thorac. Cardiovasc. Surg.*, 95:191, 1988.
126. Dasse K. A., Chipman S. D., Sherman C. N., Levine A. H., and Frazier O. H. "Clinical experience with textured blood contacting surfaces in ventricular assist devices." *Trans. Am. Soc. Artif. Intern. Organs*, 33:418, 1987.
127. Coumbe A., Salih V., Graham T. R., Keefe M. B., Reynolds P. S., and Berry C. L. "Pathological sequelae of implantation of intracorporeal left ventricular assist devices in the calf." *Am. J. Cardiovasc. Path.*, 4:302, 1993.
128. Bernhard W. F., Gernes D. G., Clay W. C., Schoen F. J., Burgeson R., Valeri R. C., Melaragno A. J., and Poirier V. L. "Investigations with an implantable, electrically actuated ventricular assist device." *J. Thorac. Cardiovasc. Surg.*, 88:11, 1984.
129. Moulopoulos S. D., Topaz S., and Kolff W. J. "Diastolic balloon pumping (with carbon dioxide) in the aorta — a mechanical assist to the failing circulation." *Am. Heart J.*, 63:699, 1962.
130. Nyilas E. "Development of blood compatible elastomers. II. Performance of Avcothane blood contact surfaces in experimental animal implantation." *J. Biomed. Mater. Res.*, 3:97, 1972.
131. Nyilas E., Leinbach R. C., Caulfield J. B., Buckley M. J., and Austen W. G. "Development of blood-compatible elastomers. III. Hematological effects of Avcothane intra-aortic balloon pumps in cardiac patients." *J. Biomed. Mater. Res. Symp.*, 3:129, 1972.
132. Tomecek J., Jaron D., Tjonneland S., and Kantrowitz A. "Phase-shift cardiac assistance with a valve balloon: experimental results." *Trans. Am. Soc. Artif. Intern. Organs*, 15:406, 1969.

133. Ashar B. and Turcotte L. R. "Analysis of longest IAB implant in human patient (327 days)." *Trans. Am. Soc. Artif. Intern. Organs,* 27:372, 1981.
134. Kabei N. "Right ventricular balloon pumping." *Life Support Systems,* 3:343, 1985.
135. Wolvek S. "The evolution of the Intra-aortic balloon: the Datascope contribution." *J. Biomater. Appl.,* 3:527, 1989.
136. Myers G. J., Landymore R. W., Leadon R. B., and Squires C. "Fracture of the internal lumen of a Datascope Percor Stat-DL balloon resulting in stroke." *Ann. Thorac. Surg.,* 57:1335, 1994.
137. Kayser K., Johnson W., and Shore R. "Comparison of driving gases for IABPs." *Med. Instrum.,* 15:51, 1981.
138. Kolff W. J., Akutsu T., Dreyer B., and Norton H. "Artificial heart in the chest and use of polyurethanes for making hearts, valves and aortas." *Trans. Am. Soc. Artif. Intern. Organs,* 5:298, 1959.
139. Mirkovitch V., Akutsu T., and Kolff W. J. "Polyurethane aortas in dogs. Three-year results." *Trans. Am. Soc. Artif. Intern. Organs,* 8:79, 1962.
140. Boretos J. W. and Pierce W. S. "Segmented polyurethane: a new elastomer for biomedical applications." *Science,* 158:1481, 1967.
141. Boretos J. W., Pierce W. S., Baier R. E., Leroy A. F., and Donachy H. J. "Surface and bulk characteristics of a polyether urethane for artificial hearts." *J. Biomed. Mater. Res.,* 9:327, 1975.
142. Kinoshita M., Mohammad S. F., and Olsen D. B. "Bacterial adhesion on Biomer and PTFE used for total artificial heart — explanted vs. non-implanted materials." *Trans. Am. Soc. Artif. Intern. Organs,* 17:108, 1991.
143. Coleman D. L., Lim D., Kessler T., and Andrade J. D. "Calcification of nontextured implantable blood pumps." *Trans. Am. Soc. Artif. Intern. Organs,* 27:97, 1981.
144. Coleman D. L. "Mineralization of blood pump bladders." *Trans. Am. Soc. Artif. Intern. Organs,* 27:708, 1981.
145. Turner S. A., Milton L. T., Poirier V. L., and Norman J. C. "Sequential studies of pseudoneointimae within long term THI E-type ALVAD's: thickness, calcification and compositional analysis." *Artif. Organs,* 5:18, 1981.
146. Berhart W. F., LaFarge C. G., Liss R. H., Szycher M., Berger R. L., and Poirier V. "An appraisal of blood trauma and the blood-prosthetic interface during left ventricular bypass in the calf and humans." *Ann. Thorac. Surg.,* 26:427, 1978.
147. Pierce W. S., Donachy J. H., Rosenberg G., and Baier R. E. "Calcification inside artificial hearts: Inhibition by warfarin-sodium." *Science* 1980:9 May:601.
148. Lemm W., Pirling E. S., and Bucherl S. "Biodegradation of some biomaterials *in vitro*." *Proc. Eur. Soc. Artif. Organs,* 7:86, 1980.
149. Lemm W., Krukenberg T., Reiger G., Gerlach K., and Bucherl E. S. "Biodegradation of some biomaterials after subcutaneous implantation." *Proc. Eur. Soc. Artif. Organs,* 8:71, 1981.
150. Hunter S. K., Gregonis D. E., Coleman D. L., Andrade J. D., and Kessler T. "Molecular weight characterization of pre- and post-implant artificial heart polyurethane materials." *Trans. Am. Soc. Artif. Intern. Organs,* 28:473, 1982.
151. Coleman D. L., Meuzelaar H. L. C., Kessler T. R., McClennen W. H., Richards J. M., and Gregonis D. E. "Retrieval and analysis of a clinical total artificial heart." *J. Biomed. Mater. Res.,* 20:417, 1986.
152. Guerin P. "Use of synthetic polymers for biomedical applications." *PACE,* 6:449, 1983.
153. Klein A. "Bioplastics and the artificial heart." ANTEC '87. 1987: 1205.
154. Dolovich J., Marshall C. P., Smith E. K. M., Shimizu A., Pearson F. C., Surgona M. A., and Lee W. "Allergy to ethylene oxide in chronic hemodialysis patients." *Artif. Organs,* 8:334, 1984.
155. Daugirdas J. T., Ing T. S., Roxe D. M., Ivanovich P. T., Kromlovsky F., Popli S., and McLaughlin M. M. "Severe anaphylactoid reactions to cuprammonium cellulose hemodialyzers." *Arch. Int. Med.,* 145:489, 1985.
156. Lee F. F., Durning C. J., and Leonard E. F. "Urethanes as ethylene oxide reservoirs in hollow-fiber dialyzers." *Trans. Am. Soc. Artif. Intern. Organs,* 31:526, 1985.
157. Ansorge W., Pelger M., Dietrich W., and Baurmeister U. "Ethylene oxide in dialyzer rinsing fluid: effect of rinsing technique, dialyzer storage time and potting compound." *Artif. Organs,* 11:118, 1987.
158. Lyman D. J. and Loo B. H. "New synthetic membranes for dialysis. IV. A copolyether-urethane membrane system." *J. Biomed. Mater. Res.,* 1:17, 1967.

159. Jayasree G. and Sharma C. P. "Permeability of PEUU membranes: their modification towards blood compatibility." *J. Biomater. Appl.,* 3:405, 1989.
160. Paul D. "Polymer hollow fiber membranes for removal of toxic substances from blood." *Prog. Polym. Sci.,* 14:597, 1989.
161. Roesler M. F., Bull C., and Ionescu M. T. "Clinical and laboratory evaluation of the Shiley S-100-A oxygenator-heat exchanger." *Cardiovasc. Surg.,* 21:271, 1980.
162. Kawanishi H., Tsuchiya T., Sugiyama M., Nishiki M., and Dohi K. "Elimination of low molecular weight proteins during hemoperfusion of dialysis patients using a urethane-sheet embedded with powdered charcoal." *Trans. Am. Soc. Artif. Intern. Organs,* 32:425, 1986.
163. Kawanishi H., Tsuchiya T., Nishiki M., Sugiyama M., and Ezaki H. "Removal of protein bound substance in hepatic failure: polyurethane sheet embedded with powdered charcoal (UPC)." *Int. J. Artif. Organs,* 7:343, 1984.
164. Zondervan G. J., Hoppen H. J., Pennings A. J., Fristchy W., Wolters G., and Schilfgaarde R. V. "Design of a polyurethane membrane for the encapsulation of islets of Langerhans." *Biomaterials,* 13:136, 1992.
165. Ward R. S., White K. A., Wolcott C. A., Wang A. Y., Kuhn R. W., Taylor J. E., and John J. K. "Development of a hybrid artificial pancreas with a dense polyurethane membrane." *ASAIO J.,*:M261, 1993.
166. Branger B. "Biocompatibility of blood tubings." *Int. J. Artif. Organs,* 13:697, 1990.
167. Barron D., Harbottle S., Hoenich N. A., Morley A. R., Appleton D., and McCabe J. F. "Particle spallation induced by blood pumps in hemodialysis tubing sets." *Artif. Organs,* 10:226, 1986.
168. Hoenich N. A., Thompson J., Varini E., McCabe J., and Appleton D. "Particle spallation and plasticiser (DEHP) release from extracorporeal circuit tubing materials." *Int. J. Artif. Organs,* 13:55, 1990.
169. Ljunggren L. "Plasticizer migration from blood lines in hemodialysis." *Artif. Organs,* 8:99, 1984.
170. Lelah M. D. and Cooper S. L. *Polyurethanes in Medicine.* CRC Press, Boca Raton, FL, 1986.
171. Bruil A., Aken W. G. V., Beugeling T., Feijen J., Stenecker I., Huisman J. G., and Prins H. K. "Asymmetric membrane filters for the removal of leukocytes from blood." *J. Biomed. Mater. Res.,* 25:1459, 1991.
172. Bruil A., Oosterom H. A., Stenecker I., Al B. J. M., Beugeling T., Aken W. G. V., and Feijen J. "Poly(ethyleneimine) modified filters for the removal of leukocytes from blood." *J. Biomed. Mater. Res.,* 27:1253, 1993.
173. Steinbach B. G., Hardt N. S., and Abbitt P. L. "Mammography: breast implants — types, complications, and adjacent breast pathology." *Curr. Prob. Diagn. Radiol.,* 22:39, 1993.
174. Pinchuk L. "A review of the biostability and carcinogenicity of polyurethanes in medicine and the new generation of 'biostable' polyurethanes." *J. Biomater. Sci., Polym. Ed.,* 6:225, 1994.
175. Ashley F. R. "A new type of breast prosthesis. Preliminary report." *Plastic Reconstr. Surg.,* 45:421, 1970.
176. Boyes D. C., Adey C. K., Bailar J. et al. "Safety of polyurethane-covered breast implants." *Can. Med. Assoc. J.,* 145:1125, 1991.
177. Hester T. R., Nahai F., Bostwick J., and Cukic J. "A 5-year experience with polyurethane-covered mammary prostheses for treatment of capsular contracture, primary augmentation mammoplasty and breast reconstruction." *Clin. Plast. Surg.,* 15:569, 1988.
178. Melmed E. P. "Polyurethane implants: A 6-year review of 416 patients." *Plastic Reconstr. Surg.,* 82:285, 1988.
179. McGrath M. H. and Burkhardt B. R. "The safety and efficacy of breast implants for augmentation mammaplasty." *Plastic Reconstr. Surg.,* 74:550, 1984.
180. Gayou R. and Rudolph R. "Capsular contraction around silicone mammary prostheses." *Ann. Plast. Surg.,* 2:62, 1979.
181. Melmed E. P. "Treatment of breast contractures with open capsulotomy and replacement of gel prostheses with polyurethane-covered implants." *Plastic Reconstr. Surg.,* 86:270, 1990.
182. Capozzi A. "Long-term complications of polyurethane-covered breast implants." *Plastic Reconstr. Surg.,* 88:458, 1991.
183. Pennisi V. R. "Polyurethane-covered silicone gel mammary prosthesis for successful breast reconstruction." *Aesthet. Plast. Surg.,* 9:73, 1985.
184. Shapiro M. A. "Smooth vs. rough: an 8-year survey of mammary prosthesis." *Plastic Reconstr. Surg.,* 84:449, 1989.

185. Handel N., Silverstein M. J., Jensen J. A., and Collins A. "Comparative experience with smooth and polyurethane breast implants using the Kaplan-Meier method of survival analysis." *Plastic Reconstr. Surg.*, 88:475, 1991.
186. Gasperoni C., Salgarello M., and Gargani G. "Polyurethane-covered mammary implants: A 12-year experience." *Ann. Plast. Surg.*, 29:303, 1992.
187. Eyssen J. E., von Werssowetz A. J., and Middleton G. D. "Reconstruction of the breast using polyurethane-coated prostheses." *Plastic Reconstr. Surg.*, 73:415, 1984.
188. Schatten W. E. "Reconstruction of breasts following mastectomy with polyurethane-covered gel-filled prostheses." *Ann. Plast. Surg.*, 12:147, 1984.
189. Cohney B. C., Cohney T. B., and Hearne V. A. "Nineteen years' experience with polyurethane foam-covered mammary prosthesis: A preliminary report." *Ann. Plast. Surg.*, 27:27, 1991.
190. Berrino P., Galli M., Rainero M. L., and Santi P. L. "Long-lasting complications with the use of polyurethane-covered breast implants." *Brit. J. Plast. Surg.*, 39:549, 1986.
191. Jabaley M. E. and Das S. K. "Late breast pain following reconstruction with polyurethane-covered implants." *Plastic Reconstr. Surg.*, 78:390, 1986.
192. Berrino P., Franchelli S., and Santi P. "Surgical correction of breast deformities following long-lasting complications of polyurethane-covered implants." *Ann. Plast. Surg.*, 24:481, 1990.
193. Dunn K. W., Hall P. N., and Khoo C. T. K. "Breast implant materials: sense and safety." *Brit. J. Plast. Surg.*, 45:315, 1992.
194. Sinclair T. M., Kerrigan C. L., and Buntie R. "Biodegradation of the polyurethane foam covering of breast implants." *Plastic Reconstr. Surg.*, 92:1003, 1993.
195. Chan S. C., Birdsell D. C., and Gradeen C. Y. "Urinary excretion of free toluenediamines in a patient with polyurethane-covered breast implants." *Clin. Chem.*, 37:2143, 1991.
196. Chan S. C., Birdsell D. C., and Gradeen C. Y. "Detection of toluenediamines in the urine of a patient with polyurethane-covered breast implants." *Clin. Chem.*, 37:756, 1991.
197. Yannas I. V. and Burke J. F. "Design of an artificial skin. I. Basic design principles." *J. Biomed. Mater. Res.*, 14:65, 1980.
198. Yannas I. V., Burke J. F., Gordon P. L., Huang C., and Rubenstein R. H. "Design of an artificial skin. II. Control of chemical composition." *J. Biomed. Mater. Res.*, 14:107, 1980.
199. Limova M. and Grekin R. C. "Synthetic membranes and cultured keratinocytes." *Am. Acad. Dermatol.*, 4:713, 1990.
200. Fabre J. "Epidermal allografts." *Immunol. Letters*, 29:161, 1991.
201. Woodley D. T., Chen J. D., Kim J. P., Sarret Y., Iwasaki T., Kim Y., and O'Keefe, E. J. "Reepithelialization. Human keratinocyte locomoton." *Dermatol. Clinics*, 11:641, 1993.
202. Margolis D. J. and Cohen J. H. "Management of chronic venous leg ulcers." *Clinics in Dermatology*, 12:19, 1994.
203. Mostow E. N. "Diagnosis and classification of chronic wounds." *Clinics in Dermatology*, 12:3, 1994.
204. Cohen F. E., Gregoret L. M., Amiri P., Aldape K., Railey J., and McKerrow J. H. "Arresting tissue invasion of a parasite by protease inhibitors chosen with the aid of computer modeling." *Biochem.*, 30:11221, 1991.
205. Eldad A., Simon G. A., Kadar T., and Kushnir M. "Immediate dressing of the burn wound — will it change its natural history?" *Burns*, 17:233, 1991.
206. Eldad A. and Tuchman I. "The use of OmidermR as an interface for skin grafting." *Burns*, 17:155, 1991.
207. Winter G. D. "Formation of scab and the rate of epithelialization of superficial wounds in the skin of the young domestic pig." *Nature*, 193:293, 1962.
208. Falanga V. "Growth factors and wound healing." *Dermatol. Clinics*, 11:667, 1993.
209. Jones B. C., Briggs C. D., and Norton D. A. "This new type of I.V. dressing can save you time." *Nursing*, December:70, 1982.
210. Leipziger L. S., Glushko V., DiBernardo B., Shafaie F., Noble J., Nichols J., and Alvarez O. M. "Dermal wound repair: Role of collagen matrix implants and synthetic polymer dressings." *J. Am. Acad. Dermatol.*, 12:409, 1985.
211. Helfman T., L. O. and Falanga V. "Occlusive dressings and wound healing." *Clinics in Dermatology*, 12:121, 1994.
212. Alvarez O. M., Mertz P. M., and Eaglestein W. H. "The effect of occlusive dressings on collagen synthesis and re-epithelialization in superficial wounds." *J. Surg. Res.*, 35:142, 1983.

213. Brown A. S. and Barot L. R. "Biologic dressings and skin substitutes." *Clin. Plast. Surg.*, 13:69, 1986.
214. Tinckler L. "A significant advance." *Nursing Mirror*,:36, 1983.
215. Eaglestein W. H. "Experiences with biosynthetic dressings." *J. Am. Acad. Dermatol.*, 12:434, 1985.
216. Eaglestein W. H., Mertz P. M., and Falanga V. "Occlusive dressings." *Am. Fam. Physician*, 35:211, 1987.
217. Pitcher D. "Sutureless skin closure for pacemaker implantation:comparison with subcuticular suture." *Postgrad. Med. J.*, 59:83, 1983.
218. Jonkman M. F., Molenaar I., Nieuwenhuis P., and Klasen H. J. "Evaporative water loss and epidermis regeneration in partial thickness wounds dressed with a fluid-retaining vs. a clot-inducing wound covering in guinea pigs." *Scand. J. Plast. Surg.*, 23:29, 1989.
219. Jonkman M. F., Bruin P., Pennings A. J., Coenen J. M. F. H., and Klasen H. J. "Poly(ether urethane) wound covering with high water vapour permeability compared with conventional tulle grass on split-skin donor sites." *Burns*, 15:211, 1989.
220. Staso M. A., Raschbaum M., Slater H., and Goldfarb I. W. "Experience with Omiderm — A new burn dressing." *J. Burn Care & Rehab.*,:209, 1991.
221. Jonkman M. F., Bruin P., Hoeksma E. A., Nieuwenhuis P., Klasen H. J., Pennings A. J., and Molenaar I. "A clot-inducing wound covering with high vapor permeability: enhancing effects on epidermal wound healing in partial-thickness wounds in guinea pigs." *Surgery*, 104:537, 1988.
222. Ramirez O. M., Granick M. S., and Futrell J. W. "Optimal wound healing under Op-Site dressing." *Plastic Reconstr. Surg.*, 73:474, 1983.
223. Behar D., Juszynski M., Ben Hur N., and Rudensky B. "Omiderm, a new synthetic wound covering: Physical properties and drug permeability studies." *J. Biomed. Mater. Res.*, 20:731, 1986.
224. Bruin P., Jonkman M. F., Meijer H. J., and Pennings A. J. "A new porous polyetherurethane wound covering." *J. Biomed. Mater. Res.*, 24:217, 1990.
225. Alling R. and North A. F. "Polyurethane film for coverage of skin graft donor sites." *J. Oral Surg.*, 39:970, 1981.
226. Nahas L. F. and Swartz B. L. "Use of semipermeable polyurethane membrane for skin graft dressings." *Plastic Reconstr. Surg.*, Jun:791, 1981.
227. Davies J. W. L. "Synthetic materials for covering burn wounds: Progress towards perfection. Part 1. Short term dressing materials." *Burns*, 10:94, 1983.
228. Young S. R., Dyson M., Hickman R., Lang S., and Osborn C. "Comparison of the effects of semi-occlusive polyurethane dressings and hydrocolloid dressings on dermal repair: 1. Cellular Changes." *J. Invest. Dermatol.*, 97:586, 1991.
229. Ostrofsky M. K. "The use of a semipermeable membrane for the handling of skin grafts in preprosthetic surgery." *J. Oral Maxillofac. Surg.*, 50:199, 1992.
230. Borenstein A., Newton E. D., Smith J. K., Goldfarb I. W., and Slater H. "Transparent polyurethane (Omiderm) dressing for free flaps." *Ann. Plast. Surg.*, 26:200, 1991.
231. Barak M., Hershkowitz S., Rod R., and Dror S. "The use of a synthetic skin covering as a protective layer in the daily care of low birth weight infants." *Eur. J. Paediatrics*, 148:665, 1989.
232. Barak J., Einav S., Tadmor A., Vidne B., and Austen W. G. "The effect of colloid osmotic pressure on the survival of sheep following cardiac surgery." *Int. J. Artif. Organs*, 12:47, 1989.
233. Zeligowski A. and Wexler M. R. "Thin polyurethane foam bandage dressing for skin-graft procedures." *Plastic Reconstr. Surg.*,:1013, 1986.
234. Poulsen T. D., Freund K. G., Arendrup K., Nyhuus P., and Pedersen O. D. "Polyurethane film (Opsite) vs. impregnated gauze (Jelonet) in the treatment of outpatient burns: a prospective, randomized study." *Burns*, 17:59, 1991.
235. Moore C. G. "Comparison of blisterfilm and gauze for peritoneal catheter exit site care." *ANNA Journal*, 16:475, 1989.
236. Blight A., Fatah M. F., Datubo-Brown D. D., Mountford E. M., and Cheshire I. M. "The treatment of donor sites with cultured epithelial grafts." *Brit. J. Plast. Surg.*, 44:12, 1991.
237. Oleske D. M., Smith X. P., White P., and Donovan M. I. "A randomized clinical trial of two dressing methods for the treatment of low-grade pressure ulcers." *J. Enteros. Ther.*, 13:90, 1986.
238. Maki D. G., Stolz S. S., Wheeler S., and Mermel L. A. "A prospective, randomized trial of gauze and two polyurethane dressings for site care of pulmonary artery catheters: Implications for catheter management." *Crit. Care Med.*, 22:1729, 1994.

239. Holland K. T., Davis W., Ingham E., and Gowland G. "A comparison of the *in vitro* anti-bacterial effect and complement activating effect of 'Opsite' and 'Tegaderm' dressings." *J. Hospital Infec.*, 5:323, 1984.
240. Wille J. C. and van Oud Alblas A. B. "A comparison of four film-type dressings by their anti-microbial effect on the flora of the skin." *J. Hospital Infec.*, 14:153, 1989.
241. Lewis D. H. and Castleberry D. J. "An assessment of recent advances in external maxillofacial materials." *J. Prosth. Dentistry*, 43:426, 1980.
242. An K. N., Gonzalez J. B., and Chao E. Y. "Standardization of a polyurethane elastomer for facial prostheses." *J. Prosth. Dentistry*, 44:338, 1980.
243. Turner G. E., Fischer T. E., Castleberry D. J., and Lemons J. E. "Intrinsic color of isophorone polyurethane for maxillofacial prosthetics.Part II: Color Stability." *J. Prosth. Dentistry*, 51:673, 1984.
244. Craven D. E., Lichtenberg D. A., Kunches L. M., and McCabe W. R. "A randomized study comparing transparent polyurethane dressing to a dry gauze dressing for peripheral intravenous catheter sites." *Infect. Control*, 6:361, 1985.
245. Aly R., Bayles C., and Maibach H. "Restriction of bacterial growth under commercial catheter dressings." *Am. J. Infect. Control*, 16:95, 1988.
246. Hoffmann K. K., Western S. A., Kaiser D. L., Wenzel R. P., and Groschel D. H. M. "Bacterial colonization and phlebitis-associated risk with transparent polyurethane film for peripheral intravenous site dressings." *Am. J. Infect. Control*, 16:101, 1988.
247. Papatheofanis R. J. and Barmada R. "The principles and applications of surgical adhesives." *Surgery Annual*, 25:49, 1993.
248. Marx M., Bettmann M. A., Bridge S., and Richie J. P. "The effects of various indwelling ureteral catheter materials on the normal canine ureter." *The Journal of Urology*, 139:180, 1988.
249. Pryor J. L., Langley M. J., and Jenkins A. D. "Comparison of symptom characteristics of indwelling ureteral catheters." *J. Urol.*, 145:719, 1991.
250. El-Faqih S. R., Shamsuddin A. B., Chakrabarti A., Atassi R., Kardar A. H., Osman M. K., and Husain I. "Polyurethane internal ureteral stents in treatment of stone patients: morbidity related to indwelling times." *J. Urol.*, 146:1487, 1991.
251. Docimo S. G. and Dewolf W. C. "High failure rate of indwelling ureteral stents in patients with extrinsic obstruction: experience at 2 institutions." *The Journal of Urology*, 142:277, 1989.
252. Cox A. J. "Effect of a hydrogel coating on the surface topography of latex-based urinary catheters: an SEM study." *Biomaterials*, 8:500, 1987.
253. Lammer J., Stoffler G., Petek W. W., and Hofler H. "*In vitro* long-term perfusion of different materials for biliary endoprostheses." *Invest. Radiol.*, 21:329, 1986.
254. Keane P. F., Bonner M. C., Johston S. R., Zafar A., and Gorman S., P. "Characterization of biofilm and encrustation on uretic stents *in vivo*." *Brit. J. Urol.*, 74:687, 1994.
255. Edleman D. A. "Nonprescription vaginal contraception." *Int. J. Gynaecol. Obst.*, 18:340, 1980.
256. Aznar R., Zamora G., Lozano M., and Levi L. "Polyurethane contraceptive vaginal sponge." *Contracept.*, 24:235, 1981.
257. Borko E., McIntyre S. L., and Feldblum P. J. "A comparative clinical trial of the contraceptive sponge and neo sampoon tablets." *Obst. Gyn.*, 65:511, 1985.
258. Quigg J. M., Miller I. F., Mack S. R., Saxena S. J., Kaminski J. M., and Zaneveld L. J. D. "Development of the polyurethane sponge as a delivery sytem for Aryl 4-Guanidinobenzoates." *Contracept.*, 38:487, 1988.
259. Burck P. J. and Zimmerman R. E. "An intravaginal contraceptive device for the delivery of an acrosin and hyaluronidase inhibitor." *Fertil. Steril.*, 41:314, 1984.
260. Drew W. L., Blair M., Miner R. C., and Conant M. "Evaluation of the virus permeability of a new condom for women." *Sexually Transmitted Diseases*, 17:110, 1990.
261. Rosenberg M. J., Waugh M. S., Solomon H. M., and Lyszkowski A. D. L. "The male polyurethane condom: a review of current knowledge." *Contracept.*, 53:141, 1996.
262. Tashev E., Shi F. Y., and Leong K. W. "Potential applications of Poly(phosphoester-urethanes) in controlled drug delivery." *RAPRA*,:43, 1991.
263. Konoplitskaya K. L., Pkhakadze G. A., and Narazayko L. F. "Biocompatibility of a prolonged-action antialcohol preparation." *Biomaterials*, 12:701, 1991.

264. Hussain M. A., DiLuccio R. C., Shefter E., and Hurwitz A. R. "Hollow fibers as an oral sustained-release delivery system using propranolol hydrochloride." *Pharmaceut. Res.,* 6:1052, 1989.
265. Hussain M. A., DiLuccio R. C., and Shefter E. "Hollow fibers as an oral sustained-release delivery system." *Pharmaceut. Res.,* 6:49, 1989.
266. Sintov A., Scott W. A., Siden R., and Levy R. J. "Efficacy of epicardial controlled-release lidocaine for ventricular tachycardia induced by rapid ventricular pacing in dogs." *J. Cardiovasc. Pharmacol.,* 16:812, 1990.
267. Badiger M. V., McNeill M. E., and Graham N. B. "Porogens in the preparation of microporous hydrogels based on poly(ethylene oxides)." *Biomaterials,* 14:1059, 1993.
268. Ikeda Y., Kohjiya S., Takesako S., and Yamashita S. "Polyurethane elastomer with PEO-PTMO-PEO soft segment for sustained release of drugs." *Ann. Plast. Surg.,* 24:80, 1990.
269. Lambert T. L., DEv V., rechavia E., Forrester J. S., Litvack F., and Eigler N. L. "Localized arterial wall drug delivery from a polymer coated removable metallic stent. Kinetics, distribution and bioactivity of Forskolin." *Circulation,* 90:1003, 1994.
270. Chithambara B., Sunny M. C., and Jayakrishnan A. "Tantalum-loaded polyurethane microspheres for particulate embolizations: preparation and properties." *Biomaterials,* 12:525, 1991.
271. Albertsson A. C., Donaruma L. G., and Vogl O. "Synthetic polymers as drugs." *Ann. N.Y. Acad. Sci.,* 446:105, 1985.
272. Merrill D. C. "Mentor inflatable penile prosthesis." *Urology,* 22:504, 1983.
273. Fein R. L. and Needell M. H. "Early problems encountered with the mentor inflatable penile prosthesis." *J. Urol.,* 134:62, 1985.
274. Lamberton P., Lipsky M., and McMillan P. "Use of semipermeable polyurethane hollow fibers for pituitary organ culture." *In Vitro Cell. Dev. Biol.,* 24:500, 1988.
275. Sternberg T., Barrau M.-B., Gangiotti L., and Thevenot D. R. "Study and development of multilayer needle-type enzyme-based glucose microsensors." *Biosensors,* 4:27, 1988.
276. Shaw G. W., Claremont D. J., and Pickup J. C. "*In vitro* testing of a simply constructed, highly stable glucose sensor suitable for implantation in diabetic patients." *Biosensors and Bioelectronics,* 6:401, 1991.
277. Hintsche R., Dransfeld I., Scheller F., Pham M. T., Hoffmann W., Hueller J., and Moritz W. "Integrated dufferential enzyme sensors using hydrogen and fluoride ion sensitive multigate FETs." *Biosensors and Bioelectronics,* 5:327, 1990.
278. Lindner E., Cosofret V. V., Ufer S., and Anderson J. M. "Ion-selective membranes with low plasticizer content: Electroanalytical characterization and biocompatibility studies." *J. Biomed. Mater. Res.,* 28:591, 1994.
279. Peterson C. J., Donachy J. H., and Kalenak A. "A segmented polyurethane composite prosthetic anterior cruciate ligament *in vivo* study." *J. Biomed. Mater. Res.,* 19:589, 1985.
280. Klompmaker J., Jansen H. W. B., Veth R. P. H., Nielsen H. K. L., de Groot J. H., Pennings A. J., and Kuijer R. "Meniscal repair by fibrocartilage? An experimental study in the dog." *J. Orthopaed. Res.,* 10:359, 1992.
281. Klompmaker J., Jansen H. W. B., Veth R. P. H., de Groot J. H., Nijenhuis A. J., and Pennings A. J. "Porous polymer implant for repair of meniscal lesions: a preliminary study in dogs." *Biomaterials,* 12:810, 1991.
282. Hoppen H. J., Leenslag J. W., Pennings A. J., and Robinson P. H. "Two-ply biodegradable nerve guide: basic aspects of design, construction and biological performance." *Biomaterials,* 11:286, 1990.
283. Bruin P., Meeuwsen E. A. J., van Andel M. V., and Pennings A. J. "Autoclavable highly crosslinked polyurethane networks in opthalmology." *Biomaterials,* 14:1089, 1993.
284. Jongebloed W. L., van der Veen G., Kalicharan D., and Worst J. G. F. "New material for low-cost intraocular lenses." *Biomaterials,* 15:766, 1994.
285. Lee C. K., Langrana N. A., Parsons J. R., and Zimmerman M. C. "Development of a prosthetic intervertebral disc." *Spine,* 16:253, 1991.
286. Ray A. R. and Bhowmick A. "Synthesis and characterization of aliphatic polyurethane fiber: A potential suture material." *J. Biomed. Mater. Res.,* 25:1249, 1991.
287. Hallock G. G. "Polyurethane Nipple Prosthesis." *Ann. Plast. Surg.,* 24:80, 1990.

288. Messner K. and Gillquist J. "Synthetic implants for the repair of osteochondral defects of the medial femoral condyle: a biomechanical and histological evaluation in the rabbit knee." *Biomaterials,* 14:513, 1993.
289. Weiss P. L., Hunter I. W., and Kearney R. E. "Rigid polyurethane foam casts for the fixation of human limbs." *Med. Biol. Eng. Comput.,* 22:603, 1984.
290. Bakker D., van Blitterswijk C. A., Hesseling S. C., Daems W. T., Kuijpers W., and Grote J. J. "The behavior of alloplastic tympanic membranes in staphylococcus aureus-induced middle ear infection. I. Quantitative biocompatibility evaluation." *J. Biomed. Mater. Res.,* 24:669, 1990.
291. Nelson R. J., White R. A., and Hirose F. M. "Neovascularity of a tracheal prosthesis/tissue complex." *J. Thorac. Cardiovasc. Surg.,* 86:800, 1983.
292. Kearfott K. J., Rottenberg D. A., and Knowles R. J. R. "A new headholder for PET, CT and NMR Imaging." *J. Computer Assisted Tomography,* 8:1217, 1984.
293. Shanahan T. G., Mehta M. P., Bertelrud K. L., and Kinsella T. J. "Minimization of small bowel volume within treatment fields utilizing customized 'Belly Boards'." *Int. J. Radiat. Oncol., Biol., Phys.,* 19:469, 1990.
294. Swanson S. K. "Handling the 'glidewire'," *J. Urol.,* 146:1339, 1991.
295. Wahl L. M. and Wahl S. M. "Inflammation." In *Wound healing: Biochemical and Clinical Aspects.* Ed. Cohen K., Dieglemann R. F., and Lindblad W. J. W. B. Saunders Co., Philadelphia, 1992.

10 Summary and Future Perspectives

In this book we have introduced the reader to polyurethane chemistry and solid state properties, their biological interactions and reviewed their performance in medical devices. Today, polyurethane elastomers are still regarded as some of the best biomaterials currently available, due to their superior mechanical properties, particularly tensile strength and fatigue resistance, and blood and tissue compatibility. As discussed in this book, the properties of polyurethanes are partially determined by the reagents selected for synthesis from the large range of possible precursors. The mechanical and interfacial characteristics of a polyurethane are also influenced by the methods used to fabricate, process and sterilize the specific device. All of these factors contribute to the performance of polyurethanes in medical devices. The optimization of polyurethanes in medical applications will be aided by further studies of the effects of polyurethane chemistry on the structure and properties of these materials. In addition, processing additives, sterilization and processing conditions also can influence the performance of a biomaterial, and this is an area of investigation where results will improve understanding of the transition from biomaterial to medical device. In particular the nature and effect of additives, whether to improve biological performance or to ease processing, on the local and systemic responses needs further investigation. The scope for materials development includes the synthesis of novel materials, the modification of those currently available, and the exploration of composite materials and blends. Cost is becoming an increasingly important issue in health care, and it may be that if a novel material is to be successful commercially, it not only has to be fabricable on a large scale but also may need to be broadly applicable to ensure that production is financially viable.

During the last few years, a number of key biomaterials, some of them polyurethanes, have been withdrawn from use in devices for long term implantation. From the standpoint of the researcher, this is quite unfortunate, as some of these materials represent polyurethane biomaterials that have been most widely studied inside and outside of the clinic. Similar materials are commercially available, although from different sources, ensuring continued provision of health care.

It has become apparent that not only can the material have an impact on the biological environment, but the biological environment also has the capacity to modify the material. This is most clearly demonstrated by the issue of biodegradation. Initially, polyetherurethanes were used in applications where hydrolysis was undesirable. Polyetherurethanes are more hydrolytically stable than polyesterurethanes, but are nevertheless prone to oxidation. New generation "biodurable" polyurethanes are being synthesized, that reduce or eliminate ether and ester linkages within the polyurethane segments, and have been designed with the goal of fabricating devices for long term implantation. The studies of polyurethane biodegradation that have been conducted since the issue came to light have served to increase our level of understanding of the degradation of polyurethanes, and aided in the design of these biodurable materials. Information on polyurethane biodegradation will also aid the development of polyurethanes for controlled release applications, through the design of matrices with specific release properties.

Traditionally, biomaterials were employed to perform singular, biologically inert roles, such as to provide a conduit for blood flow, or as membranes for solute transport. The realization that cells and tissues in the body perform many other vital regulatory and metabolic roles has highlighted the limitations of synthetic materials as tissue substitutes. Demands of biomaterials have changed from maintaining an essentially physical function without eliciting a host response, to providing a more integrated interaction with the host. This has been accompanied by increasing demands from medical devices to improve the quality of life, as well as extend the duration. Biomaterials potentially can be used as synthetic substrates for cell, tissue and organ engineering, helping the body to heal, or promoting regeneration of tissues, thus restoring physiological function. This approach is being explored in the development of synthetic vascular grafts, hybrid artificial organs for extracorporeal circulation, and encapsulation of cells for implantation into the body.

The field of biomaterials still lacks a battery of short term tests that can adequately predict the chronic biocompatibility of a device. The accelerated testing of materials to assess the physical properties in the long term is reasonably well established, and protocols have been defined and are employed by researchers. Comparable tests for the reliable biological evaluation of biomaterial performance are critical to the development and clinical acceptance of new biomaterials and medical devices. There also is a need for the adoption and widespread use of control materials, and the identification of key parameters for the measurement of biological responses to evaluate biomaterials. Continued education and increased communication among all disciplines involved in the development and utilization of biomaterials is critical to the development and evaluation of biomaterials, and the establishment of criteria for performance, remembering that the success of a biomaterial also is determined by its medical application.

Ultimately, the field of biomaterials is fundamental to advances in the performance and function of medical devices, and is a critical part of medicine and surgery. Biomaterials science is truly interdisciplinary. Thus, the development of improved biomaterials is dependent on advances in the physical and biological sciences, engineering and medicine, to increase our present understanding of synthetic materials, molecular biology and the human body. It is believed that continued research into the interactions between synthetic materials and biological systems will establish correlations between material properties and biological performance. These correlations will be useful in the design of improved materials for medical use, particularly to overcome the problems of surface induced thrombosis, device-centered infection and calcification of polyurethane materials. The challenge remains to provide safe and efficacious materials with the required mechanical properties, and ensure an acceptable level of performance throughout the lifetime of the device. Despite the limitations of synthetic materials for biological use, polyurethanes have sustained use and, by virtue of their diverse chemistry which has been creatively explored by researchers, remain one of the most broadly applied biomaterials. As the field of biomaterials finds increasing applications in cellular and tissue engineering, is likely that polyurethanes will be used in new ways as part of the therapeutic device system.

List of Abbreviations

δ — Hansen solubility parameter
ε — strain
σ — stress (force per unit area)
γ — surface tension
γ_c — critical surface tension
AFM — Atomic Force Microscopy
ASTM — American Society for Testing and Materials
ATR–FTIR — attenuated total reflectance-fourier transform infrared spectroscopy
BD — butanediol
BDDS — biphenyldisulfonic acid
CAPD — continuous ambulatory peritoneal dialysis
CFC — chlorofluorocarbon
CHDI — cyclohexyl diisocyanate
DABCO — triethylenediamine 1,4 diazo(2,2,2)bicyclooctane
DMA — N,N' dimethylacetamide
DMF — dimethylformamide
DMSO — dimethylsulfoxide
DMTA — dynamic mechanical thermal analysis
DSC — differential scanning calorimetry
E — Young's Modulus
E' — storage modulus
E" — loss modulus
ECM — extracellular matrix
ED — ethylene diamine
EG — ethylene glycol
ESC — environmental stress cracking
ESCA — Electron spectroscopy for chemical analysis (XPS)
EtO — ethylene oxide
FBGC — foreign body giant cell
FTIR — Fourier Transform infrared
GPC — gel permeation chromatography
HMDI — Hexamethylene diisocyanate
H_{12}MDI — methylene *bis* (p-cyclohexyl isocyanate)
HDI — 1,4-transcyclohexyl diisocyanate
HEBP — 2-hydroxyethane *bis* phosphonic acid
HEMA — hydroxyethylmethacrylate
HMWK — high molecular weight kininogen
HPLC — high pressure liquid chromatography
IABP — Intraaortic balloon pump
IgG — Gamma globulin
IL-1 — interleukin-1
IPDI — 3-isocyanatomethyl-3,5,5,trimethylcyclohexyl isocyanate
IR — infrared
LVAD — left ventricular assist device

M_n — number average molecular weight
M_w — weight average molecular weight
MAC — membrane attack complex
MDA — 4,4′ methylene dianiline
MDI — methylene *bis* (p-phenyl isocyanate)
MEK — methylethyl ketone
MO — metal catalyzed oxidation
NDI — 1,5-naphthalene diisocyanate
PC — polycarbonate
PCL — polycaprolactone
PDMS — polydimethylsiloxane
PEG — polyethylene glycol
PEO — polethylene oxide
PET — polyethylene terephthalate
PEU — polyetherurethane
PEUU — polyetherurethaneurea
PK — prekallikrein
PMN — polymorphonuclear leukocyte
PPG — polypropylene glycol
PPO — polypropylene oxide
PTFE — polytetrafluoroethylene
PTMA — polytetramethylene adipate
PTMEG — polytetramethyleneglycol
PTMO — polytetramethylene oxide
PVC — poly(vinyl chloride)
RGD — Arg-Gly-Asp tripeptide sequence
RIM — reaction injection molding
SALS — small angle light scattering
SAXS — small angle X-ray scattering
SEM — scanning electron microscopy
SIMS — Secondary ion mass spectrometry
SR — silicone rubber
STM — Scanning Tunnel Microscopy
TAH — total artificial heart
TDA — 2,4 toluene diamine
TDI — toluene diisocyanate
TEM — transmission electron microscopy
T_g — glass transition temperature
THF — tetrahydrofuran
T_m — melting temperature
TODI — 3,3-bitoluene diisocyanate
tPA — tissue plasminogen activator
TPU — Thermoplastic polyurethane
UHV — ultra high vacuum
UTS — ultimate tensile strength
VAD — ventricular assist device
vWF — von Willebrand factor
WAXS — wide angle X-ray scattering
XPS — X-ray photoelectron spectroscopy (ESCA)

Index

A

Abrasion resistance, 5, 49, 52
ABS (acrylonitrile butadiene styrene), 2
Absorption, *see also* Adsorption; Surface properties
    drugs, cardiac catheter materials, 208
    lipids, 104, *see also* Hydrophobicity
    water, 15, 81, 191
Acetonitrile, 108
Acquired immunity, 129–131, 139–141
Acrylics, 2
Acrylonitrile butadiene styrene (ABS), 2
Activated carbon, 228
Activation of surfaces, 150–151
Acute phase response, 132–134, 137
Acylurea, polymer synthesis, 12
Adaptive immunity, *see* Acquired immunity
Addition polymerization, 8
Additives
    antioxidants, 188–189
    plasticizers, 74, 79
    surface modifying, 29, *see also* Surface modfication
Adducts, surface modification, 152, 155
Adenosine diphosphate, 123–126
Adhesives
    applications, 239
    processing, 27–29
Adsorption, *see also* Platelet adsorption; Protein adsorption; Surface properties
    lipoproteins, 154
    protein, 22–23, 115–123, 150–158
    surface modification and, 152
Advancing contact angle, 98
Albumin, 120–121, *see also* Protein adsorption
    adsorption of, 153–154
    host-material interactions, 151–152
    passivation, 150
    surface modification, 22–23
Alicyclic diols, 228
Aliphatic isocyanates, 191–192
Aliphatic polyurethane degradation, 185, 190–192
Alkalis, 14
Alkyl chains
    albumin adsorption, 151–152, 155
    and stability, 190

Alkylene oxide, 229
Alkyl groups, surface modification, 161
Allophanate reaction
    catalysts and, 14
    low-temperature synthesis to inhibit, 17
    polymer synthesis, 11
Alternating copolymers, 5–6, 8
Alternative complement pathway, 138–139
Amides, 11–12
Amines
    degradation products, 183
    surface modifications, 109, 110
Amorphous polymers, 44
Anaphylotoxins, 128, 139
Angiogenesis, *see* Neointima formation; Vascularization
Animal testing, 148–149
Anisotropy, 34
Annealing, 71–72
Antibiotics, 23
Antibody binding, 152, *see also* Immunoglobulins
Anticoagulants, surface modification, 22, 155
Antioxidants, 188–189
Antithrombin, 122–123, 155
Aortic valve, 222
Applications, 205–241
    artificial organs, 226–230
        blood filters, 229–230
        blood tubing, 229
        heart, 226–227
        hemoperfusion, 228
        kidney, 227–228
        lung, 228
        pancreas, 229
    cardiovascular, 205–227
        artificial heart, 226–227
        assist devices, 222–226
        catheters, 205–208
        heart valves, 219–222
        pacemaker leads, 208–211
        vascular prostheses, 211–219
    tissue augmentation and prostheses, 230–240
        adhesives, 239
        artificial ducts, 239
        breast implants, 230–231
        contraceptives/prophylactics, 240
        drug delivery, 240

facial reconstruction, 238–239
miscellaneous, 241
penile prostheses, 240
wound dressings, 231–238
Arg-Gly-Asp (RGD), 121, 130, 167–168
Aromatic diols, hemodialysis membranes, 228
Aromatic isocyanates, and polymer stability, 191–192
Aromatic polyurethanes
chemical degradation, 185
degradation/stability of, 190
Arteriovenous shunts, 151
Artificial ducts, 239
Artificial organs, 226–230
blood filters, 229–230
blood tubing, 229
heart, 226–227
calcification of, 197
host response, 128
hemoperfusion, 228
kidney, 227–228
lung, 228
pancreas, 229
Atactic polymers, 43–44
Atomic force microscopy, 92–93, 109
Attenuated Total Reflection Fourier Transform Infrared Spectroscopy (ATR-FTIR), 66–68, 92–93, 105
protein adsorption, 150, 154
surface properties, 98–100
Autoclave sterilization, 228
Autooxidation, 183–185, 188–189
Avcomat products, 99
Avcothane
applications
artificial hearts, 227
intra-aortic balloon pumps, 225–226
ventricular assist devices, 224
surface properties, 97, 99, 103, 107–108

B

Bacterial adhesion, 121, see also Infection; Microorganisms; specific applications
protein adsorption and, 154
surface modification and, 152
Balloon pumps
intra-aortic, 225–226
surface properties, 99–100
Balloons, processing, 34–36
Balloon tip pulmonary artery catheters, 208
Barrier dressings, see Wound dressings
Bases, 14
Basophils, 127, 133, 139

B-cells, 127
cytokine sources and functions, 130–131
immune system, 139–141
Bentley foam filters, 230
Bilirubin removal, 228
Biobrane, 235
Bioclusive, 38–39, 235
Biocompatibility, 1, 5, see also Degradation; Host-material interactions
in vitro testing, 147–148
porosity and, 109–110
Biodegradable polymers, 199–200
Biofilm catheters, 239
Bioflex applications, 240
Biological catalysis, 185–187
Biological fluids
blood compatibility, see Blood compatibility
and fatigue behavior in, 83
Biological wound dressings, 235
Biomaterials, 1
protein adsorption, 119–122
solubility parameters, 85
Biomer products, 29, 38
applications
artificial hearts, 226–227
cardiac catheters, 208
heart valves, 222–223
ventricular assist devices, 223–224
bulk characterization, 66
calcification of, 197
degradation mechanisms, 186–187
extrusion grade, 32
fabrication process, 35
mechanical properties, 81
protein adsorption, 151, 153
solubility parameters of blood components and biomaterials, 85
surface contaminants, 105–106
surface properties, 99, 103–104, 108–109
surface tension properties, 97–98
BioSpan, 37–38, 81
Biphenyldisulfonic acid (BDDS) chain extender, 20
Birefringence, 58
3,3-Bitoluene diisocyanate (TODI), 15–16, 64, see also Toluene diisocyanate
Biuret formation
catalysts and, 14
low-temperature synthesis to inhibit, 17
polymer synthesis, 11
Bladder processing, 34–36
Blisterfilm, 39, 235, 237–238
Block copolymers, 5–6
chemical synthesis, 8

Index

intermolecular bonding in, 48
morphological models, 55–57
Blood
  and fatigue behavior, 83
  hemodynamics, 147–148
  hemoperfusion devices, 228
  Vroman effect, 156
Blood-biomaterial interactions, *see* Host-material interactions
Blood cells, *see also* Red cells; Platelets; White cells
  host defenses, *see* Cellular responses
  surface charge, 111
Blood compatibility (hemocompatibility), 1
  hemoperfusion devices, 228
  in vitro testing, 147–148
  surface properties and, 83, 109
Blood components, solubility parameters, 85
Blood filters, 128, 229–230
Blood pumps, 197, 223, 225
Blood tubing, 229
Blood vessels, *see also* Vascular grafts; Vascularization
  neointima formation, *see* Neointima formation
  surface charge, 111
Blowing agents, 32
Bonds, chemical, *see* Chemical bonds
Bowel flora, 169
Bradykinins, 133
Branched polyesters
  degradation/stability of, 190
  synthesis process, 8
Breast implants, 164, 230–231
  degradation of, 189, 192, 195–197
  inflammatory response, 165
Bubble, gastric, 189–190
Bubble microstructure, vascular grafts, 110
Bulk analysis, 104
Bulk polymer, degradation mechanisms, 181
Bulk processing, product variability, 39
Bulk properties
  modification during synthesis, 20–21
  porosity as, 109
  SEM detection, 74–75
Burns, *see* Wound dressings
1,4-Butadiene, hydroxy terminated, 18
1,4-Butanediol (BD), 17
  crosslinked polymer synthesis, 18, 20
  differential scanning calorimetry, 69

C

Calcification, 197–199
  artificial hearts, 227
  heart valves, 220–221
Calcite, 33–34
Calcium, platelet activation, 124
Calorimetry, 62–63, 68–73
Capillary rise method, 96
Caprolactone, 199
Carbodiimide formation, 12–13
Carbowax, 74, 79, 104
Carboxylation, and endothelial cell attachment, 168
Carcinogens, 17, 185, 192
Cardiomat, 38, 81, 221
Cardiopulmonary bypass, host responses, white cells, 128
Cardiothane, 38
  mechanical properties, 81
  pacemaker leads, 208
  surface characterization, 99–100
  surface contaminants, 107–108
Cardiovascular applications, 205–227
  heart, 226–227
    calcification of, 197
    host response, 128
  assist devices, 222–226
  catheters, 205–208
  complications
    calcification, 197–199
    infection, 169, 170
  heart valves, 219–222
  pacemaker leads, 208–211
    oxidation, 184
    stress cracking, 187–189
  vascular prostheses, 211–219, *see also* Vascular grafts
Cardiovascular testing, 149
Cartilage defect repair, 241
Cast Biomer, 104
Cast elastomers, 18
Casting
  balloons, bladders, catheters, 34–35
  biodegradable polymers, 200
  solvent, 28
  and surface properties, 111
Cast materials
  Biomer, 109
  and surface chemistry, 108
  tubing, 33
Catalysts, 13–14
Catheters
  cardiac, 205–208
  dressings for exit sites, 237–238
  infection, 169–170
  inflammatory response, 164
  peritoneal dialysis, 169
  polydimethylsiloxanes at surface, 106–107

Cell adhesion
   endothelial, *see* Neointima formation
   surface defects and, 83
   surface modification, 21
Cell adhesion molecules (CAMs), 121
   cell receptors, 129
   neointima formation, 167
   platelet adhesion, 124–126
Cell ingrowth
   endothelial, *see* Neointima formation
   fibroblast, 109–110
Cell-mediated immunity, 139–141
Cellular responses
   degradation mechanisms, 185–189
   host defense, 124–131
      adhesion molecules, 129
      cytokines, 129–131
      ECM, 128–129
      hemostasis and thrombosis, 131–132
      immune system, 137–141
      platelets, 124–126
      red cells, 124, 126
      white cells, 127–128
   host-material interactions, 158–171
      immunological response, 169
      neointima formation, 167–169
      platelets, 158–162
      soft tissue interactions, 164–166
      thrombus formation, 161–164
      white cells, 161
Cellulose membranes, 227–228
Chain extension, 7, 9
   catalysts and, 14
   chemical composition and physical properties, 65
   crosslinked polymer synthesis, 18, 20
   raw materials in copolymer synthesis, 15, 17, 20
Chain length, and stability, 190
Charcoal, 228
Chemical bonds
   biodegradation mechanisms, 181–182
   hydrogen bonds, 10, 59, 61–63, 70
   and polymer properties, 48
Chemical composition
   and electrical properties, 85–86
   and hydrogen bonds, 62
   and physical properties, 63–65
      chain extenders, 65
      isocyanates, 63–64
      polyols, 64–65
Chemical grafting, 21
Chemistry, 5–23
   classification criteria, 5
   crosslinked copolymers, 17–18
   degradation mechanisms, 181, 185

   history, 6–7
   linear elastomer synthesis, 17
   modification of properties, 18–22
      bulk, 20–21
      surface, 21–22
   raw materials in copolymer synthesis, 14–17
   soft and hard segments, 6–7
   synthesis, 8–14
      acylurea, 12
      allophanate reaction, 11
      biuret formation, 11
      carbodiimide formation, 12–13
      catalysts, 13–14
      isocyanates, 9–10
      isocyanurate formation, 12–13
      media for, 14
      types of polymerization reactions, 8–9
      uretidione formation, 12–13
   two-phase microdomain structure, 7–8
   types of structure, 5–6
Chemotaxis, 127, 130–131, 133–134, 138–139
Chlorofluorocarbons, 32
Cholesterol, 154
Cholesterol esterase, 193–194
Chromatography, gel permeation, 66–68
Chromic acid etching, 28
Chronic inflammation
   biopolymer material and, 164–166
   foreign body response, 134–135
ChronoFlex, 38, 217
Classification of polymers, 5
Clinical evaluation, 150, *see also* Degradation; Host-material interactions
Coagulation, 127–128, *see also* Thrombus formation
   acute phase response, 132
   electrical charge and, 111
   host defense, 122–123, 127–128
   host-material interactions, 154–155
   platelets, 124
   response to foreign materials, 136, 141
   Vroman effect, 155–157
   wound healing, 136
Coatings, 27–29, *see also* Surface modification
Cobalt naphthenate, 14
Cochlear implants, 170
Cold forming, 31
Collagen, 132
   blood pump lining, 225
   ECM, 128–129
   wound healing, 136–137, 141
Collagenase, 132
Comfeel Ulcus, 38
Commercial production, *see* Fabrication

Index

Complement system, 138–139
   host-material interactions, 155
   immune response, 138–139, 141, 169
   inflammatory mediators, 128, 133–134
Condensation polymerization, 8
Condoms, 240
Conformation of adsorbed protein, 153
Contact angle methods, 92–98
   hysteresis, 97–98
   technique, 95–97
Contact phase activation, 111
Contaminants
   commercial processing and, 39
   and contact angle measurement, 95
   SEM detection, 75
Contraceptives/prophylactics, 240
Contracture
   breast implant complications, 165–166
   wound healing, 136–137
Copolymer chemistry, *see* Chemistry
Corethane, 38, 81
Corplex, 38
Covalent bonds, 10
Cracks
   degradation and, 182, 185–186
   environmental stress, 187–189
   pacemaker leads, 209–211
   SEM detection, 75
   stress-strain properties, 78
Creep, 49, 50, 190
m-Cresol, 28
Critical surface energy, 95
Critical surface tension measurement, 96
Crosslinking, 17–18, 63
   biuret and allophanate, 11–12
   catalysts and, 14
   chain extenders, 15, 17, 20
   and crystallization, 44
   dynamic mechanical thermal analysis, 72, 74, 78
   isocyanate group, 10
   isocyanurate formation, 12–13
   synthesis process, 8
Crystalline lamella, 46–47
Crystallinity, 8, 44, 47–48, 59
   chain extenders and, 65
   dynamic mechanical thermal analysis, 72, 74, 77
   and stability, 190
   and surface properties, 108
Curing, 8
   adhesives, 239
   balloons, bladders, catheters, 36
   crosslinked polymer synthesis, 17
Cyclic extenders of urethanes, 17, 19, 65

Cycloaliphatic polyurethanes
   degradation of, 190–191
   facial reconstruction, 239
Cyclohexyldiisocyanate, 15–16
Cytokines, 127, 129
   host defense, 127, 129–131
   immune system, 139–141, 169
   inflammatory response, 132–134, 165
   sources and functions, 129–131
   wound healing, 136
Cytotoxic T-cells, 127, 139–141

D

DABCO (tri-ethylene diamine 1,4-diazo(2,2,2)bicyclooctane), 13–14
Dacron, lyethylene terephthalate
Deformation behavior, *see* Stress-strain behavior
Degradation, 181–200
   artificial hearts, 227
   biodegradable polymers, 199–200
   calcification, 197–199
   gel permeation chromatography, 66
   mechanisms of, 181–195
      biological catalysis, 185–187
      chemical degradation, 185
      hydrolysis, 181–182
      location of implant and, 194–195
      miscellaneous, 194
      oxidation, 183–184
      polymer structure and, 188–194
      sterilization, 185
   pacemaker leads, 209–211
   resistance to, 5
   SEM detection, 75
   toxicity/carcinogenicity, 195–197
DEHP (diethylhexylphthalate), 229
Delta-Tape, 237
Dentistry, 239
Derivatization, *see* Surface modification
Dextran-cibacron-blue adducts, 152
1,3-Diaminecyclohexane, 66
Diamines, chain extension reaction, 18, 20
Dibutyltin dilaurate, 14
Dielectric relaxation studies, 56–57
Diethylhexylphthalate (DEHP), 229
Differential scanning calorimetry, 62–63, 68–72, 73
Diffusion properties, degradation properties, 181–182
Dihydroxypolyester, linear elastomer synthesis, 17
Diisocyanate, 7–8, 62

Diisopropylaminoethyl methacrylate
  (DPA-EMA), 106
N,N-Dimethylacetamide (DMA), 103
Dimethylformamide (DMF), 14, 28
  linear elastomer synthesis, 17
  tubing fabrication, 33
Dimethylsulfoxide (DMSO), 14, 24
Diols, polymer synthesis, 8–9
4,4-Diphenylmethane diisocyanate (MDI), 15–16
Dipole-dipole interactions, 84
Dissipation factor, 74, 76
DMA (N,N-dimethylacetamide), 14, 28, 108
DMF, see Dimethylformamide
DMSO (dimethylsulfoxide), 14, 24
Dodecanediol (DDO), 109, 110
DPA-EMA (diisopropylaminoethyl methacrylate),
  106
Dressings
  catheter, 207–208
  wound, see Wound dressings
Drug absorption, cardiac catheter materials, 208
Drug delivery systems, 240
Ducor, 207
Ducts, artificial, 239
DuoDerm, 232
Dynamic mechanical thermal analysis, 72, 74,
  76–79

E

ECM, see Extracellular matrix (ECM)
Elastase, 132, 186
Elasticity, see also Mechanical behavior
  glass transition temperature and, 44
  tubing, 34
Elastin, 128, 136, 199
Elastomers
  cast, 18
  fabrication, 31
  synthesis, 8, 15, 17
  thermal annealing effects, 71–72
Electrical properties, 85–86, 92, 111
Electrolytes, oxidation, 183
Electron microscopy, 74–78, 79, 92,
  see also Scanning EM
Electron Spectroscopy for Chemical Analysis
  (ESCA), 100–101, 102–108
  methods, 92–93
  surface contaminants, 107–108
Electrostatic powder coating, 27
Ellagic acid, 111
Endothelium, 110
  cell adhesion molecules, 129
  and coagulation, 131–132

cytokine sources and functions, 129–131
neointima formation, see Neointima
  formation
white cell chemotaxis, 134
wound healing, 136–137
Endothermic transitions, 70–71
Enhanced ESCA methods, 92
Enka PUR products, 38
Environmental stability, 15
Environmental stress cracking,
  see Stress cracking
Enzymes, 197
  degradation of polymers, 181–187
  inflammatory response, 164
  surface modification, 23
Eosinophils, 127
Epigard, 39, 164, 238
Epolene, 35
Erythrocytes, see Red cells
Erythrothane, 81, 153
ES, see Polyesterurethanes
Estane, 29, 32, 38
  applications
    heart valves, 222
    wound dressings, 234
  degradation of, 195–197
  dynamic mechanical thermal analysis,
    74, 79
  microbiological considerations, 170
  modulus temperature curves, 78–79
Ester groups, 10, see also Polyester urethanes
  biodegradation mechanisms, 181–182
  hydrogen bonds, 61
  surface contaminants, 105
ET, see Polyether urethanes
Etching, 28
Ethers, see also Polyether urethanes
  biodegradation mechanisms, 181–182
  hydrogen bonds, 61
  linkages, 10
Ethylene diamine (ED), 17–18, 20, 192
  Biomer bulk characterization, 66
  Biomer synthesis, 104
  surface properties of polymers synthesized
    from, 103
  ventricular assist devices, 224
Ethylene glycol, 17, 20
Ethylene oxide sterilization, 33–34
E-type blood pump, 223
Expanded polytetrafluoroethylene, 211–213
Extracellular matrix (ECM)
  host defense, 128–129
  neointima formation, 167–169
  wound healing, 136, 141

Index

Extracorporeal circulation
  blood filters, 229–230
  blood oxygenation, 228
  hemoperfusion devices, 228
Extractability, 84–85
Extruded polymers
  Biomer, 109
  fabrication processes, 29–31
  tubing, 32
Extrusion Grade Biomer, 32
Ex vivo testing, 148–149

F

Fabrication, 27–39
  biodegradable polymers, 200
  commercial and experimental
    products, 37–39
  pacemaker leads, 208
  processing, 27–36
    one-dimensional, 27–29
    three-dimensional, 31–36
    two-dimensional, 29–31
  sterilization, 36–37
  and surface chemistry, 108
  and thrombogenicity, 163–164
Facial reconstruction, 238–239
Fatigue testing, 49, 50, 82–83
Feeding tubes, 169
Fenwal blood filter, 230
Ferric acetylacetonate, 14
Fibers, fabrication processes, 29, 31
Fibrils, 46–47
Fibrin, wound healing, 136
Fibrinogen, 120–121, 150, *see also* Protein
    adsorption
  adsorption of, *see* Protein adsorption
  host-material interactions, 152–153
  surface modification and, 152
  thrombus formation, 161–163
  Vroman effect, 155–157
Fibrinolytic agents, surface
    modification, 21
Fibrinolytic system
  host defense, 122–123
  host-material interactions, 155
Fibroblasts, 196
  foreign body response, 135
  inflammatory response, 132–134, 164
  wound healing, 135–137, 141
Fibronectin, 121–122, 129
  adsorption of, 153–154
  host-material interactions, 154
  wound healing, 141

Fibrosis
  biopolymer material and, 164–166
  wound healing, 109–110, 141
Fibrous tubing, 33–34
Films, 39
  dressings, 233, 235, 237–238
  hemodialysis membranes, 228
Filters, blood, 229–230
Flexibility, 44, *see also* Mechanical behavior
Flexible foams, 18
Flexural modulus, 81
Flory-Huggins solubility parameter, 54
Fluidized bed coating techniques, 27
Fluorocarbons, 100
Foams
  flexible, 18
  inflammatory response, 166
  processing, 31–32
Foreign body giant cells, 187–189
Foreign body response, 133–135, 164–166
Fourier Transform IR Spectroscopy (FTIR),
    66–68
  ATR, *see* Attenuated Total Reflectance Fourier
    Transform Infrared Spectroscopy
  bulk analysis, 104
  hydrogen bonding, 59, 62–63
  protein adsorption, 150, 154
  surface contaminants, 108
Free radicals, 133, 139. 185–186
  enzymatic degradation of polymers, 185,
    188–189
  oxidation, 183
Freundlich model of protein adsorption, 118
FTIR-ATR, *see* Attenuated Total Reflectance-FTIR
    spectroscopy
Functional groups, 5
  bulk modification, 19–21
  polymer synthesis, 10
  surface modification, 21–22
Fungal degradation of polyurethanes, 194

G

Gamma globulin, 150, *see also* Immunoglobulins
Gas plasma sterilization, 34
Gastric bubbles, 189–190
Gel permeation chromatography, 66
Glass transition temperature, 6–7
  annealing and, 71–72
  differential scanning calorimetry, 68–69
  dynamic mechanical thermal analysis, 72, 74
  and hydrogen bonds, 62
  polyols and, 64
  states of order and, 43–48

and tensile strength, 80
and viscoelasticity, 50
Glucose sensors, 241
Glutaraldehyde sterilization, 228
Glycol extended polyurethanes, 17, 20, 65
Glycosaminoglycans, 129, 141
Goniometry, contact angle measurement, 95–96
Goretex, 213–214, 219
Graft copolymers, 5–6
Graft photopolymerization, 22
Granulation tissue, 134–135
Granulocytes, 127–128, see also Neutrophils
   acute phase response, 132–134
   complement activation, 128, 138–139
Granulomas, 166
Graphite, 224
Growth factors, 127
   cytokine sources and functions, 129–131
   immune system, 139–141
   inflammatory response, 132–134, 164
   neointima formation, 167
   wound healing, 136

H

Hageman factor (FXII), 122, 154
Hamilton technique, 95
Hansen solubility parameters, 84
Hardness, 8, 81
Hard segments, 6–7
   chain packing in, 60
   facial reconstruction, 239
   morphological models, 56–57
   orientation behavior, 58–60
   size distribution, 50
HDI (1,6-hexane diisocyanate), 15, 64
Heart, see Artificial organs, heart
Heart valves, 219–222
   calcification of, 197–198
   infection, 169, 170
Helmholtz free energy, 92
Helper T-cells, 127, 141
HEMA (polyhydroxyethyl methacrylate), 22
Hemocompatibility, see Blood compatibility
Hemodialysis, 128, 227–228
Hemodynamics, testing, 147–148
Hemofiltration, 128, 229–230
Hemolysis, 219
Hemoperfusion systems, 228
Hemostasis
   host defense, 131–132
   wound healing, 141

Heparin, 155
   surface adducts, 155
   surface modification, 21–23
Heteropolymers, 5, see also Chemistry; Copolymers
Hexafluoroisopropane (HFIP), 108
1,6-Hexane diisocyanate (HDI), 15, 64
Hexanediol, 17, 20
High density polyethylene (HDPE), 2
High molecular weight kallikrein, 122, 154–157
Histamine, 133, 139
Histocompatibility, see Tissue compatibility
H12MDI, see Methylene bis (p-cyclohexyl)isocyanate
Hollow fibers
   dialysis membranes, 227–228
   drug delivery system, 240
Homopolymers, 5–6, 8
Hooke's Law, 50
Host defense, 115–141
   cells, ECM, and interactions, 124–131
      adhesion molecules, 129
      cytokines, 129–131
      ECM, 128–129
      hemostasis and thrombosis, 130, 132
      immune system, 137–141
      platelets, 124–126
      red cells, 124, 126
      white cells, 127–128
   foreign body response, 134–135
   hemostasis and thrombosis, 131–132
   immune response, 137–141
      adaptive immunity, 137, 140–141
      cellular interactions, 140–141
      complement system, 138–139
      innate immunity, 137–139, 141
   inflammatory response, 132–135
   protein adsorption, 115–123
      biomaterials, 119–122
      coagulation system, 122–123
      equilibria and isotherms, 118–119
      fibrinolytic system, 122–123
      kinetics, 117–118
   wound healing, 135–137
      fibroblast proliferation, 136
      wound closure and scar contracture, 136–137
Host-material interactions, 147–171
   assessment of, 147–150
   cellular responses, 158–171
      immunological response, 169
      neointima formation, 167–169
      platelets, 158–162
      soft tissue interactions, 164–166
      thrombus formation, 161–164
      white cells, 161

infection, 167–170
protein adsorption, 150–158
   albumin, 151–152
   coagulation system, 154–155
   complement system, 155
   fibrinogen, 152–153
   fibrinolytic system, 155
   fibronectin, 154
   lipoprotein, 154
   vitronectin, 154
   Vroman effect, 155–158
Hot coating techniques, 27
Humoral immunity, 127, 130–131, 137, 140–141
Hyaluronan, 129
Hydrocolloid, 233
Hydrogel, 208, 235
Hydrogenated polybutadiene, 19
Hydrogen bonds, 10, 59, 61–63, 70
Hydrolysis, 15, 181–182
Hydrophilic polymers, 15
Hydrophilic soft segment surface structure, 104
Hydrophobicity
   alkyl grafts, 152
   cardiac catheter materials, 208
   and coagulation, 132
   and lipoprotein adsorption, 154
   surface structure, 104
Hydroxyapatite, 197–199
2-Hydroxyethane *bis* phosphonic acid (HEBP), 199
Hydroxy groups, and mechanical properties, 17
Hydroxy terminated 1,4-butadiene, 18
Hydroxy terminated polydimethylsiloxane (PDMS), 18–19
Hysteresis, 50–51, 78
   contact angle, 97–98
   stress, 49
   tensile stress, 82–83

I

Immune response, 138–140
   adaptive immunity, 137, 140–141
   cellular interactions, 140–141
   complement system, 138–139
   cytokine sources and functions, 129–131
   host-material interactions, 169
   innate immunity, 138
Immunoglobulins, 120–121, *see also* Protein adsorption
   absorption on polymer surface, 152
   immune response, 169
   immune system, 140–141
Immunoglobulin superfamily, 129
Infection, *see also* Microorganisms; specific applications and devices
   artificial hearts, 227
   cardiac catheters, 207
   host-material interactions, 167–170
Inflammation
   biopolymer material and, 164–166
   cardiac catheters, 207
   cell adhesion molecules, 129
   cytokine sources and functions, 129–131
   host defense, 132–135
   white cells, 127–128
Infrared dichroism, 58
Infrared spectroscopy, 55, 58–59, 62–63, 66–68, *see also* Fourier Transform IR Spectroscopy
Innate immunity, 137–139, 141
Integrins, 129
Interfacial tensions, *see* Contact angle methods
Interferons, 131
Interleukins, *see* Cytokines
Intermolecular bonds, *see* Chemical bonds
Intraaortic balloon pumps, 107, 225–226
Intravaginal devices, 240
In vitro testing, biocompatibility, 147–148
In vivo testing, 148–149
Ionic groups
   and protein binding, 153
   and thrmobogenicity, 163
IPDI (isophorone diisocyanate), 15–16, 64
Irganox 10, 66
Irradiation, 185
IR spectroscopy, *see* Attenuated Total Reflectance-FTIR spectroscopy; Fourier Transform IR Spectroscopy
Islets of Langerhans, 229, 241
Isocyanates
   aromatic versus aliphatic, 191–192
   crosslinked polymer synthesis, 17–18
   chemical composition and physical properties, 63–64
   degradation products, 183
   polymer synthesis, 9–10
   raw materials in copolymer synthesis, 14–16
   and surface properties, 109
   toxicity/carcinogenicity, 195–197
Isocyanurates
   catalysts and, 14
   polymer synthesis, 12–13
Isophorone diisocyanate (IPDI), 15–16, 64

Isotactic polymers, 43–44
Isotherms, protein adsorption, 118–119

J

Jobskin, 234
Joint prostheses, 241

K

Kaolin, 111
Keratinocytes, 130, 133
Kidney dialysis, 227–228
Kinetic hysteresis, 98
Kinetics
 microphase separation, 54–55
 protein adsorption, 117–118
Kinins, 122, 133–134, 154–157

L

Lactide copolymers, 199–200
Lamellar morphology, 78
Lamination
 fabrication processes, 29, 31
 tubing, 33
Laminin, 129, 141
Langmuir model, 118–119
Left ventricular assist devices (LVAD), 223–225
 fabrication process, 35
 fatigue testing, 82–83
LeGrand model, 54
Leukocytes, *see* White cells
Leukopheresis, 128
Leukotrienes, 133
Ligament repair, 241
Light degradation, 15
Linear elastomer synthesis, 17
Lipoproteins, 121, 154
Location of implant, and degradation, 194–195
Low density polyethylene (LDPE), 2
Low-temperature properties, 15
Lumbrokinase, 155
Lung, artificial, 228
Lycra catheters, 208
Lymphocytes, 127–128
 cytokine sources and functions, 129–131
 immune system, 137–141, 169
 inflammatory response, 135, 164
 wound healing, 136
Lyofoam, 39

M

Macroglycol, 15, 17, 20
Macrophages, 127–128, 196
 cytokine sources and functions, 130–131
 enzymatic degradation of polymers, 185, 187–289
 foreign body response, 135
 immune response, 169
 immune system, 140–141
 inflammatory response, 132–133, 135, 164
 wound healing, 136
Mandrel, 34–35
Manufacturing, *see* Fabrication
Mast cells, 127, 139–141
MDI, *see* Methylene *bis* (p-phenyl) isocyanate
Mechanical behavior
 calcification and, 197
 chain chemistry and, 17, 62
 characterization of
  dynamic mechanical thermal analysis, 72, 74, 76–79
  stress-strain properties, 78, 80–84
 polymer structure and, 48–51
  hydrogen bonding, 62
  hysteresis, 50–51
  viscoelasticity, 50
Media
 linear elastomer synthesis, 17
 polymer synthesis, 14
MEK (methyl ethyl ketone), 28
Melting temperature, 73, *see also* Glass transition temperature
Membrane attack complex (MAC), 139
Meme breast implant, 189, 195–197, 230
Mentor, 240
Metal catalyzed oxidation, 183–185, 211
Methacrol, 153
Methanol, 108
N-Methyldiethanolamine, 108
4,4′-Methylene *bis* (2-chloroaniline) (MOCA), 17, 20
Methylene *bis* (p-cyclohexyl) isocyanate (H12MDI), 15–16
 degradation of, 191
 and physical properties, 64
 surface modifications, 109–110
Methylene *bis* (p-phenyl) isocyanate (MDI), 15–16
 applications
  hemodialysis membranes, 228
  ventricular assist devices, 224
 Biomer bulk characterization, 66
 Biomer synthesis, 104
 cellular response, 158, 160

degradation products, 185, 192
differential scanning calorimetry, 69
dynamic mechanical thermal analysis, 74, 78
morphological models, 56–57
and physical properties, 64
and surface chemistry, 108
surface properties of polymers synthesized from, 103
toxicity/carcinogenicity, 195–197
MDI/BD
   differential scanning calorimetry, 69
   kinetics of microphase separation, 54–55
MDI/BD/PEO, surface tension properties, 98
MDI/BD/PTMA, 74–75
MDI/BD/PTMO, 98
MDI/ED/PPO, protein adsorption, 151
MDI/ED/PTMO
   cellular response, platelets, 158
   tensile properties, 82
MDI/MDEA/PTMO, 97
MDI/PTMO/BS, 160
MDI/TDI/ED/PTMO, 158
surface tension properties, 98
Methyl ethyl ketone (MEK), 28
Mettalin, 237
Microbubbles, in synthetic vascular grafts, 110
Microfibrillar associated glyoprotein (MGAP), 128
Microorganisms, 121
   colonization of biomedical devices, 208, *see also* specific applications and devices
   degradation of polymers, 194
   host defense, 138–139
   infections, 169–170
   protein adsorption and, 154
   surface modification and, 152
Microphase mixing transition temperature, 73
Microphase separation, 10, 18, 53–55
   kinetics of phase separation, 54–55
   surface spectroscopic studies, 102–103
   thermodynamics of phase separation, 53–54
Microphase separation transition (MST), 71
Microscopic examination, 92
Microthane, 39, 192
Mitrathane, 38, 213–214
   applications
      valves, 221
      vascular prostheses, 219
   calcification of, 197
   inflammatory response, 164
MOCA, *see* 4,4′-Methylene *bis* (2-chloroaniline)
Modulus, 49
Modulus temperature curves, 78, 79
Molding, 31, 36
Molecular orientation, 57–59, 60

Molecular sequence distributions, 55
Molecular weights
   degradation and, 182
   dynamic mechanical thermal analysis, 74, 77
   and properties of polymers, 51–52
Monocytes, 127–128
   cytokine sources and functions, 130–131
   foreign body response, 135
   immune system, 140–141
Morphological models of block copolymers, 55–57
Morphology, surface, 108–111, *see also* Surface properties
Multinucleated giant cells, 135, 164, 187–189

N

N,N-dimethylacetamide (DMA), 14, 28, 108
Naphthalene diisocyanate (NDI), 15–16, 64
Natural Y prostheses, 230
NDI (naphthalene diisocyanate), 15–16, 64
Neointima formation, *see also* Vascularization
   host-material interactions, 167–169
   porosity and, 109–110
   vascular prostheses, 213–218
   ventricular assist devices, 224
Networks
   polymer synthesis, 10
   structure, 227
Neutrophils, 127–129
   complement activation, 138–139
   enzymatic degradation of polymers, 185–186, 189
   foreign body response, 134–135
   inflammatory response, 132–134, 164
   wound healing, 136
Newton's Law, 50
NK cells, 130–131, 138, 140–141
Nonpolar solvents, solubility tests, 84
Nuclear Magnetic Resonance (NMR) spectroscopy, 55
N-Vinyl pyrrolidone (NVP), 22
NVP (N-vinyl pyrrolidone), 22
Nylon, 2, 186, 206

O

Omiderm, 39, 234, 237
One-step synthesis, 8
OpSite, 39, 232, 234–235, 238
Opsonization, 138, 140
Optical methods, 92
Organ culture, 241
Organometallic catalysts, 14

Oxidation
  degradation mechanisms, 183–186
  pacemaker leads, 211
  stress cracks, 188–189
Oxygenation, extracorporeal, 228
Oxygen plasma etching, 28
Oxygen radicals, 133, 139, 185–186
Ozone sterilization, 34

P

Pacemaker leads, 32, 208–211
  oxidation, 184
  stress cracking, 187–189
Pacemakers, 169–170
Pancreas, artificial, 229
Paracrystalline domains, 59
Passivation, albumin adsorption, 150–151
PC, *see* Polycarbonates
PDMS, *see* Polydimethylsiloxanes
PEG (polyethylene glycol), 22, 103
Pellethane, 29, 32, 38
  albumin adsorption, 152
  applications
    artificial hearts, 227
    cardiac catheters, 208
    pacemaker leads, 208, 210
    valves, 221
  calcification of, 197
  degradation of, 186–188, 192
  mechanical properties, 81
  protein binding, 153
  surface tension properties, 98
Penile prostheses, 240
PEO, *see* Polyethylene oxide
Peritoneal catheter exit site dressings, 237–238
Peritoneal dialysis catheters, 169
Permeability, 84–85
Peroxides, 183, *see also* Free radicals
PET, *see* Polyethylene terephthalate
Phagocytes, 127–128, *see also* Macrophages; Neutrophils
  bacterial defenses, 169
  enzymatic degradation of polymers, 185
  immune system, 138–141
Phagocytosis, 127–128, 138–139
Phase mixing, and tensile strength, 80
Phase separation, 10, 18, 48, *see also* Microphase separation
  chain extenders and, 65
  dynamic mechanical thermal analysis, 72, 74
  hydrogen bonding and, 62
  SEM detection, 74
Phosphorylcholine moieties, 161

Photopolymerization, 22
Physical properties, *see also* Mechanical behavior; Structure-physical property relationships
  characterization of polyurethanes, 65–86
    differential scanning calorimetry, 68–73
    dynamic mechanical thermal analysis, 72, 74, 76–79
    electrical, 85–86
    electron microscopy, 74–79
    gel permeation chromatography, 66
    IR spectroscopy, 66–68
    permeability and extractability, 84–85
    solubility tests, 84, 85
    stress-strain properties and ultimate tensile strength, 78, 80–84
  chemical composition and, 17, 63–65
  fabrication methods and, 108
  modification during synthesis, 18–22
    bulk, 20–21
    surface, 21–22
  tubing, 34
Pivipol, 229
Plasma etching, 28
Plasma glow discharge technology, 22–23
Plasma polymerization, 29
Plasma sterilization of polymers, 34
Plasmin, 122–123
Plasminogen, 121
Plasminogen activator, 20–21, *see also* Tissue plasminogen activator
Plasticizers, 74, 79
Platelet activating factor (PAF), 128, 133
Platelets, 152
  adhesion to polymers, 109, *see also* specific applications
    host-material interactions, 158–162
    surface properties and, 83, 152, 155
  coagulation system, 122–123
  host defense, 116, 124–126
  inflammatory response, 132
  thrombus formation, 161–163
  Vroman effect, 155–157
  wound healing, 136, 141
Polar groups, 48
Polarized fluorescence, 58
Polarized Raman scattering, 58
Polar solvents, 17, 27–28
Poly(4-methyl pent-1-ene), 45
Polyacrylamide, 22
Polyacrylonitrile, 45
Polyaddition polymerization, 8
Polyaliphatic urethanes, degradation of, 190–191
Polyalkyldiols, soft segment, 6–7
Polyalkyl glycols, 15

Index

Polyamido side chains, 21
Polycaprolactones, 19, 190, 192
Polycarbonates (PC), 2
    degradation of, 190
    raw materials for synthesis, 15
Poly(diisopropylaminethylmethacrylate-dodecyl)methacrylate, 66
Poly(dimethylsiloxanes) (PDMS), 15
    cardiac catheters, 206–207
    degradation of, 190, 194
    FTIR studies, 68
    glass transition temperature, 45
    grafts, 216
    hydroxy terminated, 18
    and phase separation, 103
    protein adsorption, 154
    solubility parameters of blood components and biomaterials, 85
    surface contaminants, 106–108
Polyester macroglycols, 189
Polyester urethanes (ES)
    biodegradation mechanisms, 181
    degradation of, 189–190
    differential scanning calorimetry, 71
    molecular weight effects on properties, 52
    physical properties, 64–65
    raw materials for synthesis, 15
    soft segment, 6–7
    vascular prostheses, 219
Polyether urethanes (ET)
    biodegradation mechanisms, 181
    degradation/stability of, 190
    differential scanning calorimetry, 69, 71
    linear elastomer synthesis, 17
    molecular weight effects on properties, 52
    proteolytic enzymes and, 186
    raw materials for synthesis, 15
    soft segment, 6–7
Polyetherurethane urea elastomers, degradation mechanisms, 188–190
Polyethylene adipate (PEA), 18
    degradation/stability of, 190
    stress lifetime curve, 49, 50
Polyethylene glycol (PEG), 22, 103, 190
Polyethylene oxide (PEO), 15, 18, 21
    applications
        hemodialysis membranes, 228
        valves, 221
    FTIR studies, 68
    glass transition temperature, 45
    platelets and, 158
    protein adsorption, 152–155
    protein binding, 152, 153
    proteolytic enzymes and, 186
    surface modification, 22, 109
    thrombogenicity, 151, 155, 163
Polyethylene oxide (PEO) hydrogel, 240
Polyethylene oxide (PEO-PTMO-PEO) system, 240
Polyethylenes, 2
    cardiac catheters, 206
    glass transition temperature, 45
    Vroman effect, 156
Polyethylene terephthalate (PET), 2
    proteolytic enzymes and, 186
    surface properties, 109
    vascular prostheses, 211–213, 219
Polyhexamethylene carbonate glycol, 19
Polyhydroxyethyl methacrylate (HEMA), 22
Polylactide, 216
Polymer families, 2
Polymerization
    plasma, 29
    types of reactions, 8–9
Polymethylmethacrylate
    facial reconstruction, 239
    glass transition temperature, 45
    hemodialysis membranes, 228
    proteolytic enzymes and, 186
Polymorphonuclear leukocytes, *see* Neutrophils
Polyols, 6–7, 18–19
    chemical composition and physical properties, 64–65
    crosslinked polymer synthesis, 18
    raw materials in copolymer synthesis, 15, 18–19
Poly(oxytetramethylene) glycol (PTMEG), 18
    physical properties, 65
    solubility parameters of blood components and biomaterials, 85
Polypropylene (PP), 2
    extracorporeal blood oxygenator, 228
    glass transition temperature, 45
    stereoisomers, 44
Polypropylene glycol (PPG), 103
Polypropylene oxide (PPO), 15, 18
    cellular response, 158
    FTIR studies, 68
    kinetics of microphase separation, 55
    protein adsorption, 151
    stereoisomers, 44
    stress lifetime curve, 49–50
    thrombogenicity, 163
    toxicity/carcinogenicity of degradation products, 195–196, 197
Polypropylene oxide (PPO-PEO), 55
Polysiloxanes, thrombogenicity, 163–164
Polystyrene, 2, 45
Polytetrafluoroethylene (PTFE), 2

applications
    cardiac catheters, 206–207
    extracorporeal blood oxygenator, 228
    inflammatory response, 164
Polytetramethylene adipate (PTMA), 19
  differential scanning calorimetry, 69
  stress lifetime curve, 49–50
Poly(tetramethylene oxide) (PTMO), 15, 18, 224
  Biomer bulk characterization, 66
  Biomer synthesis, 104
  differential scanning calorimetry, 69–70
  FTIR studies, 68
  kinetics of microphase separation, 55
  morphological studies, 78
  and phase separation, 103
  physical properties, 65
  platelets and, 158, 160
  protein adsorption, 151–154
  and surface chemistry, 108
  thrombogenicity, 163
  ventricular assist devices, 224
Polyurethaneurea, 9
Polyvinyl alcohol (PVA), 45
Polyvinylchloride (PVC), 2
  applications
    blood tubing, 229
    cardiac catheters, 206–207
    complement system, 155
  glass transition temperature, 45
Polyvinylchloride acetate (PVCA), 196
Polyvinyl pyrrolidone (PVP), 22
Polyvinyls, facial reconstruction, 239
Pore size, hemodialysis membranes, 228
Porosity
  and biocompatibility, 109–111
  degradation mechanisms, 186
  and inflammatory response, 165
  SEM detection, 74
  vascular prostheses, 213–218
Porous polymers, Biomer, 109
Porous tubing, 33–34
Post forming, 31
PP, see Polypropylene
PPG (polypropylene glycol), 103
Prekallikrein, 122, 154
Prepolymer method, 9
Pressure sores, 238
Processing, 27–36
  one-dimensional, 27–29
  three-dimensional, 31–36
    balloons, bladders, and other devices, 34–36
    foams, 31–32
    tubing, 32–34
  two-dimensional, 29–31
Production, see Fabrication
Propane sulfone, surface modifications, 109
Properties, see Mechanical behavior; Physical properties; Structure-physical property relationships
Prophylactics, 240
Prostacyclin, 22
Prostaglandins/prostanoids, 22, 123
  inflammatory mediators, 133, 164
  surface modification, 161
Prostheses, see Tissue augmentation and prostheses
Prosthetic heart valves, see Valves
Protein adsorption
  conformation of adsorbed protein, 153
  host defense, 115–123
    biomaterials, 119–122
    coagulation system, 122–123
    equilibria and isotherms, 118–119
    fibrinolytic system, 122–123
    kinetics, 117–118
    white cell adhesion, 128
  host-material interactions, 150–158
    albumin, 151–152
    coagulation system, 154–155
    complement system, 155
    fibrinogen, 152–153
    fibrinolytic system, 155
    fibronectin, 154
    lipoprotein, 154
    vitronectin, 154
    Vroman effect, 155–158
  thrombus formation, 161–163
Proteolytic enzymes, 186, 197
Prothrombin, 122
Prothrombinase, 125
Pseudomonas aeruginosa, 170
Pseudoneointima, 215, 224
PTFE (polytetrafluoroethylene), 2
PTMEG, see Poly(oxytetramethylene) glycol
PTMO, see Poly(tetramethylene oxide)
Pulmonary artery catheters, 208
PVP (polyvinyl pyrrolidone), 22
PYUA products, 81

Q

Quaternary ammonium groups, 21

R

Radiation sterilization, 34, 185
Raman scattering, polarized, 58

Random copolymers, 5–6, 8
Raw materials, copolymer synthesis, 14–17
Reaction injection molding (RIM), 31
Rearrangement polymerization, 8
Receding contact angle, 97–98
Reconstructive surgery, 238–239, 241
Red cells
  coagulation process, 131
  host defense, 124, 126–127
Renal dialysis, 227–228
Renal Embolus Test, 149
Renathane, 153
Revascularization, see Neointima formation; Vascularization
RGD (Arg-Gly-Asp), 121, 129, 167–168
Rigidax, 35
Rimplast, 38, 81
Roughness, see also Surface properties
  categories of, 109
  and contact angle measurement, 95

S

Santowhite, 189
Scanning EM, 74–75, 92–93
  cardiac catheters, 207
  degradation studies, 191
  intra-aortic balloon pumps, 225–226
  stress cracks, 188
  surface evaluation, 109
  vascular prostheses, 213–217
  wound dressing, 234
Scanning probe microscopy, 92
Scanning tunneling microscopy, 109
Scar contracture, 136–137
Scott prosthesis, 240
Secondary Ion Mass Spectroscopy (SIMS), 92–93, 101–108
Segmented polyurethanes, morphological model of, 59–60
SEM, see Scanning electron microscopy
Semicrystalline polymers, 44–48
  hard segment, 7
  stability, 190
Serotonin, 124, 133
Sheet forming, 31
Shiley S-100, 228
Side chains, surface modification, 21
Side reactions, crosslinked polymer synthesis, 17
Silastic, cardiac catheters, 207
Silicon contamination, 104–105
Silicone oil, 85

Silicone rubber, 2
  applications
    artificial hearts, 227
    cardiac catheters, 206
    extracorporeal blood oxygenator, 228
  solubility parameters of blood components and biomaterials, 85
  thrombogenicity, 151
Silicones, 2
  Cardiothane-51, 100
  facial reconstruction, 239
  inflammatory response, 165
Siliconized latex, cardiac catheters, 207
Siloxanes, thrombogenicity, 163–164
SIMS, see Secondary Ion Mass Spectroscopy
Skin dressings, see Wound dressings
Small Angle Light Scattering (SALS), 58
Small Angle X-Ray Scattering (SAXS), 54–55, 58, 71
Smoothness, 5, see also Surface properties
Sodium dodecyl sulfate elution, 152
Soft segment, 6–7
  degradation processes, 189–190
  morphological models, 56–57
  orientation behavior, 58
  surface structure, 104
Soft tissue interactions, host-material interactions, 164–166
Solubility tests, 84–85
Solution grade Biomer (SB), 103, 104
Solvent casting, 33–35
Solvent coating, 27–28
Solvents
  fiber production, 29
  linear elastomer synthesis, 17
  solubility tests, 84
  and surface chemistry, 108
  tubing fabrication, 33
Spandex fibers, 29
Spectroscopic methods, 66–68, 92
Spherulites, 46–47
Spray coating, 27
Staphyloccus aureus, 170
Staphylococcus epidermidis, 170
Static SIMS methods, 92–93
Steam sterilization, 36, 192
Stepwise synthesis, 50–51
Stereoisomers, polypropylene, 44
Steric factors, 44
Sterilization
  and degradation, 185
  degradation products, 192
  fabrication process, 36–37
  hemodialysis membranes, 228

Stiffness, 8
Storage modulus, 72, 74–75
Streaming potential, 111
Stress cracking
    oxidation and, 188–189
    pacemaker leads, 210–211
Stress cracking, environmental, 187–189
Stress-crystallized soft segment, 59
Stress relaxation, 49–50
Stress-strain properties, 78, 80–84
    structure and, 48–49
    vascular prostheses, 218–219
Structure
    and degradation, 188–194
    surface modification, see Surface modification
Structure-physical property relationships, 43–86
    characterization of polyurethanes, 65–86
        differential scanning calorimetry, 68–73
        dynamic mechanical thermal analysis, 72, 74, 76–79
        electrical, 85, 86
        electron microscopy, 74–78, 79
        gel permeation chromatography, 66
        IR spectroscopy, 66–68
        permeability and extractability, 84–85
        solubility tests, 84, 85
        stress-strain properties and ultimate tensile strength, 78, 80–84
    chemical composition and physical properties, 63–65
        chain extenders, 65
        isocyanates, 63–64
        polyols, 64–65
    crosslinking, 63
    hydrogen bonding, 59, 61–62
    intermolecular bonding, 48
    mechanical behavior, 48–51
        hysteresis, 50–51
        viscoelasticity, 50
    microphase separation, 53–55
    molecular orientation, 57–60
    molecular weight, 51–52
    morphological models of block copolymers, 55–57
    states of order and thermal transition of polymers, 43–48
Sulfonation, 20–21
    and phase separation, 62
    and protein binding, 153, 155
    surface modifications, 109–110
    and thrombogenicity, 163
Superoxide radical, 128, 185
Superthane, 153
Suppressor T-cells, 127–128

Surethane, 39
Surface modification, 19–20, 152, 155
    albumin adsorption, 151–152
    endothelial cell attachment, 168
    heart valve materials, 221
    product variability, 39
    with prostaglandins, 161
Surface-modifying additives (SMA), 29
Surface properties, 5, see also Hydrophobicity
    blood filters, 230
    and coagulation, 131–132
    and contact angle measurement, 95
    degradation and, 182
    electric charge, blood vessels, 111
    fabrication methods and, 36
    fatigue and, 83
    and inflammatory response, 165–166
    modification during synthesis, 21–22
    protein activation versus passivation, 150–151
    and thrombogenicity, 163–164
    vascular prostheses, 213–218
Surface properties, characterization of, 91–111
    ATR-FTIR spectroscopy, 98–100
    electrical properties, 111
    morphology, 108–111
    spectroscopic techniques, 100–108
        Secondary Ion Mass Spectroscopy (SIMS), 101–108
        X-Ray Photoelectron Spectroscopy (XPS), 100–108
    surface energy and surface tension, 91–98
        contact angle, 94–95
        contact angle hysteresis, 97–98
        contact angle measurement, 95–97
Surfactants
    foam production, 32
    surface modification, 20–21
Surgical adhesives, 349
Surgitek, 197
Sutures, 241
Switchboard model, 46
Syndiotactic polymers, 43–44
Synthesis, 8–14
    acylurea, 12
    allophanate reaction, 11
    biuret formation, 11
    carbodiimide formation, 12–13
    catalysts, 13–14
    isocyanates, 9–10
    isocyanurate formation, 12–13
    linear elastomers, 17
    media for, 14
    types of polymerization reactions, 8–9
    uretidione formation, 12–13

T

Tacticity, 43–44
T-cells, 127
   cytokine sources and functions, 129–131
   cytotoxic, 127, 139–141
   helper, 127, 139, 141
   immune system, 138, 141–142, 169
   inflammatory response, 134
   suppressor, 127–128
TDA, *see* Toluene diamine
TDI, *see* Toluene diisocyanate
TDMAC (tridodecylmethylammonium chloride), 21
Tear strength, 49
Tecoflex, 36, 38, 66, 234, 240
   applications
      artificial hearts, 227
      pacemaker leads, 208
   degradation of, 190–191
   mechanical properties, 81
Teflon
   applications, 239
      cardiac catheters, 207
      heart valves, 222
   fabrication process, 36
   thrombogenicity, 151
   tubing, 33
   Vroman effect, 156
Tegaderm, 39, 232, 235, 238
Temperature, *see also* Glass transition temperature
   adhesive curing, 239
   and hydrogen bonds, 62
   and tensile strength, 80
Tendon repair, 241
Tensile properties, 5, 49, 78, 80–84
   commercial products, properties of, 81
   molecular weight effects on properties, 52
   structure and, 48–49
Tertiary amines, 13
Tetrahydrofuran (THF), 14, 27–28
   linear elastomer synthesis, 17
   and surface chemistry, 108
Texane, 81
Thermal degradation, 15, 183
Thermal transition temperature, 43–48, *see also* Glass transition temperature
Thermedics, 224
Thermodynamic hysteresis, 98
Thermodynamics of phase separation, 53–54
Thermomechanical spectra, dynamic mechanical thermal analysis, 72, 74
Thermoplastic polymer classes, 2, 5
Thermosetting polymer classes, 2, 5
THF, *see* Tetrahydrofuran
Thoratec, 81
Three-dimensional processing, 31–36
Three-dimensional structure, synthesis process, 8
Thrombin, 122–125
Thromboglobulin-beta, 124
Thromboxanes, 123, 124
Thrombus formation, *see also* specific applications
   albumin adsorption and, 151–152, 155
   calcification and, 198
   electrical charge and, 111
   host defense, 131–132
   host-material interactions, 161–164
      protein ratios as indicator of thrombogenicity, 150–151
      testing, 149
   surface modification and, 152
   surface properties, 95
   vascular graft surface properties and, 110
   Vroman effect, 155–157
   wound healing, 141
Tin-containing (organotin) catalysts, 14
Tissue augmentation and prostheses, 230–240
   adhesives, 239
   artificial ducts, 239
   breast implants, 230–231
   contraceptives/prophylactics, 240
   drug delivery, 240
   facial reconstruction, 238–239
   miscellaneous, 241
   penile prostheses, 240
   wound dressings, 231–238
Tissue compatibility (histocompatibility), 1
   in vitro testing, 147–148
   porosity and, 109–110
Tissue culture, 241
Tissue in growth, *see also* Fibrosis
   biopolymer material and, 164–166
   neointima formation, *see* Neointima formation
   porosity and, 109–110
   wound healing, 109–110, 135–136, 141
Tissue plasminogen activator (tPA)
   host defense, 122–123
   surface modification, 20–21
Toluene, 28
Toluene diamine (TDA), 183, 192
   breast implant degradation, 230
   degradation products, 183, 192
   toxicity/carcinogenicity, 195–197
Toluene diisocyanate (TDI), 15–16, 192
   degradation products, 183, 193
   differential scanning calorimetry, 70

and physical properties, 64
TDI/PCL/ED degradation products, 193
toxicity/carcinogenicity, 195–197
Toluene isocyanate amine (TIA)
 toxicity/carcinogenicity, 195–197
Total artificial heart, 226–227
 calcification of, 197
 neointima formation, 167–169
Toughness, 5
Toxicity, 195–197
Toyobo, 38, 224
Tracheal prostheses, 241
Transferrin, 121
Transmission electron microscopy, 75–78, 92
Tridodecylmethylammonium chloride (TDMAC), 21
Tubing
 blood, 229
 processing, 32–34
Tumor necrosis factor, 128, 130
Two-phase morphology, 78
Two-step polymerization, 9
Two-step synthesis, 50

U

Ulcers, 238
Underwater contact angle measurement, 96
Uniflex, 238
Urea bonds, 181–182
Urea formation, 11
Ureas
 catalysts and, 14
 hydrogen bonds, 61, 63
Urethane bonds, 61, 181–182
Urethane linkage, 5–6
Urethanes, 8
Uretidione formation, 12–13
Urokinase, 155

V

Vacuum forming, 31
Vaginal sponges and condoms, 240
Valves, 197–198, 219–222
Vascugraft, 213–214
Vascular grafts, 211–219
 infection, 169–170
 inflammatory response, 164
 neointima formation, 167–169
 porosity, 109–110
 surface properties, 110–111
Vascularization, *see also* Neointima formation
 host-material interactions, 167–169
 porosity and, 109–110
 wound healing, 135–136, 141
Vascular prostheses, 211–219
Vascular shunts, 155
Vena Cava Ring Test, 149
Ventricular cannula, 208
Ventriculoperitoneal shunts, 169
Vialon, 38, 97, 207
Viasorb, 38
N-Vinyl pyrrolidone (NVP), 22
Viscoelasticity, 47–48, 50, 78
Vitronectin, 154
von Willebrand factor, 121, 125
Vroman effect, 155–158

W

Water absorption, 15
 aliphatic polyurethanes, 191
 commercial products, properties of, 81
Water absorption characteristics, 85–86
Water resistance, 15
White cells
 coagulation process, 131
 complement activation, 138–139
 cytokine sources and functions, 129–131
 enzymatic degradation of polymers, 185–186, 189
 foreign body response, 134–135
 host defense, 127–128
 host-material interactions, 161
 immune response, 138–141
 inflammatory response, 132–134
 types and functions of, 127–128
 wound healing, 136–137
Wide angle X-ray scattering, 56, 58
Wilhemy plate balance, 95–96
Wound dressings, 137, 189–190, 231–238
 commerical products, 235–237
 infections, 238
 occlusive and semi-occlusive, 232, 234–238
 types of wounds, 231–233
Wound healing, 135–137, 164
 breast surgery, 231

Index

cell adhesion molecules, 129
fibroblast proliferation, 136
inflammatory response, 132–134
surface properties and,
 165–166
wound closure and scar contracture,
 136–137
Woven polymers, 109

X

Xeroform, 237
X-ray diffraction studies, 59
X-Ray Photoelectron Spectroscopy (XPS),
 92–93, 100–101, 102–108
X-ray scattering techniques, 54–56, 58, 71

Y

Young's equation, 94
Young's modulus, 48, 54, 82, 218

Z

Zeta potential, 111
Zisman method, 96